Dialectical Behavior Therapy
in Clinical Practice

Dialectical Behavior Therapy *in* Clinical Practice

APPLICATIONS ACROSS DISORDERS AND SETTINGS

EDITED BY

Linda A. Dimeff
Kelly Koerner

Foreword by Marsha M. Linehan

THE GUILFORD PRESS
New York   London

Printed in the United States of America

This book is printed on acid-free paper.

Last digit is print number: 9 8 7 6 5 4 3 2 1

The authors have checked with sources believed to be reliable in their efforts to provide information that is complete and generally in accord with the standards of practice that are accepted at the time of publication. However, in view of the possibility of human error or changes in medical sciences, neither the authors, nor the editor and publisher, nor any other party who has been involved in the preparation or publication of this work warrants that the information contained herein is in every respect accurate or complete, and they are not responsible for any errors or omissions or the results obtained from the use of such information. Readers are encouraged to confirm the information contained in this book with other sources.

Library of Congress Cataloging-in-Publication Data

Dialectical behavior therapy in clinical practice : applications across disorders and settings / edited by Linda A. Dimeff, Kelly Koerner ; foreword by Marsha M. Linehan.
     p. ; cm.
   Includes bibliographical references and index.
   ISBN-10: 1-57230-974-1 ISBN-13: 978-1-57230-974-6 (cloth : alk. paper)
   1. Dialectical behavior therapy. I. Dimeff, Linda A. II. Koerner, Kelly, 1964–
   [DNLM: 1. Behavior Therapy—methods. 2. Professional–Patient Relations. 3. Psychology, Clinical. WM 425 D536 2007]
   RC489.B4D515 2007
   616.89′142—dc22

                                                                    2007024869

For
Cynthia J. Sanderson
and
Marsha M. Linehan

About the Editors

Linda A. Dimeff, PhD, is Chief Scientific Officer for Behavioral Tech Research, Inc., an organization devoted to the dissemination of evidence-based practices. She is also on the clinical faculty in the Department of Psychology at the University of Washington. Dr. Dimeff received her doctorate in clinical psychology from the University of Washington, where she specialized in prevention and treatment of addictive behaviors and in dialectical behavior therapy (DBT). She collaborated with Marsha Linehan in the development of an adaptation of DBT for substance-dependent individuals with borderline personality disorder, and is currently coauthoring a book with Dr. Linehan that describes this treatment. Dr. Dimeff currently has eight dissemination research grants through the National Institutes of Health. Over the years, she has written numerous theoretical and empirical papers in the areas of addictive behaviors, DBT, and dissemination. Dr. Dimeff's experience includes providing extensive training, supervision, and consultation to treatment providers affiliated with large public-sector systems in their implementation of DBT, as well as to individuals in private practice.

Kelly Koerner, PhD, is a clinical psychologist and clinician, clinical supervisor, and trainer in DBT. She is Creative Director of the Evidence-Based Practice Institute, which provides online communities and continuing education for practitioners who strive to combine science and compassion in their work. Dr. Koerner has served as Director of Training for Marsha Linehan's research investigating the efficacy of DBT for suicidal and drug-abusing individuals with borderline personality disorder; Creative Director for Behavioral Tech Research, Inc., where she developed e-learning and other technology-based methods to disseminate evidence-based practices; and cofounder and first CEO of Behavioral Tech, LLC, a company that provides training in DBT. She is on the clinical faculty in the Department of Psychology at the University of Washington and maintains a consulting and psychotherapy practice in Seattle.

Contributors

Gwen Abney-Cunningham, LMSW, InterAct of Michigan, Kalamazoo, Michigan

Bradley Beach, BA, Echo Glen Children's Center, Snoqualmie, Washington

Elisabeth Bellows, MD, Behavioral Medicine Clinic of the Peninsula, Redwood City, California

Martin Bohus, MD, Department of Psychosomatic Medicine and Psychotherapy, Central Institute of Mental Health, University of Heidelberg, Mannheim, Germany

Jennifer S. Cheavens, PhD, Department of Psychiatry and Behavioral Sciences, Duke University Medical Center, Durham, North Carolina

Eunice Chen, PhD, Department of Psychiatry, University of Chicago Medical Hospitals, Chicago, Illinois

Katherine Anne Comtois, PhD, Harborview Medical Center, Seattle, Washington

Elizabeth T. Dexter-Mazza, PsyD, Department of Psychology, University of Washington, Seattle, Washington

Linda A. Dimeff, PhD, Behavioral Tech Research, Inc., Seattle, Washington

Anthony P. DuBose, PsyD, Dialectical Behavior Therapy Center of Seattle, Seattle, Washington

Alan E. Fruzzetti, PhD, Department of Psychology, University of Nevada–Reno, Reno, Nevada

Arielle R. Goldklang, PsyD, Cognitive and Behavioral Consultants of Westchester, LLC, White Plains, New York

Perry D. Hoffman, PhD, National Education Alliance for Borderline Personality Disorder, Rye, New York

André Ivanoff, PhD, Columbia University School of Social Work, New York, New York

Soonie A. Kim, PhD, Portland DBT Program, Portland, Oregon

Kelly Koerner, PhD, Evidence-Based Practice Institute and Department of Psychology, University of Washington, Seattle, Washington

Cedar R. Koons, MSW, LISW, Santa Fe DBT Consultation, Santa Fe, New Mexico

Marsha M. Linehan, PhD, Department of Psychology, University of Washington, Seattle, Washington

Thomas R. Lynch, PhD, Department of Psychiatry and Behavioral Sciences, Duke University Medical Center, and Department of Psychology and Neurosciences, Duke University, Durham, North Carolina

Sharon Y. Manning, PhD, Behavioral Tech, LLC, Behavioral Tech Research, Inc., Chapin, South Carolina

Robin A. McCann, PhD, Colorado Mental Health Institute, Pueblo, Colorado

Shelley McMain, PhD, Centre for Addiction and Mental Health, Department of Psychiatry, University of Toronto, Toronto, Ontario, Canada

Alec L. Miller, PsyD, Department of Psychiatry and Behavioral Sciences, Montefiore Medical Center/Albert Einstein College of Medicine, Bronx, New York

Maria Monroe-DeVita, PhD, The Washington Institute for Mental Illness Research and Training, University of Washington, Seattle, Washington

Kimberly Patterson, MSW, Allegheny HealthChoices, Inc., Pittsburgh, Pennsylvania

Jill H. Rathus, PhD, Department of Psychology, Long Island University, Brookville, New York

Sarah K. Reynolds, PhD, Western Psychiatric Institute and Clinic, Department of Psychiatry, University of Pittsburgh Medical Center, Pittsburgh, Pennsylvania

Shireen L. Rizvi, PhD, Department of Psychology, New School for Social Research, New York, New York

Debra Safer, MD, Department of Psychiatry, Stanford University Medical Center, Stanford, California

Daniel A. Santisteban, PhD, Center for Family Studies, University of Miami, Miami, Florida

Jennifer H. R. Sayrs, PhD, Dialectical Behavior Therapy Center of Seattle, Seattle, Washington

Henry Schmidt, PhD, Washington State Juvenile Rehabilitation Administration, Olympia, Washington

Charles R. Swenson, MD, Department of Psychiatry, University of Massachusetts Medical School, Worcester, Massachusetts, and private practice, Northampton, Massachusetts

Lucene Wisniewski, PhD, Cleveland Center for Eating Disorders, Beachwood, Ohio

Suzanne Witterholt, MD, Anoka-Metro Regional Treatment Center, Anoka, Minnesota

Randy Wolbert, MSW, InterAct of Michigan and Western Michigan University School of Social Work, Kalamazoo, Michigan

Foreword

The 20th century saw an explosion of new, innovative, and highly effective psychosocial therapies, each carrying a promise of reducing the pain and suffering of millions of people afflicted with debilitating mental health problems. Effective therapies were developed to successfully treat major depression (in fewer than 20 sessions), panic disorder (in fewer than 15), posttraumatic stress disorder, obsessive–compulsive disorder, substance use disorders, and eating disorders, to name just a few. Dialectical behavior therapy (DBT), a treatment I have spent my career developing and investigating, offered the promise of a life worth living for highly suicidal people with borderline personality disorder (BPD), a group previously considered "untreatable"—and for good reason. These individuals were viewed by most as notoriously difficult to treat and they typically had very poor clinical outcomes.

We arrived at the 21st century facing a serious problem: We now had a number of effective therapies, but few tools and strategies to disseminate and implement them. Clinicians were leaving graduate school without training in many (if not most) of these evidence-based therapies, and there were scant opportunities to fully learn them once working as a social worker, psychologist, or psychiatrist. Those who did read the treatment manuals for an evidence-based therapy often struggled to figure out how to actually *implement* the treatment in their unique setting. We have learned over the years that implementing an evidence-based therapy in a unique, non-research-supported clinical practice is not as simple as "plug and play."

When I disseminated the original version of my (yet unpublished) DBT treatment manuals in 1984, I thought I had said enough about how DBT works *and* how to apply it. I discovered the error of my thinking when I first began teaching DBT workshops to clinicians in various communities. When I published the DBT treatment manuals (1993a, 1993b), I thought I had added enough information to allow easy access to the treatment. As I continued to train individuals across various clinical settings, many would say to me that they simply could not do DBT in their clinical settings. In 1999 I published a paper in which I outlined the functions of any comprehensive clinical intervention (Linehan, 1999). I had figured out these functions in my many interactions with the community therapists I was teaching (Linehan, Cochran, & Kehrer, 2001). My intent at the time was to help DBT teams implement comprehensive DBT in their own settings. When DBT cannot be fully adopted because the setting in no way resembles the outpatient clinic where it was developed, how is this done in a fashion that preserves fidelity to the treatment method? Even when all the modes are offered, how can you be sure it actually *is* DBT? Distinguishing the functions from the modes of treatment created an important tool in evaluating whether a program was really *doing* DBT. For example, meeting 1 hour a week as a team and reviewing cases is not a DBT team meeting unless there is explicit discussion of what the therapists need in order to be more skillful and/or more motivated to provide DBT to their clients.

This book is personally very exciting to me for a number of reasons. First, this is a book on how to transfer DBT to your own setting if there ever was one: It is filled with very specific tools, strategies, and recommendations for building and sustaining your DBT programs. It reflects two decades of learning about how best to disseminate and implement DBT across a wide array of settings and client populations and how to adapt it in a fashion that best preserves its fidelity. The principles applied throughout this book arise directly from the treatment itself. This book will, without doubt, have an impact on the field—it will certainly influence clinicians wishing to build or sustain a DBT program, but I hope it will also provide a set of tools that may be helpful to the field as a whole as we focus our efforts and energies on improving our capability to transfer what we have developed in the lab to the front lines of treatment.

Second, this book was inspired, conceived of, organized, and edited by two of my students at the University of Washington, Drs. Linda A. Dimeff and Kelly Koerner. Both Linda and Kelly were with me at the Behavioral Research and Therapy Clinics (BRTC), my clinic at the University of Washington, long before DBT was a popular, "in-demand" treatment. Kelly was part of the very first DBT treatment team at the BRTC. She, along with the other students on the team, provided critical feedback that ultimately influenced the development of DBT. Linda joined my lab just as I was pioneering my first adaptation of DBT to a population of polysubstance-dependent individuals with BPD. Linda and other members of my drug-treatment team made significant contributions to the development of DBT for substance abusers (described in Chapter 6) and she has been my chief coauthor of the articles and papers that describe that treatment. Both Linda and Kelly helped form what is now Behavioral Tech, LLC—Kelly as an initial founder with me and the organization's very first President and CEO. Linda was the very first Director of Research and Development at what is now Behavioral Tech Research, Inc. Both Linda and Kelly are experts in DBT and have extensive expertise in training and consulting to teams who are building their DBT programs. Indeed, many of the contributors to this book are also my students and chief research collaborators. As their teacher, mentor, friend, and colleague, nothing gives me greater delight than to see them each actively extend my work in this fashion.

I wish to offer two words of wisdom as I conclude. The first is about how to approach this book and the second is about how to approach your work in applying DBT. About the first, I recommend that you read widely, and not limit yourself to only those chapters that have the greatest relevance to you and your program. It may be by carefully reading a chapter that appears to have no direct relevance to your work that you have the greatest "ah-ha" moment of all: You'll see the DBT principles at play in a new light; you'll have a creative brainstorm around a particular programmatic roadblock; and you'll feel part of a large DBT community that is thinking creatively, compassionately, and scientifically about how to solve complex problems in the service of improving the lives of some of the most challenging of clients.

About the second, I encourage you to know and follow the data on both CBT (cognitive-behavioral therapy) and DBT, and to keep your allegiance not to DBT, but to what is most effective based on the empirical literature. After nine randomized controlled published trials, we know DBT is effective. We are at just the beginning of what promises to be an important and exciting area of research where we can identify the active ingredients of DBT. What is abundantly clear is that for severely disordered individuals with BPD and other complex behavioral problems, comprehensive DBT (i.e., all DBT functions and modes) is effective. As more is empirically known about what is and is not effective in DBT, I expect that the treatment itself will change—to be in sync with the empirical literature.

Best wishes to you in your further development and mastery of DBT.

MARSHA M. LINEHAN, PhD
Seattle, Washington

REFERENCES

Linehan, M. M. (1993a). *Cognitive-behavioral treatment of borderline personality disorder*. New York: Guilford Press.

Linehan, M. M. (1993b). *Skills training manual for treating borderline personality disorder*. New York: Guilford Press.

Linehan, M. M. (1999). Development, evaluation, and dissemination of effective psychosocial treatments: Levels of disorder, stages of care, and stages of treatment research. In M. G. Glantz & C. R. Hartel (Eds.), *Drug abuse: Origins and interventions* (pp. 367–394). Washington, DC: American Psychological Association.

Linehan, M. M., Cochran, B., & Kehrer, C. A. (2001). Borderline personality disorder. In D. H. Barlow (Ed.), *Clinical handbook of psychological disorders* (3rd ed., pp. 470–522). New York: Guilford Press.

Preface

This book is intended to save you grief.

We have spent many years as trainers and consultants helping people use dialectical behavior therapy (DBT). What we have learned is that even across very different clinical settings and populations, the questions and challenges in implementing DBT are remarkably similar.

This means two things. First, it means that sharing the concise set of information we present here will help you avoid common pitfalls as you adopt and adapt DBT to your particular setting. We suggest you read Chapters 1, 2, and 12 first. Chapter 1 provides an overview of DBT and clarifies some of its more confusing elements. It is a great chapter to share with colleagues as a first introduction to DBT. Chapter 2 helps you decide whether to adopt DBT's standard model or to adapt it to better fit your situation. Chapter 12 provides a step-by-step method to evaluate your implementation of DBT. These chapters address many of the questions and challenges common across settings and populations.

Second, it means that no matter how seemingly unique the barriers of your setting, it is likely that someone in the broader DBT community has faced them too. When we teach and consult to teams implementing DBT, we repeatedly find ourselves saying, "Do you know so-and-so? Let me put you in touch with them! They faced the same issue and what they did was. . . . " This book puts you in touch with many gifted clinicians and program directors who offer you hard-won, firsthand experience of successfully adopting and adapting DBT. We asked authors, most of whom themselves teach and consult to other teams, "What do you wish someone had told you as you began to use DBT? What difficulties did you face and what advice would you offer so that others can benefit from your experience?" The quality of creative problem solving you will find in these chapters will save you from reinventing many wheels!

After reading Chapters 1, 2, and 12, we suggest that you next read Chapters 3 and 4, followed by any chapters that address specific populations or settings of interest to you. If you are looking for ideas about how to solve a particular problem, you might use the index to see solutions across different settings and populations (e.g., look up "telephone coaching" and "crisis calls" for all the creative ways to make this important mode of DBT work).

Early drafts of each chapter were critiqued by readers like you to make sure authors responded to their nitty-gritty practical questions. Then each chapter draft was critiqued by experts in DBT adherence, that is, by people whose job it is to ensure that specific instances of DBT stay true to the researched model and its principles. Integrating all of this feedback was an arduous process for all involved. But the resulting chapters offer you the state of the art: the combined wisdom, innovation, and rigor of some of DBT's best clinicians and researchers as they deliberately anticipate and address the questions you will have as you use DBT.

May this work be of benefit to you.

KELLY KOERNER
LINDA A. DIMEFF
June 27, 2007

Acknowledgments

Sometimes you undertake a project that you think will be straightforward, and it instead takes a very different path, leaving you finally, at the end, grateful and wizened. The untimely death of Cindy Sanderson, the original lead editor for this project, was a terrible loss. Cindy was a gifted writer and rigorous thinker; her quirky, hilarious, and rabidly curious intellect and charismatic teaching encouraged hundreds of dialectical behavior therapy (DBT) teams in their work. To this day, Cindy's vast kindness and compassion remain with many of us who contributed to this book. Her influence on our work has been invaluable. Her long-time collaboration with Charles Swenson is an unacknowledged root and catalyst for much of the successful dissemination of DBT; their work is a ground note for many. The impact of Cindy's death strongly reverberated throughout the DBT community, as had her life, deeply affecting those who knew her. This book is dedicated, with great respect, to her life and memory.

The authors in this book similarly have been change agents. The work they describe and the advice they offer distill years of personal and professional struggle and leadership. It takes deep courage to be the first to adopt and implement a new treatment, particularly one like DBT that is intended, by design, for the most severe, high-risk, and out-of-control clients. Writing a chapter for this particular book posed its own unique set of challenges. Unlike many writing projects where the authors complete their draft, receive a few critiques, and make a few revisions, authors for this book received extensive, complex critiques and requests for substantial changes. These requests came from multiple stakeholders: front-line clinicians who wanted even greater detail about *what* to do; senior scientists who wanted greater review of the research literature; DBT experts who pushed for revisions and clarification to ensure that the text conveyed fully adherent DBT. We are grateful beyond words to all the contributing authors of this book for their patience with the process, their own high standards for excellence, and their willingness to enter into often extensive conversations about our requested revisions. We are particularly grateful to the chapter leads (Alan E. Fruzzetti, Alec L. Miller, André Ivanoff, Cedar R. Koons, Charles R. Swenson, Jennifer H. R. Sayrs, Katherine Anne Comtois, Lucene Wisniewski, Robin A. McCann, Thomas R. Lynch, Sarah K. Reynolds, Shelley McMain, and Shireen L. Rizvi) for overseeing the total efforts and ultimately assuming the burden and hardship of delivering.

We thank Meredith Byars, who served as a managing editor before she left for law school. Her commitment to social justice for underserved populations, her tenacity, her resourcefulness, and her organizational prowess have taken many forms in her career. We deeply appreciate her early contributions to launching this book.

Many colleagues reviewed early drafts to ensure that each chapter addressed the specific needs of other clinicians working in comparable settings and/or with comparable clients. We appreciate the thoughtfulness of their critiques, which often helped identify the most important issues of all when it comes to implementing DBT in clinical practice. We are indebted to Kathryn E. Korslund, Associate Director of the Behavioral Research and Therapy Clinic at the University of Washington, who provided extensive and invaluable feedback on each chapter in this book regarding its adherence to DBT. She has an amazing capacity to share her expertise in a concise, pointed, generous fashion, remaining gracious regardless of time pressures. Sharon Y. Manning, President/CEO of Behavioral Tech, LLC, and Behavioral Tech Research, Inc., also reviewed each chapter to ensure adherence to DBT. Dr. Manning is herself an early adopter of DBT who has extensive experience implementing it in a wide variety of settings and with diverse clients, which proved invaluable in her critique. Andrew Paves served as our steadfast and exceptionally competent research assistant, who provided the administrative support to editors and authors—from reformatting tables and finding citations to managing multiple versions of drafts, people, and timelines. Eric Woodcock beautifully provided further administrative assistance at the project's end, as we made the final mad dash to the finish line.

We would like to thank Kitty Moore, Executive Editor at The Guilford Press, for guiding the development and evolution of this book and providing the occasional nudges that kept it moving forward. We are also very grateful to Jennifer DePrima, our production editor at Guilford, for ensuring that the final product reflected the effort we devoted to this project over the past several years.

Finally, we would like to express our sincere appreciation to our mentor and DBT treatment developer, Marsha M. Linehan. The field has repeatedly recognized her contributions. For us, however, as her students, we feel a depth of gratitude that is hard to put into words. We have seen the great personal sacrifice, professional integrity, and courage her work has required: the fight through then-dominant clinical opinion and ad hominem attacks in her early years to insist that a compassionate, scientific approach be brought to help those with borderline personality disorder who struggle with suicidal behaviors; the ongoing struggle to provide training for graduate students and professionals, ensuring that no clinician is left without the necessary capabilities to care for those who are most in need; the spirit of contemplation in action that makes science, clinical practice, and mindfulness inseparable. Her dedication has inspired our own, and it is with joy that we dedicate this book to her.

LINDA A. DIMEFF
KELLY KOERNER

Contents

CHAPTER 1

Overview of Dialectical Behavior Therapy

Kelly Koerner *and* Linda A. Dimeff

In this chapter we provide an overview of standard outpatient dialectical behavior therapy (DBT) and its evidence base. Our purpose is to describe DBT in enough detail to help you determine whether adopting DBT will meet the needs of your setting or population. This chapter also serves as an anchor and reference point on the standard outpatient model of DBT so that you can easily compare and contrast it with variations of DBT described in subsequent chapters. This chapter is also meant to be one you could share with colleagues as an introduction to DBT.

DBT in a Nutshell

DBT is a cognitive-behavioral treatment originally developed by Marsha M. Linehan, PhD, as a treatment for chronically suicidal individuals, and first validated with suicidal women who met criteria for borderline personality disorder (BPD). Those with BPD represent 14–20% of inpatients (Widiger & Frances, 1989; Widiger & Weissman, 1991), include 8–11% of outpatients (Widiger & Frances, 1989; Kroll, Sines, & Martin, 1981; Modestin, Abrecht, Tschaggelar, & Hoffman, 1997), and consume a disproportionate amount of mental health resources, often up to 40%. Adequately addressing the needs of individuals with BPD poses several challenges. Individuals with BPD typically require therapy for multiple, complex, and severe Axis I problems, often in the context of unrelenting crises and management of high-risk suicidal behavior. With many of these clients, the sheer number of serious (at times life-threatening) problems that therapy must address makes it difficult to establish and maintain a treatment focus. Following the concern most pressing to the client can result in a different crisis management focus each week. Therapy can feel like a car veering out of control, barely averting disaster, with a sense of forward motion but no meaningful progress.

Treatment decisions are made yet more complicated because clients with chronic suicidal behavior and extreme emotional sensitivity often act in ways that distress their therapists. Suicide attempts, threats of suicide attempts, and anger directed at the therapist can be very stressful. Regardless of their training and experience, therapists can struggle with their own emotional reactions when a client is recurrently suicidal and both rejects the help that the therapist offers and demands help that therapist cannot give. Even when the therapist is on the right track, progress can be slow and sporadic. All these factors increase the chance of therapeutic errors, including making premature changes to the treatment plan, and may contribute to the fact that those with BPD have high rates of treatment failure (Perry & Cooper, 1985; Tucker, Bauer, Wagner, Harlam, & Sher, 1987). Intense distress, treatment failure, and repeated suicidal behavior, in turn, contribute to the high use of psychiatric services by this population. Individuals who meet criteria for BPD typically have sought help repeatedly and from multiple sources; in one study, 97% of those seeking treatment had received prior outpatient treatment from a mean of 6.1 previous therapists and 72% had had at least one psychiatric hospitalization (Skodol, Buckley, & Charles, 1983; Perry, Herman, Van der Kolk, & Hoke, 1990; Bender et al., 2001). Legal and ethical concerns about suicide make it difficult to limit hospital use, even when "revolving door" use of involuntary inpatient facilities may itself inadvertently cause harm (i.e., be iatrogenic). The experience for individuals who meet criteria for BPD and their treatment providers has historically been a discouraging path of recurrent treatment failures despite their best efforts.

It was within this context that DBT evolved. As Linehan began to use standard clinical behavior therapy (Goldfried & Davison, 1976), she was led by the nature of her clients' problems to balance and complement behavior therapy's change orientation with other therapeutic strategies. Linehan's careful observation of successes and failures resulted in treatment manuals (1993a, 1993b) that organize strategies into protocols and that structure therapy and clinical decision making so that therapists can respond flexibly to an ever-changing clinical picture. Although DBT shares elements with the psychodynamic, client-centered, gestalt, paradoxical, and strategic approaches to therapy (cf. Heard & Linehan, 1994), it is the application of behavioral science, mindfulness, and dialectical philosophy that are its defining features.

DBT has evolved into a sophisticated treatment, yet most of its concepts are quite straightforward. For example, DBT emphasizes an organized, systematic approach in which members of the treatment team share fundamental assumptions about therapy and clients. DBT considers suicidal behavior to be a form of maladaptive problem solving and uses well-researched cognitive-behavioral therapy (CBT) techniques to help clients solve life problems in more adaptive ways. DBT therapists take every opportunity to strengthen clients' valid responses, which alone and in combination with CBT interventions facilitate change (e.g., Linehan et al., 2002). Because difficult clinical problems naturally provoke strong differing opinions among treatment providers, and because DBT clients' problems themselves include dichotomous, rigid thinking and behavioral and emotional extremes, dialectical philosophy and strategies offer a means of reconciling differences so that conflicts in therapy are met with movement rather than with impasse. Below we discuss each of these in turn as a way to lay out DBT in a nutshell.

DBT as Framework

A number of elements of DBT provide a structure or conceptual frame for the therapist and client. DBT case conceptualization is based on biosocial theory and level of disorder. These in turn translate into a basic collaborative therapeutic stance and into treatment goals and targets that are hierarchically organized according to importance. These targets are clearly assigned to modes of services delivery (weekly individual psychotherapy and skills training, and as-needed phone consultation for clients; weekly peer consultation for therapists) so that specific duties and roles are assigned and each mode has specific targets it is responsible for treating. We next sketch each of these in turn.

Biosocial Theory

According to Linehan (1993a), the primary problem of BPD is pervasive disorder of the emotion regulation system. This idea guides all treatment interventions and is used as a psychoeducational frame so that clients and therapists share a common understanding of problems and interventions. From this perspective, BPD criterion behaviors function to regulate emotions (e.g., suicidal behavior) or are a consequence of failed emotion regulation (e.g., dissociative symptoms or transient psychotic symptoms).

This pervasive emotion dysregulation is hypothesized to be developed and maintained by both biological and environmental factors. On the biological side, individuals are thought to be more vulnerable to difficulties regulating their emotions due to differences in the central nervous system (e.g., due to genetics, events during fetal development, or early life trauma). Emerging research suggests that those with BPD do experience more frequent, more intense, and longer-lasting aversive states (Stiglmayr et al., 2005), and that biological vulnerability may contribute to their difficulties in regulating their emotions (e.g., Juengling et al., 2003; Ebner-Priemer et al., 2005). Because, normatively, many capabilities depend on adequate emotion regulation, difficulties here result in instabilities in an abiding sense of self, resolution of interpersonal conflict, goal-oriented action, and the like.

Problems arise when a biologically vulnerable individual is in a pervasively invalidating environment. Invalidating environments communicate that the individual's characteristic responses to events (particularly his or her emotional responses) are incorrect, inappropriate, pathological, or not to be taken seriously. Not understanding how debilitating it is to struggle with emotion regulation, those in the environment oversimplify the ease of solving problems and fail to teach the individual to tolerate distress or to form realistic goals and expectations. By punishing communication of negative experiences and only responding to negative emotional displays when they are escalated, the environment teaches the individual to oscillate between emotional inhibition and extreme emotional communication.

Childhood sexual abuse is a prototypical invalidating environment related to BPD, given the correlation observed among BPD, suicidal behavior, and reports of childhood sexual abuse (Wagner & Linehan, 1997). However, because not all individuals who meet BPD criteria report histories of sexual abuse and because not all victims of childhood sexual abuse develop BPD, it remains unclear how to account for individual differences. Interesting findings suggest that negative affect intensity/reactivity is a stronger predictor of BPD symptoms than childhood sexual abuse and that higher thought suppression may mediate the relationship between BPD symptoms and childhood sexual abuse (Rosenthal, Cheavens, Lejuez, & Lynch, 2005).

The resulting pervasive emotion dysregulation interferes with problem solving and creates problems in its own right. For example, a client comes into her therapy session after having been fired because she lost her temper with a coworker. When the therapist asks what happened, the client is overwhelmed with shame, becomes mute, and curls up in the chair, banging her head against the armrest. This response derails any help the therapist might have offered about managing anger at work and creates a new situation about which the client feels shame (i.e., how she acted in therapy). Such maladaptive behaviors, including extreme behaviors such as suicidal behavior, function to solve problems and, in particular, dysfunctional behaviors solve the problem of painful emotional states by providing relief. For clients, it is difficult to know whether to blame oneself or others: either one is able to control one's own behavior (as others believe and expect) but won't, and therefore one is "manipulative," or one is unable to control one's emotions, as a lifetime of experiences shows, which means that life will always be a never-ending nightmare of dyscontrol. When the person tries to fulfill expectations that are out of line with true capabilities, he or she may fail, feel ashamed, and decide that being punished or even being dead is what is deserved. When the person adjusts his or her own standards to accommodate vulnerability but others do not, the client can become angry that no one offers needed help.

This is a key dilemma in therapy. When the therapist focuses on accepting vulnerability and limitations, this sets off despair that problems will never change; focusing on change, however, may trigger panic because clients who have struggled with pervasive emotion dysregulation know that there is no way to consistently meet expectations. The DBT therapist must understand and reckon with the intense pain involved in living without "emotional skin" and directly target reduction in painful emotions and solutions to problems that give rise to painful emotions. For example, in response to intense emotional reactions during therapeutic tasks (e.g., talking about an event from the previous week), the therapist validates the uncontrollable, helpless experience of emotional arousal, and teaches the individual to modulate emotion in session, balancing, moment to moment, the use of supportive acceptance and confrontive change strategies.

Levels of Disorder and Stages, Goals, and Targets of Treatment

In DBT the current extent of disordered behavior determines what treatment tasks are relevant and feasible. For example, what is relevant and feasible for a homeless client with out-of-control heroin use, who has angrily "blown out" of multiple methadone treatment programs, and who has recently attempted suicide, is different than what is relevant and feasible for a nurse, also addicted to opiates, who avoided a suspended license for stealing drugs from work and has a supportive family and an employer who is willing to take him back when he's drug-free. While many of the interventions for addiction will be the same, the first person needs more comprehensive help. Treating some of her behaviors (e.g., suicide attempts) will take precedence over treating others. Multiple problems (e.g., drug abuse, homelessness, out-of-control anger) may need to be solved simultaneously. In a commonsense way, DBT's stage model of treatment (Linehan, 1993a, 1996) prioritizes the problems that must be addressed at a particular point in therapy according to the threat they pose to the client's reasonable quality of life.

The first stage of treatment with all DBT clients is pretreatment, followed by one to four subsequent stages. The number of subsequent stages depends on the extent of behavioral disorder when the client begins treatment. In the pretreatment stage, as with other CBT approaches, the client and the therapist explicitly and collaboratively agree to the essential goals and methods of treatment. While it is not important to have a written contract, it is important to have a mutual verbal commitment to treatment agreements. Specific agreements may vary by setting and clients' problems, but for the client might include agreeing to work on the Stage 1 treatment targets for a specified length of treatment and attend all scheduled sessions, pay fees, and the like. For the therapist, they might include agreeing to provide the best treatment possible (including increasing his or her own skills as needed), to abide by ethical principles, and to participate in consultation. Such agreements should be in place before beginning formal treatment. Because DBT requires voluntary rather than coerced consent, both the client and the therapist must have the choice of committing to DBT over some other non-DBT option. So, for example, in a forensic unit or when a client is legally mandated to treatment, he or she is not considered to have entered DBT until a considered verbal commitment is obtained. In pretreatment, once the therapist commits to the client, the priority is to obtain engagement in therapy.

Stage 1 of DBT is for the most severe level of disorder. Stage 1 of therapy targets behaviors needed to achieve reasonable (immediate) life expectancy, control of action, and sufficient connection to treatment and behavioral capabilities to achieve these goals. To reach these goals, treatment time is allocated to give priority to targets in the following order of importance: (1) suicidal/homicidal or other imminently life-threatening behavior; (2) therapy-interfering behavior by the therapist or the client; (3) behavior that severely compromises the client's quality of life (e.g., Axis I problems as well as serious problems with relationships, the legal system, employment/school, illness, and housing); and (4) deficits in behavioral capabilities needed to make life changes. DBT assumes that certain deficits are particularly relevant to BPD and provides training to help clients (1) regulate emotions; (2) tolerate distress; (3) respond skillfully to interpersonal situations; (4) observe, describe, and participate without judging, with awareness and focusing on effectiveness; and (5) manage their own behavior with strategies other than self-punishment. These skills are linked to the particular BPD criterion behaviors with mindfulness intended to decrease identity confusion, emptiness, and cognitive dysregulation; interpersonal effectiveness addressing interpersonal chaos and fears of abandonment; emotion regulation skills reducing labile affect and excessive anger; and distress tolerance helping to reduce impulsive behaviors, suicide threats, and intentional self-injury. It's important to note that DBT actively targets therapy-interfering behaviors of both the client and the therapist, viewing it as second only to life-threatening behavior. In other words, client behaviors that interfere with receiving therapy such as not attending, noncollaboration, and noncompliance, or that push therapist limits or reduce his or her motivation to treat the client are viewed on an equal footing as behaviors of the therapist that unbalance therapy such as being extremely accepting or extremely change-focused, too flexible or too rigid, too nurturing or too withholding, and so on. Specific targets are mutually identified and then are monitored and provide the main agenda for individual therapy sessions along with helping the client reach individual goals. In DBT it is important to communicate that the goals of therapy are not simply to suppress severe dysfunctional behavior, but rather to build a life that any reasonable person would consider worth living.

Many clients who are not out of control still experience tremendous emotional pain due to either posttraumatic stress responses or other painful emotional experiences that leave them alienated or isolated from meaningful connections to other people or to a vocation. They suffer lives of quiet desperation, where emotional experience is either too intense (although behavioral control is maintained) or the person is numbed. Therefore, with these clients, the Stage 2 goals of therapy are to have nontraumatizing emotional experience and connection to the environment. In Stage 3 the client synthesizes what has been learned, increases his or her self-respect and an abiding sense of connection, and works toward resolving problems in living. Targets here are self-respect, mastery, self-efficacy, a sense of morality, and an acceptable quality of life. Stage 4 (Linehan, 1996) focuses on the sense of incompleteness that many individuals experience, even after problems in living are essentially resolved. For many, Stage 4 goals fall outside the realm of traditional therapy and within a spiritual practice that gives rise to the capacity for freedom, joy, or spiritual fulfillment.

Although the stages of therapy are presented linearly, progress is often not linear and the stages overlap. It is not uncommon to return to discussions like those of pretreatment to regain commitment to the treatment goals or methods. The transition from Stage 1 to Stage 2 is also difficult for many, because exposure work can lead to intense, painful emotions and consequent behavioral dyscontrol. Like other trauma approaches (cf. Follette & Ruzek, 2006), DBT encourages acquisition of skills to a sufficient level that one has a reasonable quality of life/stability of behavioral control prior to systematic exposure to the cues that are associated with past traumas. The infrequency of Stage 1 behaviors as well as the speed of reregulation (rather than the presence of any one instance of behavior) defines the differences between stages. Readiness for Stage 2 work is idiosyncratic. In general, the client is ready for transition when he or she is no longer engaging in severe dysfunctional behavior, can maintain a strong therapy relationship, and has demonstrated to his or her own and the therapist's satisfaction the ability to cope with cues that used to set off problem behavior. Stage 3 is often a review of the same issues from a different vantage point.

Level of disorder and stages of treatment have implications for service delivery. Many clinics have different levels of care contingent on the severity of behavioral dyscontrol. What's required is to have reinforcers (e.g., more and more in-depth services) available contingent on progress rather than on continuation of maladaptive behavior. For example, if it is the case that someone can only get individual therapy by being completely out of control or that clients lose access to individual therapists as soon as they are out of crisis, then the contingencies favor lack of progress and continued crises.

As mentioned earlier, responsibility for treating specific targets is assigned to modes. For example, the individual psychotherapist is assigned the role of treatment planning, ensuring that progress is made on all DBT targets, helping to integrate other modes of therapy, consulting to the client on effective behaviors with other providers, and management of crises and life-threatening behaviors. This allows the primary therapist—who is often the person who best knows the client's capabilities—to teach, to strengthen, and to generalize the client's new responses to crises without reinforcing client dysfunctional behavior. This also prevents multiple alternative treatment plans being run at once.

The skills trainer's role is to ensure that the client acquires new skills. To maximize learning and keep roles from conflicting, he or she only minimally targets behaviors that interfere with skills training (e.g., dissociating in group, coming late), referring the client back to the primary individual therapist to work on the bulk of those problems. Similarly, in suicidal and other crises, the skills trainer refers the client back to the individual therapist, after conducting requisite suicide risk assessment and providing the intervention needed to get the client in contact with the primary therapist.

DBT as Problem Solving

As mentioned earlier, DBT uses empirically supported behavior therapy protocols to treat Axis I problems. As do other CBT approaches, it emphasizes use of behavioral principles and behavioral assessment to determine the controlling variables for problem behaviors. It uses standard CBT interventions (e.g., self-monitoring, behavioral analysis and solution analysis, didactic and orienting strategies, contingency management, cognitive restructuring, skills training, and exposure procedures). Rather than describe such CBT interventions in depth, we assume that the reader is already familiar with them. Here we highlight those that are unique to or emphasized in DBT. For example, all CBT approaches include psychoeducation and place a strong emphasis on orienting the client to the treatment rationale and treatment methods. However, because the emotional arousal of clients with BPD often interferes with their information processing and collaboration, their DBT therapist frequently must do what could be called "micro-orienting," instructing the client specifically about what to do in the particular treatment task at hand.

As the primary therapist and client identify and commit to goals for therapy in the first several sessions, the therapist gathers the history needed to accurately assess suicide risk and begins to identify situations that evoke suicide ideation and intentional self-injury in order to manage suicidal crises. In particular, the therapist identifies the conditions associated with near-lethal suicide attempts, suicidal behavior with high intent to die, and other medically serious intentional self-injury.

After the client and the therapist develop their goals and agreements, the client begins to monitor those behaviors they've agreed to target. Whenever one of the targeted problem behaviors occurs, the therapist and the client conduct an in-depth analysis of events and situational factors before, during, and after that particular instance (or set of instances) of the targeted behavior. The goal of this *chain analysis* is to provide an accurate and reasonably complete account of the behavioral and environmental events associated with the problem behavior. As the therapist and the client discuss a chain of events, the therapist highlights dysfunctional behavior, focusing on emotions, and helps the client gain insight by recognizing the patterns between this and other instances of problem behavior. Together they identify where an alternative client response might have produced positive change and why that more skillful alternative did not happen. This process of identifying the problem and analyzing the chain of events moment to moment over time to determine which variables control/influence the behavior occurs for each targeted problem behavior as it occurs.

As in other CBT approaches, the absence of adaptive behavior is considered to be due to one of four factors linked to behavior therapy change procedures: skills training, exposure procedures, contingency management, and cognitive restructuring. If chain analysis reveals a capability deficit (i.e., the client does not have the necessary skills in his or her repertoire), then skills training is emphasized. When the client does have the skill, but emotions, contingencies, or cognitions interfere with his or her ability to act skillfully, the therapist uses basic principles and strategies from exposure procedures, contingency management, and cognitive restructuring to help the client overcome barriers to using his or her capabilities.

Similarly, when cognitive-behavioral therapists generate solutions, they typically also preemptively figure out what would prevent the use of the solution or troubleshoot. In DBT this troubleshooting takes on added emphasis because the client often has severe mood-dependent behaviors and one cannot assume generalization in the same way one would with a less mood-dependent person.

Treating clients with multiple severe and chronic disorders requires the therapist to know treatment protocols for specific disorders but also requires the therapist to have some cohesive way of integrating them to treat an ever-changing clinical picture. The complexity of the task is further complicated because of the work one must do to establish and keep a collaborative and productive therapeutic relationship. One could treat the presenting or major problem first, see what resolves, and then proceed to treat the multiple other Axis I disorders sequentially. However, even if one had enough time (and enough insurance coverage) to do so, between one session and the next a typically dysregulated client has had a major life crisis. For example, last week a client took home readings to orient her to treatment for panic disorder. The therapist came to the session ready to discuss the treatment rationale. However, as she looked over the diary card and asked how the week went, the session agenda radically shifted. In the intervening week the client had had a fight with her boyfriend, who kicked her out of his apartment. She was on the street and had been staying in a homeless shelter for the past 2 days. While at the shelter she was sexually harassed, setting off nightmares and some dissociative symptoms. Because of all the chaos in her life, she skipped skills training group and she now doubts that she can make it to group this week either. Living on the street she ran into some of her old drug buddies and she used heroin. She describes the week in a matter-of-fact tone of voice, yet her diary card shows high ratings on misery and suicidal ideation. When the therapist assesses suicidality, she discovers that the client has her preferred means in her car. As the session continues, the client dissociates to the point where she is not talking.

As mentioned earlier, DBT was developed for people with multiple disorders who are often in crisis. DBT interventions will hierarchically target behaviors so that the immediate focus will be to assess and treat suicide risk. However, in addition to getting rid of the immediate means and addressing the problems associated with suicidal behavior, the therapist may also need to address the problems of housing, going to skills group, not using heroin again, managing dissociative behaviors, and processing the end of the romantic relationship (and perhaps shame and despair at not starting treatment for panic). This requires the therapist to apply mini-interventions drawn from effective behavioral protocols to problems as they arise. The required improvisation is akin to jazz—it is built upon sound mastery of one's instrument and understanding of music but tightly linked to the exact moment and players. This flexible application of strategies results from overlearning of behavior therapy protocols and also from dialectical philosophy and strategies that help at therapeutic impasses.

Skills Training

Comprehensive DBT includes skills training as a treatment mode dedicated to enhancing skills capabilities in areas where many individuals with BPD have behavioral deficits. With its focus on teaching and strengthening DBT skills (Linehan, 1993b, in press), DBT skills training is provided on a weekly basis for approximately 2½ hours. Linehan's *Skills Training Manual for Borderline Personality Disorder* (1993b), as well as its second edition (Linehan, in press), provide extensive instructions for therapists in how to teach the DBT skills, explicit instructions for practicing the skills in group, and numerous reproducible client handouts and homework sheets. Four skills training modules are taught over the course of approximately 6 months, allowing for completion of all skills twice within a standard DBT outpatient group. DBT skills training modules include skills to regulate emotions (emotion regulation skills), to tolerate emotional distress when change is slow or unlikely (distress tolerance skills), to be more effective in interpersonal conflicts (interpersonal effectiveness skills), and to control attention in order to skillfully participate in the moment (mindfulness skills). *Emotion regulation* training teaches a range of behavioral and cognitive strategies for reducing unwanted emotional responses as well as impulsive dysfunctional behaviors that occur in the context of intense emotions by teaching clients how to identify and describe emotions, how to stop avoiding negative emotions, how to increase positive emotions, and how to change unwanted negative emotions. *Distress tolerance* training teaches a number of impulse control and self-soothing techniques aimed at surviving crises without using drugs, attempting suicide, or engaging in other dysfunctional behavior. *Interpersonal effectiveness* teaches a variety of assertiveness skills to achieve one's objective while maintaining relationships and one's self-respect. *Mindfulness skills* include focusing attention on observing oneself or one's immediate context, describing observations, participating (spontaneously), assuming a non-judgmental stance, focusing awareness, and developing effectiveness (focusing on what works).

Although all CBT pays attention to generalization, this goal is particularly emphasized in DBT. To generalize newly acquired skills across situations in daily life, therapists employ phone consultation and *in vivo* therapy (i.e., therapy outside the office as needed). While skills acquisition and strengthening is the domain of the skills trainers in the context of the skills training group, it is the task of the individual therapist to help generalize these skills in all relevant contexts.

Validation

DBT shares elements with other supportive treatment approaches (Heard & Linehan, 1994). Exquisite emotional sensitivity, proneness to emotional dysregulation, and a long history of failed attempts to change either this intense emotionality or the problem behaviors associated with it make supportive treatment elements important. All clients benefit from validation, but validation is essential for the success of change-oriented strategies with those who are particularly emotionally sensitive and prone to emotional dysregulation (Linehan, 1993a). DBT validation strategies are meant not only to communicate empathic understanding but also to communicate the validity of the client's emotions, thoughts, and actions. In DBT these strategies are important in and of themselves, as well as in combination with change strategies. Validation is also used to balance the pathologizing to which both clients and therapists are prone. Clients often have learned to treat their own valid responses as invalid (as "stupid," "weak," "defective," "bad"). Similarly, therapists also have learned to view normal responses as pathological. Validation strategies balance this viewpoint by requiring the therapist to search for the strengths, normality, or effectiveness inherent in the client's responses whenever possible and by teaching the client to self-validate. Even patently invalid behavior may be valid in terms of being effective. When a client says she hates herself, hatred might be valid because it is a justifiable response if the person acted in a manner that violates important values (e.g., she had deliberately harmed another person out of anger). Cutting one's arms in response to overwhelming emotional distress is valid (i.e., makes sense), given that it often produces relief from unbearable emotions: It is an effective emotion regulation strategy. Cutting is simultaneously invalid: It is not normative, it prevents developing other means of emotion regulation, it causes scars, and it alienates others. The same behavior can be both valid and invalid at the same time. From this perspective, all behavior is valid in some way. The DBT therapist strives to identify and communicate what is valid with the client.

In nearly all situations, the DBT therapist may validate that the client's problems are important, that a task is difficult, that emotional pain or a sense of being out of control is understandable, and that there is wisdom in the client's ultimate goals, even if not the particular means he or she might use to achieve them. Similarly, it is often useful for the therapist to validate the client's views about life problems and beliefs about how changes can or should be made. Unless the client believes that the therapist truly understands his or her dilemma (e.g., exactly how painful, difficult to change, or important a problem is), he or she will not trust that the therapist's solutions are appropriate or adequate, and therefore collaboration and consequently the therapist's ability to help the client change will be limited. In this way, validation is essential to change: The therapist must simultaneously deeply understand the client's perspective as well as maintain hope and clarity about how to effect change.

DBT as Dialectics

Dialectical philosophy has been influential across the sciences (Basseches, 1984; Levins & Lewontin, 1985). In DBT it provides the practical means for the therapist and the client to retain flexibility and balance. Dialectics is both a method of persuasion and a worldview or set of assumptions about the nature of reality. In both, an essential idea is that each thesis or statement of a position contains within it its antithesis or opposite position. For example, suicidal clients often simultaneously want to live and want to die. Saying aloud to the therapist, "I want to die," rather than killing oneself in secrecy, contains within it the opposite position of wanting to live. However, it is not the case that wanting to live is "more true" than wanting to die. The person genuinely does not want to live his or her life as it currently is—few of us would trade stations with our clients with BPD. Nor does the low lethality of a suicide attempt mean that the person really did not want to die. It's not even that the person alternates between the two—the client simultaneously holds both opposing positions. Dialectical change or progress comes from the resolution of these opposing positions into a synthesis. The whole dialogue of therapy constructs new positions where the quality of one's life doesn't give rise to wanting to die. Suicide is one way out of an unbearable life. However, building a life that is genuinely worth living is an equally valid position. The constant refrain in DBT is that a better solution can be found. The best alternative to suicide is to build a life that is worth living.

Cognitive modification strategies in DBT are based on dialectical persuasion. Although the DBT therapist may sometimes challenge problematic beliefs with reason or through hypothesis-testing experiments, as do other cognitive-behavioral therapies, there is a special emphasis on cognitive modification through conversations that create the experience of the contradictions inherent in one's own position. For example, a client who experiences immediate relief from intense emotional pain when she burns her arms with cigarettes is reluctant to give it up. As the therapist assesses the factors that led up to a recent incident, the client nonchalantly says, "The burn really wasn't that bad this time."

THERAPIST: So what you're saying is that if you saw a person in a lot of emotional pain, say your little niece, and she was feeling as badly as you were the night you burned your arm, she was feeling as devastated by disappointment as you were that night, you'd burn her arm with a cigarette to help her feel better.

CLIENT: No I wouldn't.

THERAPIST: Why not?

CLIENT: I just wouldn't.

THERAPIST: I believe you wouldn't, but why not?

CLIENT: I'd comfort her or do something else to help her feel better.

THERAPIST: But what if she was inconsolable, and nothing you did made her feel better? Besides, you wouldn't burn her that badly.

CLIENT: I just wouldn't do it. It's not right. I'd do something, but not that.

THERAPIST: That's interesting, don't you think?

The client simultaneously believes that one should not burn someone else under any circumstances and that burning herself to get relief is no big deal. In dialectical persuasion, the therapist highlights the inconsistencies among the client's own actions, beliefs, and values. The dialogue focuses on helping the client reach a viewpoint that is more whole and internally consistent with her values.

A dialectical worldview permeates DBT. A dialectical perspective holds that one can't make sense of the parts without considering the whole, that the nature of reality is holistic even if it appears that one can talk meaningfully about an element or part independently. This has a number of implications. Clinicians never have a "whole" perspective on a client. Rather, therapists are like the blind wise men each touching a part of an elephant and each being certain that the whole is exactly like the part they are touching. "An elephant is big and floppy"; "No, no, an elephant is long and round and thin"; "No, no, an elephant is solid like a wall." The therapist who interacts with the client in a one-to-one supportive relationship sees incremental progress. The nurse whose sole contact consists of arguments declining requests for benzodiazepines, the crisis worker who sees the person over and over only at her worst, and the group leader who has to repair the damage of the person's sarcastic comments to another group member have alternative perspectives. Each perspective is true, but each is also partial.

Applying a dialectical perspective further implies that it is natural and to be expected for these differing and partial perspectives to be radically in opposition. The existence of "yes" gives rise to "no," "all" to "nothing." Whether it is the nature of reality or simply the nature of human perception or language, this process of oppositional elements in tension with each other regularly occurs. As soon as someone on the inpatient unit thinks the client can be reasonably discharged, someone else on the team will bring forward the reasons why that is not a good idea. One person voices the position of holding a hard line on program rules, which elicits someone else's description of why in this case an exception to the rule should be made. Both opposing positions may be true or contain elements of the truth (e.g., there are valid reasons to discharge *and* to delay discharge). From this point of view, polarized divergent opinions should be expected when a client has complex problems that generate strong emotional reactions in his or her helpers.

A related idea is that one cannot make sense of elements without reference to the whole, that is, that identity is relational. The only reason he looks old is because she looks younger; the only reason I look rigid is because you are so flexible. Furthermore, the way we might identify or define a part changes and is changed by changes in other parts of the whole. The client we have all come to think of as "the Critic" in a skills training group, who is a constantly pointing out how unhelpful the skills and skills trainer are, suddenly becomes a joy when a new member joins the group. They share the same blend of humor and skepticism, but where the one is caustic, the other is wry—their chemistry together takes the sting out of the criticism and creates a lighter but still pointed feedback loop for the lead skills trainer. The group leader, released from her siege mentality and genuinely seeing the Critic's humor now, becomes more creative and likable herself. Taking a dialectical perspective means that words like *good* or *bad* or *dysfunctional* are merely snapshots of the person in context, not defining qualities inherent in the person. It also draws one into considering a web of causation rather than linear causation. Sometimes the connection is obvious: A change in *A* leads to a change in *B*, as in a man-to-man defense where the defender tracks the opponent closely, guarding against a shot. Sometimes the connection is less obvious, however, more like a zone defense, where a person's shifting leads to some change but not as much as in a man-to-man defense. And sometimes the connection is not obvious at all, such as the "butterfly effect," in which a butterfly flapping its wings in Peru results in a snowstorm in Seattle. Or the previously submissive Aunt Mary finally hitting the end of her rope and for the first time in a 20-year marriage insisting that Uncle Maurice get his own dinner and later that week young cousin Maylin deciding to apply for college. This idea translates into a clinical understanding that everything is caused and could not be otherwise, even if you cannot come up with the causes at the moment. From a dialectical perspective, the attention is not on the client alone but rather on the relationships among the client, the client's community, the therapist, and the therapist's community.

Taken together, these views lead to the stance that truth evolves. On a treatment team, this means that no one person has a lock on the truth and any understanding is likely partial and likely to leave something important out. Therefore, DBT puts a strong emphasis on dialogues that lead to synthesis rather than on an individual reasoning by him- or herself from immutable facts.

This philosophy is most easily seen in action during a team conflict. For example, an individual therapist has a client who enters therapy in a suicide crisis because he is being asked to leave his supported housing arrangement and has damaged the relationship with the residential counselor with whom he had been closest. He is so ashamed of how he's acted that even getting the details about what's going on rather than suicide threats and hopelessness is nearly impossible in the sessions. The client will become homeless if new housing is not arranged soon and the residential counselor who would have handled this problem in the past is not in the mood to help. In the consultation team, the group skills trainers mention that the client has missed two groups already and they want the therapist to work on getting him to group. The individual therapist agrees, but says there is no time in session to do it. It is all she can do simply to manage the "crisis of the week" and keep the person alive, let alone deal with therapy-interfering behaviors like not going to group. The skills trainers, however, know that unless the person learns some new skills and gets hooked up with the group, they are likely to lose the client to dropout. Both sides have valid points: The individual therapist is the one who is "supposed to" work on the therapy-interfering behavior of not going to group, and has bigger fish to fry (suicide crisis behavior); but the client must learn new skills and will lose the entire treatment program if he does not get to group. Any solution must take into account the valid points of the dialogue in order to be effective. The solution may be for the individual therapist to move her session time to just before group time to make the transition easier. The individual therapist may need more support to regulate her fear that the client is going to kill himself (perhaps she is overestimating the client's suicide risk because she is afraid). The skills trainers, similarly, may work to make group more appealing to the client or offer a reminder call early in the day of skills group. It would not be a dialectical solution for either position to capitulate—for example, for the skills trainers to back down on attendance or for the individual therapist to target therapy-interfering behavior at the expense of treating suicide crises. Adoption of a dialectical philosophy leads other team members to notice and comment on the polarization as an expected phenomenon, and them to direct the dialogue to what is left out and what is valid in each position.

Dialectical Strategies

A number of strategies are included in DBT that serve the function of keeping polarized positions from remaining polarized. The first of these is that core strategies are used to balance acceptance and change. For example, DBT requires the therapist to have a balanced communication style. On the acceptance side, the therapist employs a responsive style in which the client's agenda is taken seriously and responded directly to rather than interpreted for its latent meaning. For example, if a client asks something personal about the therapist, the therapist is more likely to use self-disclosure, warm engagement, and genuineness either to answer the question or to matter-of-factly decline to answer based on his or her own limits.

However, this style alone or an imbalance toward this style can lead to impasse. When the glum client who has told the same story of grievance many times has a therapist who simply paraphrases in the same monotone as the client, the probability is that the client's mood will stay the same or worsen. Consequently, reciprocal communication is balanced by irreverence that jolts the person off track to allow the client to resume the therapeutic task at hand. For example, the therapist might use an unorthodox, offbeat manner. The therapist, who had just been as engaged as the client in a power struggle, suddenly shifts tone and laughs, "You know, this moment is just not as black and white as I had hoped." Similarly, the therapist may plunge in where angels fear to tread. For example, he might say matter of factly to the woman whose major precipitant to suicidal crises is the threat of losing her husband, "Look, cutting yourself and leaving blood all over the bathroom is destroying any hope of having a real relationship with your husband." Or the therapist might say to a new client, "Given that you've assaulted two of your three last therapists, let's start off with what led up to that and how it's not going to happen with me. I'm going to be of no use to you if I'm afraid of you." Using an irreverent style of communication includes using a confrontational tone, using humor or unconventional phrasing, oscillating intensity, or at times expressing omnipotence or impotence in the face of the client's problems.

Another way that DBT balances acceptance and change is in case management strategies. Individuals who meet criteria for BPD often have multiple treatment providers and consequently a number of strategies have been developed to help the client–therapist dyad manage the relationships with other clinicians and family members. DBT is weighted toward a consultation-to-the-client strategy that emphasizes change. The DBT therapist consults with the client about how to handle relationships with other treatment providers and family members, rather than consulting with other treatment providers and family members about how to deal with the client. So, for example, this means that the therapist does not meet with other professionals about the client, but rather that the client is present at treatment planning meetings (and preferably has set them up him- or herself). Rather than meet with another provider without the client present, a conference call might be scheduled during an individual session. If the therapist has to meet without the client present for some practical reason, the conversation is shared with the client or discussed in advance. This same principle holds for conversations with the client's family. Even in a crisis, the spirit of consulting to the client is maintained whenever possible. If the client shows up in the emergency room, and the triage nurse or resident on call contacts the therapist to ask the therapist what he or she would like done, the DBT therapist is likely to first ask to speak with the client in order to discuss with the client how going in the hospital does and does not coincide with the client's long-term goals and their agreed-upon treatment plan. The therapist might then coach the client on how to interact skillfully with the emergency room (ER) staff or have the client communicate the plan to the ER staff and then simply confirm that with the staff, if that is required for credibility. If the hospital staff were concerned about suicide risk and were reluctant to release the person, the DBT therapist would not "tell" the hospital staff to release the client, but instead might coach the client on what was needed to decrease the legitimate worries of the ER staff.

The DBT therapist will intervene in the environment on the client's behalf when the short-term gain is worth the long-term loss in learning—for example, when the client is unable to act on his or her own and the outcome is very important; when the environment is intransigent and high in power; to save the life of the client or to avoid substantial risk to others; when it is the humane thing to do and will cause no harm; or when the client is a minor. In these cases, the therapist may provide information, advocate, or enter the environment to give assistance. However, the usual role is as consultant to help the client become more skillful in personal and professional relationships.

Other dialectical strategies include use of metaphor or assuming the position of devil's advocate in order to prevent polarization. The therapist may call a client's bluff or use extending—for example, when a client on an inpatient unit threatens suicide in an angry or blasé manner, the therapist might say, "Listen, this is really serious. We should go right now and put you on line-of-sight observation and get you into a suicide gown." Informed by dialectical philosophy, the therapist and the treatment team assume that their case formulations are partial and therefore move to assess what is left out when there is an impasse (dialectical assessment). The therapist may view a discouraging event as an opportunity to practice distress tolerance (making lemonade out of lemons) or allowing rather than preventing natural change (such as a group leader leaving and being replaced), knowing that this too is an opportunity to practice acceptance of reality as it is.

Research on DBT

Despite the public health significance, little research is available on the psychosocial treatment of suicidal behavior and less still on the treatment of suicidal behavior and other severe dysfunctional behavior among clients meeting criteria for BPD (Linehan, 1997; Linehan, Rizvi, Shaw-Welch, & Page, 2000). Clinical lore and literature about effective treatment of BPD is vast, while the empirical literature is small. Other than a promising 18-month partial hospital program (Bateman & Fonagy, 1999, 2001), DBT is the only other treatment to our knowledge with demonstrated efficacy for reducing suicidal behavior among chronically suicidal clients with BPD and multidisorders. Of the two treatments, DBT has the most empirical support. To date, there are nine published randomized controlled trials (RCTs) conducted across five research institutions that support

DBT's efficacy across a number of behavioral problems, including suicide attempts and self-injurious behaviors (Linehan, Armstrong, Suarez, Allman, & Heard, 1991; Linehan, Heard, & Armstrong, 1993; Koons et al., 2001; Verheul et al., 2003; van den Bosch et al., 2005; Linehan et al., 2006), substance abuse (Linehan et al., 1999; Linehan et al., 2002), bulimia (Safer, Telch, & Agras, 2001), binge eating (Telch, Agras, & Linehan, 2001), and depression in the elderly (Lynch, Morse, Mendelson, & Robins, 2003). These and other studies also demonstrated the cost effectiveness of DBT compared to treatment as usual (TAU) in reducing hospitalization, emergency room visits, medical severity of suicide attempts, and utilization of crisis/respite beds (American Psychiatric Association, 1998; Linehan & Heard, 1999; Linehan, Kanter, & Comtois, 1999).

In the most recently published research, Linehan and colleagues compared DBT to non-behavioral treatment-by-experts (Linehan, Comtois, Murray, Brown, Gallop, et al., 2006). Their findings replicated those in previous studies and suggest that DBT's effectiveness is unlikely to be due simply to general factors found in any expert psychotherapy—instead, DBT may be uniquely effective in reducing suicide attempts.

Conclusion

In this chapter we have described the comprehensive outpatient model of DBT to help you begin to evaluate whether adopting it makes sense for your setting or population. For chronically suicidal individuals who meet criteria for BPD, the accumulated scientific evidence regarding the efficacy of standard DBT makes it the treatment of choice. Particularly in those settings that are mandated to provide evidence-based care and that also need a cost-effective approach for consumers who disproportionately use expensive psychiatric emergency services, adopting standard DBT is an obvious decision. Yet for many readers, questions arise as they consider differences between the needs and constraints of their particular setting or patient population versus those of standard outpatient DBT as it has been researched. Subsequent chapters address these common questions and illustrate the successful adaptations of DBT to new patient populations and settings.

REFERENCES

American Psychiatric Association. (1998). Gold Award: Integrating dialectical behavior therapy into a community mental health program. *Psychiatric Services, 49,* 1338–1340.

American Psychiatric Association. (2001). Practice guideline for the treatment of clients with borderline personality disorder: American Psychiatric Association Practice Guidelines. *American Journal of Psychiatry, 158*(Suppl.), 1–52.

Basseches, M. (1984). *Dialectical thinking and adult development.* Norwood, NJ: Ablex.

Bateman, A., & Fonagy, P. (1999). Effectiveness of partial hospitalization in the treatment of borderline personality disorder: A randomized controlled trial. *American Journal of Psychiatry, 156,* 1563–1569.

Bateman, A., & Fonagy, P. (2001). Treatment of borderline personality disorder with psychoanalytically oriented partial hospitalization: An 18-month follow-up. *American Journal of Psychiatry, 158,* 36–42.

Bender, D. S., Dolan, R. T., Skodol, A. E., Sanislow, C. A., Dyck, I. R., McGlashan, T. H., et al. (2001). Treatment utilization by clients with personality disorders. *American Journal of Psychiatry, 158,* 295–302.

Bohus, M., Haaf, B., Stiglmayr, C., Pohl, U., Bohme, R., & Linehan, M. M. (2000). Evaluation of inpatient dialectical behavioral therapy for borderline personality disorder: A prospective study. *Behaviour Research and Therapy, 38*(9), 875–887.

Comtois, K. A., Elwood, L. M., Holdcraft, L. C., & Simpson, T. L. (2002). *Effectiveness of DBT in a community mental health center.* Poster presented at the 36th annual meeting of the Association for Advancement of Behavior Therapy, Reno, NV.

Ebner-Priemer, U. W., Badeck, S., Beckmann, C., Wagner, A., Feige, B., Weiss, I., et al. (2005). Affective dysregulation and dissociative experience in female patients with borderline personality disorder: A startle response study. *Journal of Psychiatric Research, 39,* 85–92.

Follette, V. M., & Ruzek, J. I. (Eds.). (2006). *Cognitive-behavioral therapies for trauma* (2nd ed.). New York: Guilford Press.

Goldfried, M. R., & Davison, G. C. (1976). *Clinical behavior therapy.* New York: Holt, Rinehart & Winston.

Heard, H. L., & Linehan, M. M. (1994). Dialectical behavior therapy: An integrative approach to the treatment of borderline personality disorder. *Journal of Psychotherapy Integration, 4,* 55–82.

Juengling, F. D., Schmahl, C., Hesslinger, B., Ebert, D., Bremner, J. D., Bohus, M., et al. (2003). Positron emission tomography in female patients with borderline personality disorder. *Journal of Psychiatric Research, 37,* 109–115.

Koons, C. R., Betts, B. B., Chapman, A. L., O'Rourke, B., Morse, N., & Robins, C. J. (in press). Dialectical behavior therapy adapted for the vocational rehabilitation of significantly disabled mentally ill adults. *Cognitive and Behavioral Practice.*

Koons, C. R., Robins, C. J., Tweed, J. L., Lynch, T. R., Gonzalez, A. M., Morse, J. Q., et al. (2001). Efficacy of dialectical behavior therapy in women veterans with borderline personality disorder. *Behavior Therapy, 32,* 371–390.

Kroll, J. L., Sines, L. K., & Martin, K. (1981). Borderline personality disorder: Construct validity of the concept. *Archives of General Psychiatry, 39,* 60–63.

Levins, R., & Lewontin, R. (1985). *The dialectical biologist.* Cambridge, MA: Harvard University Press.

Linehan, M. M. (1993a). *Cognitive-behavioral treatment of borderline personality disorder.* New York: Guilford Press.

Linehan, M.M. (1993b). *Skills training manual for treating borderline personality disorder.* New York: Guilford Press.

Linehan, M. M. (1996). Dialectical behavior therapy for borderline personality disorder. In B. Schmitz (Ed.), *Treatment of personality disorders* (pp. 179–199). Munich, Germany: Psychologie Verlags Union.

Linehan, M. M. (1997). Behavioral treatments of suicidal behaviors: Definitional obfuscation and treatment outcomes. In D. M. Stoff & J. J. Mann (Eds.), *Neurobiology of suicide: From the bench to the clinic* (pp. 302–328). New York: Annals of the New York Academy of Sciences.

Linehan, M. M. (in press). *Skills training manual for treating borderline personality disorder* (2nd ed.). New York: Guilford Press.

Linehan, M. M., Armstrong, H. E., Suarez, A., Allmon, D., & Heard, H. (1991). Cognitive-behavioral treatment of chronically parasuicidal borderline clients. *Archives of General Psychiatry, 48,* 1060–1064.

Linehan, M. M., Comtois, K. A., Brown, M. Z., Heard, H. L., & Wagner, A. W. (2006). Suicide Attempt Self-Injury Interview (SASII): Development, reliabililty, and validity of a scale to assess suicide attempts and intentional self-injury. *Psychological Assessment, 18,* 303–312.

Linehan, M. M., Comtois, K. A., Murray, A. M., Brown, M. Z., Gallop, R. J., Heard, H. L., et al. (2006). Two-year randomized trial + follow-up of dialectical behavior therapy vs. therapy by experts for suicidal behaviors and borderline personality disorder. *Archives of General Psychiatry, 63*(7), 757–766.

Linehan, M. M., Dimeff, L. A., Reynolds, S. K., Comtois, K., Shaw-Welch, S., Heagerty, P., et al. (2002). Dialectical behavior therapy versus comprehensive validation plus 12-step for the treatment of opioid dependent women meeting criteria for borderline personality disorder. *Drug and Alcohol Dependence, 67,* 13–26.

Linehan, M. M., & Heard, H. L. (1999). Borderline personality disorder: Costs, course, and treatment outcomes. In N. Miller & K. Magruder (Eds.), *The cost effectiveness of psychotherapy: A guide for practitioners* (pp. 291–305). New York: Oxford University Press.

Linehan, M. M., Heard, H. L., & Armstrong, H. E. (1993). Naturalistic follow-up of a behavioral treatment for chronically parasuicidal borderline clients. *Archives of General Psychiatry, 50,* 971–974.

Linehan, M. M., Kanter, J. W., & Comtois, K. A. (1999). Dialectical behavior therapy for borderline personality disorder: Efficacy, specificity, and cost-effectiveness. In D. S. Janowsky (Ed.), *Psychotherapy: Indications and outcomes* (pp. 93–118). Washington, DC: American Psychiatric Press.

Linehan, M. M., Rizvi, S. L., Shaw-Welch, S., & Page, B. (2000). Psychiatric aspects of suicidal behaviour: Personality disorders. In K. Hawton & K. van Heeringen (Eds.), *International handbook of suicide and attempted suicide* (pp. 147–178). London, UK: Wiley.

Linehan, M. M., Schmidt, H., III, Dimeff, L. A., Craft, J. C., Kanter, J., & Comtois, K. A. (1999). Dialectical behavior therapy for clients with borderline personality disorder and drug-dependence. *American Journal of Addiction, 8,* 279–292.

Lynch, T. R., Morse, J. Q., Mendelson, T., & Robins, C. J. (2003). Dialectical behavior therapy for depressed older adults: A randomized pilot study. *American Journal of Geriatric Psychiatry, 11*(1), 33–45.

Modestin, J., Abrecht, I., Tschaggelar, W., & Hoffman, H. (1997). Diagnosing borderline: A contribution to the question of its conceptual validity. *Archives Psychiatrica Nervenkra, 233,* 359–370.

Perry, J. C., & Cooper, S. H. (1985). Psychodynamics, symptoms, and outcome in borderline and antisocial personality disorders and bipolar type II affective disorder. In T. H. McGlashan (Ed.), *The borderline: Current empirical research* (pp. 21–41). Washington, DC: American Psychiatric Press.

Perry, J. C., Herman, J. L., van der Kolk, B. A., & Hoke, L. A. (1990). Psychotherapy and psychological trauma in borderline personality disorder. *Psychiatric Annals, 20,* 33–43.

Rathus, J. H., & Miller, A. L. (2002). Dialectical behavior therapy adapted for suicidal adolescents. *Suicide and Life-Threatening Behavior, 32*(2), 146–157.

Rosenthal, M. Z., Cheavens, J. S., Lejuez, C. W., & Lynch, T. R. (2005). Thought suppression mediates the relationship between negative affect and borderline personality disorder symptoms. *Behaviour Research and Therapy, 43,* 1173–1185.

Safer, D. L., Telch, C. F., & Agras, W. S. (2001). Dialectical behavior therapy for bulimia nervosa. *American Journal of Psychiatry, 158*(4), 632–634.

Skodol, A. E., Buckley, P., & Charles, E. (1983). Is there a characteristic pattern to the treatment history of clinic outpatients with borderline personality? *Journal of Nervous and Mental Disease, 171,* 405–410.

Stiglmayr, C. E., Grathwol, T., Linehan, M. M., Ihorst, G., Fahrenberg, J., & Bohus, M. (2005). Aversive tension in patients with borderline personality disorder: A computer-based controlled field study. *Acta Psychiatrica Scandinavica, 111,* 372–379.

Telch, C. F., Agras, W. S., & Linehan, M. M. (2001). Dialectical behavior therapy for binge eating disorder. *Journal of Consulting and Clinical Psychology, 69*(6), 1061–1065.

Tucker, L., Bauer, S. F., Wagner, S., Harlam, D., & Sher, I. (1987). Long-term hospital treatment of borderline clients: A descriptive outcome study. *American Journal of Psychiatry, 144,* 1443–1448.

van den Bosch, L. M. C., Maarten, W. J., Koeter, M. W. J., Stijen, T., Verjeul, V., & van den Brink, K. (2005). Sustained efficacy of dialectical behaviour therapy for borderline personality disorder. *Behaviour Research and Therapy, 43,* 1231–1241.

Verheul, R., van den Bosch, L. M. C., Koeter, M. W. J., de Ridder, M. A. J., Stijnen, T., & van den Brink, W. (2003). Dialectical behaviour therapy for women with borderline personality disorder: 12-month, randomised clinical trial in the Netherlands. *British Journal of Psychiatry, 182,* 135–140.

Wagner, A. W., & Linehan, M. M. (1997). Biosocial perspective on the relationship of childhood sexual abuse, suicidal behavior, and borderline personality disorder. In M. Zanarini (Ed.), *The role of sexual abuse in the etiology of borderline personality disorder* (pp. 203–223). Washington, DC: American Psychiatric Association.

Widiger, T. A., & France, A. J. (1989). Epidemiology, diagnosis, and comorbidity of borderline personality disorder. In A. Tasman, R. E. Hales, & A. J. Frances (Eds.), *American Psychiatric Press review of psychiatry* (Vol. 8, pp. 8–24). Washington, DC: American Psychiatric Press.

Widiger, T. A., & Weissman, M. M. (1991). Epidemiology of borderline personality disorder. *Hospital Community Psychiatry, 42*, 1015–1021.

CHAPTER 2

Adopt or Adapt?
FIDELITY MATTERS

Kelly Koerner, Linda A. Dimeff, *and* Charles R. Swenson

As you consider using dialectical behavior therapy (DBT) and certainly when you begin to implement it, questions will arise about whether to adopt the standard, comprehensive model of DBT defined in Linehan (1993a, 1993b) or instead to adapt or modify DBT to fit the needs and constraints of your setting. For example, it is natural to ask, "Should I consider using DBT if my setting or patients differ from those in the research?" Or "What if it doesn't seem possible to include every DBT mode in our setting?" Maybe you lack enough therapists to offer weekly individual psychotherapy, or productivity demands make an unreimbursed therapists' consultation team meeting too costly, or perhaps your individual therapists do not want to provide after-hours phone coaching. When the empirically supported model of DBT isn't a perfect match to the needs and constraints of a local setting, it is almost inevitable to think "We can't use the standard model of DBT."

Differences between a defined model and your particular situation can push and pull for innovation or *adaptation* of the defined model. In fact, some have argued that "local adaptation, which often involves simplification, is a nearly universal property of *successful* dissemination" (Berwick, 2003, p. 1971). Hypothetically, such adaptation could result in a creatively streamlined version of DBT that better fits a service setting or better serves consumers' needs. Yet there are four implications that should be considered before adapting rather than adopting the standard model of DBT.

1. *A particular modification may or may not work as well as the standard model.* The first implication of modifying the standard model of DBT is that modifications may or may not retain the active ingredients required to get good clinical outcomes. At this point, little is known about the specific active ingredients of DBT (or, for that matter,

about any psychosocial interventions). Consequently, one cannot *assume* that the clinical outcomes of an adapted version of DBT will be equivalent to or better than the standard model. For example, even a straightforward line of reasoning—such as, a *little* DBT is better than *no* DBT—is not unequivocally true. Although it is reasonable to think that using the DBT skills training component but not using the other elements of the comprehensive model should still offer some benefit, this has yet to be demonstrated. As discussed in Chapter 1, adding DBT skills training to non-DBT individual psychotherapy (i.e., skills training without DBT individual psychotherapy, phone coaching, and a consultation team) did not add any benefit. In fact, when patients were taught only a subset of DBT skills in a brief group format that did not abide by DBT's proscription against discussion of intentional self-injury in the group, there was actually evidence of harm (Springer, Lohr, Buchtel, & Silk, 1996). These data show that one can't *assume* that a partial implementation or adaptation will be effective (or ineffective): Assessing clinical outcomes is necessary. Modifying without assessing outcomes is a risky strategy.

The conclusion from the broader literature on fidelity to treatment is that "when two programs offer a practice of care that is known to be effective, the program with higher fidelity to the defined practice model tends to produce superior outcomes" (Drake et al., 2001, p. 180). Add this research (e.g., Jerrel & Ridgely, 1999; McDonnell, Nofs, Hardman, & Chambless, 1989; McHugo, Drake, Teague, & Xie, 1999) to the small body available on fidelity to the standard DBT model and you have a strong argument against *assuming* that a modified version of DBT will have equally positive outcomes. To the extent that an intervention's benefits are caused by its active ingredients, omitting the active ingredients (or enough of the active ingredients) results in a treatment that fails to produce the intended benefits. A watered-down version of a psychosocial intervention is like a sugar pill: all form, no function. The first consideration, therefore, before undertaking adaptation of DBT is that good clinical outcomes may require adopting and implementing the standard model, the form and the functions of DBT, so that "enough" of the effective elements are active in your setting.

2. *Offering an untested modification of DBT complicates the process of informed consent.* A second implication of adaptation is that modification requires appropriate informed consent to treatment. There is an ethical obligation to be certain that what is offered does no harm and is beneficial. One cannot be certain about the benefits of an untested modification of DBT. Given the current uncertainty regarding which features are the essential features of DBT, one cannot with confidence tell consumers and funders that a particular adaptation being described as "DBT" has the essential ingredients or principles that account for DBT's effectiveness. What exactly are they consenting to receive and pay for? Without data about the efficacy of a modification, it is difficult to accurately inform clients about risks and benefits. Such concerns have led Linehan and colleagues to define a process for program accreditation in DBT (Witterholt, 2006) that will serve as something of a quality control measure so that stakeholders can accurately tell what services are offered.

3. *Implementing an untested modification may present problems with reimbursement.* A third implication of adapting rather than adopting the standard model is that there are and will increasingly be practical problems with getting reimbursed for versions of DBT that deviate from the empirically validated model. As reimbursement for services becomes increasingly tied to documented adherence and program fidelity, and especially once a process of DBT program accreditation is in place, partial or blended models that are untested or unaccredited may become ineligible for reimbursement. The fact that many funding sources have been willing to reimburse for DBT has created pressure for

programs to say that they are providing DBT, regardless of how close to the defined model those services actually are. If modification or partial implementation is called "DBT" and that modification fails to produce benefit or actually causes harm, it can poison the local waters, turning off consumers and funders to a treatment that could have been of great benefit if provided with high fidelity.

4. *Adapting (rather than adopting) DBT can heighten risk and legal liability.* The fact that DBT is used with high-risk suicidal populations exposes those who use it to legal risk. Experts in the treatment of suicidal behavior and management of liability following a patient suicide emphasize that the best protection for the clinician or agency is to have provided good clinical care that followed acceptable standards of practice (Silverman et al., 1998). Documenting that one attempted to apply comprehensive DBT and thereby met acceptable standards of practice is likely to be more credible than trying to justify an untested modification of DBT.

Considerations of clinical effectiveness, informed consent, reimbursement, and legal liability all weigh heavily on the side of adopting the proven standard comprehensive DBT model rather than adapting it. Ethical and practical issues also argue for sticking with a validated model. However, on the other hand, real needs and constraints in your setting may be incompatible with the model exactly as defined. Adopting the standard model of DBT may be exactly the *wrong* decision. For example, in an acute psychiatric hospital with a 2-week average length of stay it is not feasible to teach all the DBT skills; paraprofessional staff at a residential "halfway" house do not have the requisite clinical skills and credentials to provide the individual therapy mode of DBT. Similarly, if you want to see if DBT can help a patient population yet to be researched (e.g., fetal alcohol-effected individuals), the only choice is to adapt.

This tension—"we must adopt" versus "we must adapt"—is the inherent dilemma many teams face as they begin to implement DBT. It has prompted this book. We think that in fact both statements are simultaneously true; these seeming opposing truths stand side by side. If one fails to adhere to DBT as manualized, then there is the risk that the treatment will be less effective, and perhaps even have ill effects—you won't know until you test it. *And* simultaneously, it can be true that needs or setting constraints are such that one can't do DBT exactly as it has been defined in research. Several tips may help in working with this dilemma, or "dialectic."

Tip 1: Radically Accept the Dialectical Tension and Search for a Synthesis

Our first piece of general advice, regardless of your setting or population, is to expect this basic dialectical tension between adopting versus adapting to arise repeatedly as you explore and begin to implement DBT. Problem solving during implementation should be rooted in the fact that both positions are true: It's true that the best chance of obtaining good clinical outcomes is to adopt and implement the defined model and it's simultaneously true that the model has to meet the needs and fit the constraints of your setting and the population you serve. Rather than abandoning fidelity to standard DBT to meet the local conditions and rather than shoehorning the needs and constraints of your setting or population to fit the defined model of DBT, insist that any solution actually incorporate both of these valid positions. In other words, apply dialectical thinking to the implementation process itself. The ongoing dialogue between the two poles of adoption and adaptation, between adherence to the standard model and creativity, will yield the synthesis of a workable, high-fidelity implementation.

Of course, the devil is in the details! In the rest of this chapter and those that follow we provide guidance about how to stay true to the defined model of DBT while simultaneously adapting the model to meet local needs. In this chapter we provide principles that can guide problem solving across settings and populations. In subsequent chapters, authors who have adopted and adapted DBT in outpatient public community mental health and private practice (outpatient and ACT) and for a variety of nonoutpatient settings (Chapters 4 and 5) and with new populations (Chapters 6 through 10) describe in detail how they have creatively negotiated conflicts between adherence and local needs and constraints. What is common to the adaptations in this book is that each team simultaneously emphasized adherence to the defined model yet in meaningful ways reinvented the model to solve local problems. They have done so in structured yet creative ways, with openness to peer and expert review along the way, as well as through the collection of program evaluation data, the final arbiter of whether the particular adaptations were effective.

Tip 2: Clearly Identify If You Plan to Adopt or Adapt

Another point of general advice is to be as clear as you can, with yourself and with your stakeholders, about whether you intend is to adopt the standard comprehensive model of DBT or to adapt DBT. The "right" answer for your DBT program may not be simple or straightforward. A useful starting point is to recognize your predisposition toward adopting versus adapting and to consciously decide which course you will take. Figure 2.1 shows various possibilities of how one might offer DBT or variations of DBT as well as what to call these services in order to accurately represent them to consumers and other stakeholders.

What you offer can be described both categorically (i.e., the treatment offered is DBT or it is not DBT, indicated by a strong black bar in Figure 2.1) and along a continuum of comprehensiveness (more or less comprehensive and adherent DBT). If you

Not DBT		**DBT-Informed Treatment** *(less comprehensive/adherent)*		**DBT**
Either No Elements of DBT or Technical Eclecticism	**A d o p t**	Elements of DBT	Some Modes of DBT but Not Entire Model	Comprehensive DBT
	A d a p t	Elements of DBT	Systematic Innovation and Evaluation of New Treatment	Model-Advancing Team/ Research DBT: Systematic Innovation and Evaluation of Comprehensive DBT for New Populations or Settings

FIGURE 2.1. Using fidelity to name what we offer.

decide not to do DBT at all or you decide to offer comprehensive DBT according to the defined model, then it's clear how to describe your services. On one end, there is no DBT: there either is no intention to use elements of DBT or techniques are eclectically adopted independent of adoption of principles, assumptions, or theory and the treatment is not called DBT. On the other end of the spectrum, DBT is comprehensive and all modes fully adhere to DBT principles, assumptions, and theory. The latter system includes teams offering standard DBT as well as teams who are systematically modifying and advancing the treatment model. Grounded in adherence, they are creatively improving DBT's fit to new populations and settings. However, it is less clear what to call services in the grey zone between these two anchor points. When should (or should not) a program be called "DBT"? What is the minimum number of DBT elements required to expect good clinical outcomes?

Defining DBT in the Gray Zone of Partial Implementation

In this gray zone of partial implementation are both those whose ultimate goal is the adoption of comprehensive DBT and those whose ultimate goal is an adaptation. In the case of the former, they may be in the gray zone simply due to lack of resources at the moment. Such a program might implement some of the modes of DBT, as true to the standard model as possible, but omit other modes for the time being (e.g., a program might start up with a skills training group and a consultation team, but not with individual therapy or phone consultations). It is not unusual for teams to take a step-by-step route to a comprehensive version of DBT. Alternatively, also in the gray zone of partial implementation are individuals and teams where partial implementation is the stopping point. Here we would differentiate "DBT-informed treatment" from technical eclecticism (not DBT). We reserve the term "DBT-informed" to designate the intent to significantly anchor adoption or adaptation in DBT's treatment principles, strategies, and modes. For example, Turner (2000) investigated a DBT-informed treatment in which he systematically implemented all modes and strategies of DBT and most of its principles and theory, but left case formulation psychodynamic. This kind of DBT-informed treatment stands in contrast to "technical eclecticism" (not DBT) where one selectively adds elements of DBT to his or her therapeutic toolkit as one might take an engine or wheels from one vehicle to customize another vehicle.

Also in the gray zone is the more reactive or haphazard stance toward adopting or adapting where one may be pushed into partial implementation to accommodate pressures of the treatment environment or personal preferences (e.g., "Given productivity pressures, we don't have time for a DBT consultation team, so let's drop that" or "I like the skills group idea, but I'd rather continue with the psychoanalytic frame I use in individual therapy"). This stance can be contrasted with a DBT-informed partial implementation in which setting constraints or needs lead to offering only one or two fully adherent modes. For example, practical considerations might lead a clinic to offer only a fully adherent DBT skills group, but not other modes. (Clients nonetheless might receive comprehensive DBT even in this case if they simultaneously have an individual DBT therapist elsewhere in the community who offers skills coaching and participates in a consult team.) Regardless of intent to adopt or adapt and regardless of being en route to comprehensive DBT or not, it is not known whether any of such partial implementations retain enough of DBT's active ingredients to result in good clinical outcomes.

To accurately describe your program to stakeholders, we suggest that you describe it as a DBT program *only* when it is comprehensive. If a partial implementation of

DBT is offered, particular care should be given to accurately describing services and to collecting and providing clinical outcome evaluation data to stakeholders to enable appropriate informed consent. We suggest that if your adoption or adaptation is well anchored in the principles and theory that guide DBT, you refer to your program as "DBT-informed treatment." Here, too, what is needed is to be clear about how the treatment differs from comprehensive DBT and to provide program evaluation data. As mentioned before, when partial implementations have been mislabeled as DBT and fail to produce benefits or actually causes harm, such results can effectively turn off consumers and funders for years to a treatment that could have been of great benefit if it had been provided with high fidelity. If elements or strategies are adopted or adapted relatively independently of DBT principles, the resulting program should not be called DBT.

Tip 3: Start with a Small, Tightly Focused Pilot Program

We also strongly suggest, because most of us are not in a position to carefully develop and evaluate the infinite variety of possible partial implementations, that the most ethical and practical course is to first learn and deliver the defined, standard model of DBT within a small, tightly focused pilot program and to evaluate clinical outcomes in your setting and with your population. Guidance about program evaluation is provided in Rizvi, Monroe-DeVita, & Dimeff, Chapter 12, this volume). Such continuous monitoring of program fidelity and valued outcomes has been recommended as essential by the Implementing Evidence-Based Practices Project (Torrey et al., 2001). To follow this advice, for example, you might begin by forming a consultation team of three or more colleagues to meet as a study group to learn DBT using the treatment manuals. To facilitate learning the treatment and establish a structure for the process of program development, you might consider attending a 10-day DBT intensive training session (*www.behavioraltech. com*). In the next section, we will help you think through typical questions and problems encountered in the implementation of DBT.

Tip 4: Think Through Typical Questions and Problems Using Functions, Principles, and Adherence

In the process of implementing DBT, common questions and problems unfold. These typical issues are listed in Figure 2.2. During early exploration and implementation two questions typically come up: "To whom will we offer DBT?" and "Will we adopt and offer comprehensive DBT?"

Who Is Your Target Population—BPD and Suicidal Behavior?

Several principles can guide decisions about to whom you will offer DBT. The first is to stay close to the evidence base. As discussed in Koerner and Dimeff (Chapter 1, this volume), the evidence of DBT's efficacy is strongest for those who are chronically suicidal and meet criteria for BPD. If you want or need to serve a broader or wholly different pop-

Who is your target population?		
Will match a population validated in research.	Will offer to broader patient group or use different selection criteria than has been researched.	
	Specify targets and theory of psychopathology.	
Will you offer comprehensive DBT?		
Yes. We'll offer all modes and functions of DBT.	*No*. We'll offer non-DBT or non-DBT-informed treatment.	
Is your setting currently amenable to standard modes of DBT?	Systematically determine modifications and evaluate outcomes. Accurately represent how services differ from comprehensive DBT.	
Yes	*No*	See Rizvi et al. (Chapter 12, this volume)
Adopt standard modes.	Determine which modes to provide. Use functions, principles, and adherence to guide decision making	
Do you/your team have the requisite professional skill set for DBT?		
Yes.	*No.* Develop and begin to implement a plan to acquire needed skills.	
Proceed to develop a small pilot project implementing comprehensive DBT. Evaluate outcomes.		
Adopting the defined model fits setting needs and constraints?		
Yes, adopting model works.	*No, adaptation seems needed.*	
Continue to monitor outcomes.	Systematically make modifications and evaluate outcomes.	

FIGURE 2.2. Typical questions and problems.

ulation, then you must carefully consider the theories of disorder and change that guide DBT. For example, research and theory make it logical to consider DBT for populations whose problems arise from pervasive emotional dysregulation. Adaptations for individuals with substance abuse disorders, eating disorders, antisocial personality disorder, and comorbid depression and personality disorder in the elderly all stem from the key role emotion dysregulation is considered to play in those disorders. Some settings offer DBT to individuals who disproportionately use psychiatric services and have repeatedly failed treatment as usual regardless of diagnosis. However, DBT is not a panacea and should not be used as a first-line treatment if there is already another evidence-based practice for the problem or population. For example, it would be a mistake to offer DBT to patients with anxiety disorders or with bipolar disorder who had apparently failed at conventional treatment before being certain that *in fact* the evidence-based treatments for these disorders had been provided with good fidelity to those protocols.

If you plan to offer DBT to a group for whom there is as yet little evidence, there are two essential steps to follow. First, use available research and theory on the disorder or population of interest to delineate the disorder-specific targets to be treated and clearly assign these targets to whichever mode(s) of DBT will be responsible for treating them. A common mistake is to assume that all sorts of adaptations will be necessary for a new population before trying and evaluating the standard version of DBT. Another mistake is to reorder the target hierarchy to place disorder-specific targets above life-threatening behavior and therapy-interfering behavior. Instead, retain the commonsense priority of life-threatening behavior and therapy-interfering behavior and make disorder-specific targets the highest priority among the quality-of-life targets. See McMain, Sayrs, Dimeff, and Linehan (Chapter 6, this volume) and Wisniewski, Safer, and Chen (Chapter 7, this volume) (on substance abuse and eating disorders) for prototypes of how this can be done well. Second, again, it is essential to carefully evaluate your outcomes when using DBT with a new population.

Comprehensive DBT and Standard DBT Modes?

Another early and common dilemma arises about whether to offer comprehensive DBT in your setting and how to respond to obstacles one encounters implementing DBT's standard modes. DBT as it has been manualized and researched for Stage 1 clients is a comprehensive outpatient treatment—that is, it is meant to provide all the treatment clients need to address all the targets and goals that lead to behavioral control and an acceptable quality of life. As discussed in Chapter 1, a key idea here is that the level of disorder determines the comprehensiveness of treatment needed to accomplish treatment goals. To be comprehensive, a treatment should (1) enhance clients' capabilities, (2) motivate clients to use these capabilities, and (3) ensure that clients can generalize these capabilities to all relevant situations. A comprehensive treatment should also (4) enhance therapists' skills and motivation and (5) structure the environment of both clients and therapists in a manner that facilitates clinical progress. In DBT, these primary tasks, called the *functions* of comprehensive treatment (see Table 2.1), are allocated across the standard modes of DBT service delivery (i.e., weekly individual psychotherapy, weekly skills training, as-needed skills-coaching phone calls, and a consultation team for treatment of the therapist). Linehan (Linehan, 1995, 1997; Linehan, Kanter, & Comtois, 1999) articulated this distinction between functions and modes to help treatment developers consider the special needs of clients in Stage 1 and to help early adopters implement DBT in new settings and with new populations when the needs or constraints in the local setting interfered with adopting DBT's standard modes. For example, both a solo private practitioner and a prison setting might find it difficult to run a standard DBT skills group (e.g., because of no suitable room, difficulty getting six to eight clients in the room at once for a 2½-hour session). Yet because each DBT mode has specific targets and functions for which it is responsible, simply dropping a mode because it was difficult to implement meant that its functions and targets were not accomplished, potentially undermining treatment effectiveness.

Although the particulars of the mode of skills training might be difficult in the example of a private practice or a prison setting, the function to be accomplished—enhancing client capabilities—can still be accomplished. Enhancing clients' capabilities means that treatment helps clients to acquire cognitive, emotional, physiological, and overt behavior-

TABLE 2.1. Functions and Modes of Comprehensive Treatment

Functions	Modes
Enhancing client capabilities: help clients acquire repertoires needed for effective performance.	Skills training (individual or group) Pharmacotherapy Psychoeducation
Improving motivation: strengthen clinical progress and help reduce factors that inhibit and/or interfere with progress (e.g., emotions, cognitions, overt behavior, environment).	Individual psychotherapy Milieu
Ensuring generalization: transfer skillful response repertoire from therapy to client's natural environment and help integrate skillful responses within the changing natural environment.	Skills coaching, milieu treatment, therapeutic communities, *in vivo* interventions, review of session tapes, involvement of family/friends
Enhancing therapist skill and motivation: acquire, integrate, and generalize the cognitive, emotional, and overt behavioral and verbal repertoires necessary for effective application of treatment. As well, this function includes the strengthening of therapeutic responses and the reduction of responses that inhibit and/or interfere with effective application of treatment.	Supervision, therapist consultation meeting, continuing education, treatment manuals, adherence and competency monitoring, and staff incentives
Structuring the environment through contingency management within the treatment program as a whole as well as through contingency management within the client's community.	Clinic director or via administrative interactions, case management, and family and marital interventions

al response repertoires, and to integrate these response repertoires for effective performance. In standard outpatient DBT, a once-a-week 2½-hour skills training group is the primary service mode that accomplishes this function. But by thinking creatively about other ways to accomplish the treatment functions of the blocked mode, one need not abandon what is essential. Other modes of service delivery such as psychoeducation, bibliotherapy readings and handouts, and pharmacotherapy can also accomplish this function of enhancing capability. Skills training can be conducted individually or via peer-to-peer groups (Swenson, personal communication, March 15, 2007). Skills-training videotapes might be made available to clients. In some settings, perhaps splitting skills training time into a 1-hour lecture on new material and then individual homework review might be a more feasible way to accomplish this function.

Similarly, in standard outpatient DBT, individual psychotherapy is the mode of service delivery that has primary responsibility for improving motivation, the second function of comprehensive treatment. This means that the individual therapist is the primary person who strengthens clinical progress and who helps the client to reduce factors that inhibit and/or interfere with his or her progress (e.g., by reducing factors that interfere such as emotions/physiological responses, cognitions/cognitive style, overt behavior patterns, and environmental events). But say, for example, that you are in a setting that lacks individual psychotherapy. Again, thinking of functions as independent of modes helps clinicians to discover other ways a function can be accomplished. For example, in Comtois et al. (Chapter 3, this volume) and McCann, Ivanoff, Schmidt, and Beach (Chapter 5, this volume), the authors suggest creative ways for this function to be accomplished by the milieu in settings where lengths of stay or staffing patterns make individual psychotherapy infeasible.

The third function of ensuring generalization to all relevant environments demands ensuring transfer of a skillful response repertoire from therapy to the client's natural environment and helping the integration of skillful responses within the changing natural environment to result in effective performance. In standard DBT with highly suicidal and emotionally dysregulated clients, crisis calls and skills coaching is considered essential. In addition to employing after-hours and crisis phone coaching, generalization can also be accomplished through milieu skills coaching and treatment(s), therapeutic communities, *in vivo* interventions (including case management), review of session tapes, and systems interventions. This function of generalization takes on particular importance with adolescents; consequently, a major modification in the form of additional involvement of family members has been created to help ensure generalization (Fruzzetti, Santisteban, & Hoffman, Chapter 8, and Miller, Rathus, DuBose, Dexter-Mazza, & Goldklang, Chapter 9; both, this volume).

As DBT was transported into routine outpatient settings, some early adopters encountered setting constraints that blocked the individual therapists from taking after-hours calls to provide coaching for their clients. This is a significant and controversial departure from standard DBT. If crisis calls are handled by whoever happens to be on call, that person may or may not know how to coach DBT skills and may or may not be trained to offer needed help while avoiding reinforcing suicidal crisis behavior. In other words, the therapist's DBT training and intimate knowledge of the client is thought to be needed to walk the tightrope of prompting new behavior in a crisis, particularly with individuals who are chronically suicidal and highly lethal. In DBT it is considered optimal for the person who knows the client best to manage suicidal crises. But, say, system constraints preclude individual therapists from managing crises after hours. Then what? Some teams who have run into absolute barriers to the individual therapist taking call have used the relevant functions and principles to guide them. They prioritize that, first, the client has assistance generalizing skills to crisis situations, and, second, that reinforcers are aligned to support preferred skillful behaviors over old suicidal crisis behaviors. Then they consider all the ways that the client can get needed assistance in a suicidal crisis without inadvertently being reinforced. For example, maybe the client herself learns to share an up-to-date analysis of the controlling variables for her suicide crises and to convey skills that are most useful or relevant to her. Crisis staff can be trained to coach DBT skills and to use DBT's suicide crisis protocol. Teams can continue to communicate and document for administrators their belief that failing to provide clients with this skilled assistance in suicide crises violates the DBT protocol, could be a source of liability, and so on. Again, a problem that arises here is that there is no evidence one way or another about the empirical effects of providing or failing to provide this standard of care. However, at this point it is considered the standard of care in DBT for individual therapists to be available and willing to provide skills coaching.

This idea of using the functions of comprehensive treatment to help negotiate obstacles to implementing DBT is helpful not just during start-up or initial adoption of a mode, but also useful throughout the implementation process. So, for example, the fourth function is enhancing therapist capabilities and motivation. The idea is that comprehensive treatment requires that therapists acquire, integrate, and generalize their own cognitive, emotional, and overt behavioral and verbal repertoires needed for effective application of treatment. In addition, this function includes the strengthening of therapeutic responses and reduction of responses that inhibit and/or interfere with effective application of treatment. This is usually accomplished through supervision, therapist consultation meetings, continuing education, treatment manuals, adherence and competency monitoring, and staff incentives. A well-functioning team creates conditions that facilitate looking at one's own reactions and problematic behavior in therapy. The function of the consultation team as being "therapy for the therapist" can be challenged as teams grow to add new members. Too large a group, an imbalance between inexperienced and experienced members, significant differences in commitment to the treatment philosophy, or irregular attendance can all interfere with this function. By keeping the function to be served in mind, however, the clinician will be able to recognize drift and find a direction for problem solving.

The fifth function is structuring the environment through contingency management within the treatment program as a whole as well as by contingency management within the client's community. This function is typically accomplished by the clinic director or via administrative interactions, case management, and family and marital interventions (see Fruzzetti et al., Chapter 8, this volume). So, for example, in the inpatient and forensic chapters, you'll find a detailed description of what structuring the environment means in that setting that can also serve as a more general template for other settings. The authors illustrate how DBT principles inform everything from unit rules, program schedules, and use of physical space to how basic assumptions and agreements are adapted to the setting. With adolescents, structuring the environment is a particularly important function. Thoughtfulness is needed to facilitate confidentiality while the youth, the therapist, and the family jointly manage high-risk behaviors.

These five functions of comprehensive treatment are a first set of principles for thinking through obstacles that arise when implementing a particular DBT mode. As tensions arise, you can ask yourself, "What is the function we are trying to accomplish? Given that we want to offer genuinely comprehensive treatment, is there a way to work around the setting constraint without compromising this function? Is there another way to accomplish this function if we can't do it 'by the book'?"

Does Adopting the Standard Model Fit Setting Needs?

A next set of questions emerges as one gets into the nitty-gritty of implementing DBT. Do the details of the defined model (strategies, protocols, assumptions, agreements, treatment philosophy, change procedures, etc.) fit your setting needs and constraints? DBT is defined not only in terms of its comprehensive functions. It is also defined by its particular form, those broad classes of elements as well as the specific strategies and protocols that differentiate DBT from other approaches to treatment. It's not DBT unless both the form *and* the functions are present.

But what is the consequence of partial adherence within a mode? For example, what if only some of the team understand dialectics or mindfulness? What if program directors or mental health authorities are not willing to stick to the arbitrary rules? What if individual therapists fail to use diary cards or ignore the target hierarchy to organize sessions? What if the spirit of voluntary commitment and consultation to the patient are absent? What if the skills group fails to cover all the skills? No data as yet identify the elements of DBT that are responsible for outcomes. Therefore, it can be complicated to think through what elements to be especially careful to adhere to. One way to help organize your thinking is to consider the broad categories that might be responsible for DBT's effectiveness. For example, if DBT were a tree, then its unchangeable roots would be dialectics, mindfulness, and behaviorism, and its trunk would be a biosocial theory appropriate to the particular disorder being treated. Also constant would be the large branches of levels of disorder/stages of treatment, functions of comprehensive treatment, and core strategies of validation, problem solving, and dialectics. Smaller branches such as modes, agreements, or particular protocols that combined DBT's core strategies might differ according to local conditions in order to suit a program or population while remaining conceptually well integrated with DBT's core principles and strategies.

Using broad categories to describe what might be responsible for DBT's effectiveness, for example, gives rise to different hypotheses that can help you stay clear about fidelity.

1. *Clearly structure treatment.* One hypothesis is that DBT is effective because it clearly structures treatment. Teams can actively self-monitor how well they know and use behavioral theory and science, dialectics, mindfulness, and biosocial theory to organize case formulation; and they can also monitor whether the level of disorder, stages of treatment, and the target hierarchy are used to organize their interactions with clients. They can self-assess the clarity of agreements, assumptions, and therapist roles. Teams can scan to ensure that consultation-to-patient strategies and contingencies in the treatment program support skillful behavior on the part of therapists and clients (e.g., the four miss rules that activates therapists; the culture feels like a community of therapists helping a community of clients, who are all in it together; more good things flow to those who improve).

2. *Apply behavior therapy.* Another hypothesis is that DBT has its effects because it applies behavior therapy to suicidal behavior and other intentional self-injury. Research evidence would suggest that this active problem-solving stance is effective (Linehan, 2000). Therefore, you can self-assess and do your utmost to develop competence with cognitive-behavioral protocols and strategies.

3. *Add validation.* A third hypothesis is that DBT has its effects because it adds validation, which in and of itself offers a powerful mechanism of change (Linehan et al., 2002). Again, you can self-assess and strengthen the use of validation across modes.

4. *Add dialectics.* Similarly, a fourth hypothesis is that the dialectical stance and strategies are essential—that the constant balance of change and acceptance and ways out of therapeutic impasse contribute to DBT's effects.

5. *Integrate mindfulness practice across modes.* A fifth hypothesis is that DBT's emphasis on the therapist's use of mindfulness as a practice that is integrated throughout all modes contributes to DBT's efficacy.

Each of these is a defining aspect of DBT. Without its presence, one could not call the therapy DBT. Thinking in this way provides directions for you to evaluate and strengthen these elements of your program and in each mode to optimize the potential mechanisms of change.

Again, we encourage the adoption of strategies and protocols as close to the defined model as possible. In terms of objectively measuring your adherence in each mode, there is not yet an adherence scale widely available for this purpose. Until such a measure is available, we suggest you use checklists in Linehan's (1993a) *Cognitive Behavioral Treatment for Borderline Personality Disorder.* You can consider whether your program is progressing over time by comparing yourself to yourself (e.g., "Compared to where we were 6 months ago, are we getting closer to the defined model?") and/or you can compare yourself to a specific ideal (e.g., "Our goal is to have 90% of all elements listed in the manual in place in each mode").

While adopting most of the DBT strategies and protocols is noncontroversial, there are particular areas that pull for adaptation or drift from the defined model that we cover in detail now. We look first at the program level and then at common concerns with particular modes.

Suicidal Behavior and Hospitalization Protocols

DBT's suicidal behavior and hospitalization protocols can differ from the practices of the wider network. For example, chronically suicidal clients whose use of the hospital interferes with their quality of life often have inadvertently been reinforced for crisis behavior and fragility—they learn that help is more forthcoming as their extreme behavior escalates. In DBT, treatment goals and agreements minimize the link between crisis behavior and additional contact by providing regular noncontingent help and after-hours coaching with strong encouragement to get help before a crisis. In this context DBT has a 24-hour rule: For 24 hours after a client's intentional self-injury, the primary therapist keeps already scheduled contacts but does not increase client contact. This system can be at odds with the expectations of family members and other professionals in the client's network. Consequently, DBT therapists consult to their clients about how to best orient the client's network to the treatment rationale and instruct the network about what is most likely to be helpful. This may be accomplished by having the client draft a letter to all treatment providers that orients them, by holding conjoint meetings where the client and the therapist orient family members, and so on. This stance of insisting that the client assume an active competent stance in his or her own treatment plan may also be at odds with past experiences and need to be explained to those in the client's network.

Similarly, crisis and suicidal behavior protocols can conflict with usual practices because DBT allocates the central role of managing these to the primary therapist. In some systems, the person assigned the role of individual therapist may lack the training or authority needed to make decisions regarding management of suicidal behavior and hospitalization. In some cases, this responsibility is always held by the psychiatrist even if he or she is not the primary therapist or even on the DBT team. Sometimes authority is distributed in such a way that administrators who manage risk also exert influence and may inadvertently reinforce the client when crises escalate. Again, in these situations, orienting the network and consultation to the patient are the primary strategies to use. (See Reynolds, Wolbert, Abney-Cunningham, & Patterson, Chapter 11, this volume, for useful scripts and ideas about orienting the network in such cases.)

Arbitrary Rules Regarding Attendance

Another source of conflict can arise regarding the arbitrary rules about attendance in DBT. Standard DBT has the rule that if a client misses four consecutive sessions of individual or group skills training, then the client is discharged from the program for the remainder of the contracted treatment period (after which time the client could negotiate reentry into the program). However, some systems are set up such that they are either legally mandated or in some other way obligated to continue to provide service to the client regardless of his or her participation or improvement. In these situations, a DBT program within a nonprogram may help maintain this principle. See Comtois et al. (Chapter 3, this volume) and Swenson et al. (Chapter 4, this volume) for further discussion of this topic.

Challenges Specific to Modes: Skills Training

Several common obstacles can arise when adopting the format of DBT skills training defined in Linehan (1993b). First, the standard format is a year-long, 2½-hour, once-a-week group. In some settings this may not work. What is important is acquiring, strengthening, and generalizing new skills—that is why standardly the skills are taught twice, that homework is reviewed and new skills are taught, and that the target hierarchy in skills training is used as a guide to keep focused on teaching skills. Consequently, if your client's length of stay is briefer, we would suggest teaching fewer skills but retaining the emphasis on acquiring and strengthening skills by teaching each skill twice with many practice opportunities rather than covering more materials in less depth. Second, the standard format typically has two skills trainers. The purpose here too is to aid clients in acquiring and strengthening their skills: One trainer functions as lead and ensures that material is covered; the other tracks process and provides support to assist clients and the lead skills trainer in emotion regulation so that skills can be learned. Having two leaders means skills training continues even in the toughest circumstances. If there were to be a clinical emergency such as a life-threatening suicide crisis with one of the group members, one skills trainer can handle it, while the other continues to teach. If, for some reason, you can have only one therapist, attention should be paid to how to otherwise accomplish these tasks. A third frequently faced issue has to do with offering skills training to individuals who do not have a DBT therapist or even any therapist. Here we return to the principle of Stage 1 clients requiring comprehensive treatment. Early research suggests that a skills-only component may not offer benefits. Yet for less-disordered individuals it may be that a skills group format is sufficient (e.g., see Wisniewski et al., Chapter 7, this volume).

Consultation Team

Many challenges arise in the context of the consultation team. First, at some point, teams typically need to add new members. New members may not have as much formal DBT training, they have not shared the formative experiences of the founding members of the team, and they may not share basic assumptions about clients or therapy (e.g., not viewing it as important to learn cognitive-behavioral interventions). What to do? Many teams successfully recruit team members in ways similar to enrolling new clients. The enrollment process includes a clear commitment from the new member, with clarity around expectations and agreements and how these do and do not fit with his or her professional goals. Second, part of the team's function is to help team members observe their personal and professional limits. This can usefully be expanded as needed to include attending to program limits too. For example, team members may have competing roles (i.e., DBT is part-time work) or program leaders may get spread too thin so that they falter in important duties or the aversives outweigh the reinforcement. Growing the program too quickly in response to need and pressure, resulting in more referrals than the team can handle, can also be a struggle. Just as therapy-interfering behavior is prioritized, so too should team-interfering behavior be prioritized. In addition to adopting a dialectical problem-solving approach and applying DBT strategies to ourselves, we also advise an attentive and active effort to maximize the reinforcing aspects of the team. In other words, thoughtful and regular attention should be given to how the team serves its function to enhance therapists' skills and motivation and solve any problems that interfere with these goals. This will vary by team and individual member, but may include ensuring that adequate time is spent on cases and not diverted by discussion of ever-present administrative issues or tangential topics; that the size of the team doesn't grow so large that members have too little time to get help on tough cases; that new members are integrated in a way that balances their needs to learn basics without compromising more senior members' needs for more sophisticated discussion; and so on.

Tip 5: Use the Dissemination of Innovation Literature to Increase Your Success

Our final piece of advice is to look to the dissemination of innovation literature for ideas on how to help structure the environment to increase your success with implementing DBT. Here is a quick synopsis of tips:

1. *Intensity of effort is associated with practice change.* First, implementing DBT can often require significant changes in clinicians' behavior. Research shows that education alone leads to little change clinicians' behavior (Davis, Thomson, Oxman, & Haynes, 1995; Oxman, Thomson, Davis, & Haynes, 1995). Instead, practice behaviors are strongly affected by factors such as consumer demand for services, financial incentives and penalties, administrative rules and regulations, and feedback on practice patterns (Greco & Eisenberg, 1993; Handley, Stuart, & Kirz, 1994). Practice improvements become more likely as more of these factors are used to mobilize change. In other words, it is intensity of effort that seems most directly related to practice change (Davis, Thomson, Oxman, & Haynes, 1995; Schulberg, Katon, Simon, & Rush, 1998). Because intensity of effort is related to clinicians' practice change, you should not expect in-services or off-site training alone to be sufficient to actually produce DBT program implementation. Instead, use multiple strategies to support change in practice. Care and attention should be given to structuring the environment to support implementation in as many ways as possible. This leads to our second point.

2. *Enlist stakeholders via social marketing and tailored messages.* Implementing a new evidence-based practice such as DBT can require significant support from various stakeholders in the system. Lomas (1993) talks about the effective use of social marketing as a means for developing support of innovations. Social marketing would advise selecting an influential person to be the spokesperson for the innovation, using personalized interactions and local anecdotes or experiences as the message, seeking out opinion leaders among stakeholders, and using informal environments to communicate about the innovation.

Consequently, early in your program development, we suggest that you identify your most effective spokesperson(s) and create presentations and materials that can be used to communicate with therapists, clients, administrators, and funders about DBT and your program. You might also consider tailoring your message to colleagues based on whether they are more or less likely to be interested in innovative practices. What has appealed to you as an "early adopter" of a new practice such as DBT may be different than others in your setting who adopt it later. For example Berwick (2003) suggests that those in the early majority of adopting an innovation are

> . . . quite local in their perspectives. They learn mainly from people they know well, and they rely on personal familiarity, more than on science or theory, before they decide to test a

change. They are most interested in information regarding how to solve local problems (not general ones or general background info). (p. 1972)

Those in the late majority wait for local proof that innovation is the new status quo before adopting the change, so they may need to hear from a respected program leader who provides evidence to show that DBT is indeed working and becoming the new standard of care.

3. *Maximize stakeholders' ability to evaluate: Benefit, compatibility, simplicity, trialability, and observability.* Berwick (2003) suggests that "changes spread faster when they have these five perceived attributes: benefit, compatibility, simplicity, trialability and observability" (p. 1971). In your presentations, highlight the perceived *benefit* of change by presenting information that decreases the uncertainty of the consequences of an innovation. For example, include summaries of research and estimates of the nature and costs of implementation and training along with the data on treatment as usual within your system and cost of treatment failures. Increase the felt *compatibility* of DBT with the stakeholders' "values, beliefs, past history and current needs" (Berwick, 2003, p. 1971). As suggested by Swenson (2000; Swenson, Torrey, & Koerner, 2002), your presentation might highlight the need for a new approach via discussion of high-profile treatment failures. You might highlight how DBT fits with what stakeholders are already doing and how DBT is compatible with both the recovery and the consumer movements. Depending on your audience, you might mention how DBT is attractive to managed care, pragmatic and immediate in focus as well as comprehensive and long term, and is applicable to other populations. *Trialability* means creating ways for potential adopters to test the change on a small scale without implementing it everywhere at first. Examples of trialability include hosting an open-case consultation meeting where DBT team members offer to consult on difficult cases so that potential new team members can try on the concepts; hosting an open-skills group where therapists or consumers can try out and see the skills; and making skills sheets and posters readily available in common rooms. Finally, *observability* also helps innovations spread more quickly. Make the changes you are proposing highly observable so that potential adopters can watch others try the change first. Toward this end you might present cases during meetings such as grand rounds to explain what interventions are being tried with high-profile cases. You might also host open houses for your program for new clients and administrators.

Summary and Conclusions

Our advice is to take a dialectical stance toward the inevitable tension between adopting versus adapting DBT in your setting. The best chance of obtaining good clinical outcomes is to adopt and implement the defined model and to simultaneously look for ways to fit the model to meet the needs and constraints of your setting and population. Insist that any solution provide a synthesis of these two positions so that you have a workable, high-fidelity implementation. Again, the evidence to date supports adopting the standard model (unless one is adopting an adaptation that has itself become evidence-based). We suggest that the goal should be implementing the standard model of DBT (until [if] we learn more clearly which elements cause positive outcomes so that research can guide modification). We suggest that you first develop a small, tightly focused pilot program that is "by the book." As you encounter conflicts implementing standard DBT, use functions of treatment to creatively think through potential solutions. If you encounter conflicts about particular strategies or protocols, focus on adherence and apply the treatment principles themselves to solving these problems. Monitor your outcomes against benchmarks of published outcomes and treatment as usual in your own setting. During implementation remember to focus attention on garnering support from stakeholders so that the environment becomes increasingly structured to sustain your efforts.

Using This Book

After reading the first two chapters, the best way to use this book is to next read Chapters 3 and 4, followed by any particular chapters that address specific populations or settings of interest to you. Comtois et al. (Chapter 3, this volume) highlights pragmatic strategies for implementing outpatient DBT both in private practice and in public-sector communities. This chapter weaves in solutions to barriers and misunderstandings common across settings and populations. It also includes an overview of new innovations (Comtois, Elwood, Holdcraft, & Simpson, 2006) for aiding patients with BPD to get off public assistance and into productive work. Similarly, Swenson, Witterholt, and Bohus (Chapter 4, this volume) detail the oldest adaptation of DBT and the first application of DBT in a milieu setting, and provide a terrific example of how to preserve DBT principles at every turn despite obstacles to the standard model of DBT. Rizvi et al. (Chapter 12, this volume) describe all the how-tos of program evaluation. Our suggestion is that program evaluation be undertaken in tandem with program development, rather than treated as an add-on once the program is already underway. These five chapters will provide you with the basics you will need to think through most difficulties with implementation you will encounter. We hope that we can save you the energy of reinventing the wheel, and that some of the materials we present here will be useful to you.

REFERENCES

Berwick, D. M. (2003). Disseminating innovation in healthcare. *Journal of the American Medical Association, 289,* 1969–1975

Comtois, K. A., Elwood, L. M., Holdcraft, L. C., & Simpson, T. L. (2006). Effectiveness of dialectical behavior therapy in a community mental health center. *Cognitive Behavioral Practice.*

Davis, D. A., Thomson, M. A., Oxman, A. D., & Haynes, G. (1992). Evidence for the effectiveness of CME: A review of 50 randomized controlled trials. *Journal of the American Medical Association, 268,* 1111–1117.

Davis, D. A., Thomson, M. A., Oxman, A. D., & Haynes, G. (1995). Changing physician performance: A systematic review of the effect of continuing medical education strategies. *Journal of the American Medical Association, 274,* 700–705.

Drake, R. E., Goldman, H. H., Leff, H. S., Lehman, A. F., Dixon, L., Mueser, K. T., et al. (2001). Implementing evidence-based practices in routine mental health service settings. *Psychiatric Services, 52,* 179–182.

Greco, P. J., & Eisenberg, J. M. (1993). Changing physician practices. *New England Journal of Medicine, 329,* 1271–1274.

Handley, M. R., Stuart, M. E., & Kirz, H. L. (1994). An evidence-based approach to evaluating and improving clinical practice: Implementing practice guidelines. *HMO Practice, 8,* 75–83.

Jerrel, J. M., & Ridgely, M. S. (1999). Impact of robustness of program implementation on outcomes of clients in dual diagnosis programs. *Psychiatric Services, 50,* 109–112.

Linehan, M. M. (1993a). *Cognitive-behavioral treatment for borderline personality disorder.* New York: Guilford Press.

Linehan, M. M. (1993b). *Skills training manual for treating borderline personality disorder*. New York: Guilford Press.

Linehan, M. M. (1995). Combining pharmacotherapy with psychotherapy for substance abusers with borderline personality disorder: Strategies for enhancing compliance. In *NIDA Research Monograph Series: Integrating behavioral therapies with medications in the treatment of drug dependence* (pp. 129–142). Rockville, MD: National Institute of Mental Health.

Linehan, M. M. (1997). Special feature: Theory and treatment development and evaluation: Reflections on Benjamin's "models of treatment." *Journal of Personality Disorder, 11*(4), 325—335.

Linehan, M. M. (2000). Behavioral treatment of suicidal behavior: Definitional obfuscation and treatment outcomes. In R. W. Maris, S. S. Canetto, J. L. McIntosh, & M. M. Silverman (Eds.), *Review of suicidology, 2000* (pp. 84–111). New York: Guilford Press.

Linehan, M. M., Comtois, K. A., Murray, A. M., Brown, M. Z., Gallop, R. J., Heard, H. L., et al. (2006). Two year randomized trial + follow-up of dialectical behavior therapy vs. treatment by experts for suicidal behaviors and borderline personality disorder. *Archives of General Psychiatry, 63*, 757–766.

Linehan, M. M., Dimeff, L. A., Reynolds, S. K., Comtois, K. A., Shaw-Welch, S., Heagerty, P., & Kivlahan, D. R. (2002). Dialectical behavior therapy versus comprehensive validation plus 12-step treatment of opioid-dependent women meeting criteria for borderline personality disorder. *Drug and Alcohol Dependence, 67*, 13–26.

Linehan, M. M., Kanter, J., & Comtois, K. A. (1999). Dialectical behavior therapy for borderline personality disorder: Efficacy, specificity, and cost effectiveness. In D. Janowsky (Ed.), *Psychotherapy indications and outcomes* (pp. 93–118). Washington, DC: American Psychiatric Press.

Lomas, J. (1993). Diffusion, dissemination, and implementation: Who should do what? *Annals of the New York Academy of Science, 703*, 226–237.

McDonnell, J., Nofs, D., Hardman, M., & Chambless, C. (1989). An analysis of the procedural components of supported employment programs associated with employment outcomes. *Journal of Applied Behavior Analysis, 22*, 417–428.

McHugo, G. J., Drake, R. E., Teague, G. B., & Xie, H. (1999). Fidelity to assertive community treatment and client outcomes in the New Hampshire Dual Disorders Study. *Psychiatric Services, 50*, 818–824.

Oxman, A. D., Thomson, M. A., Davis, D. A., & Haynes, R. B. (1995). No magic bullets: A systematic review of 102 trials of interventions to improve professional practice. *Canadian Medical Association Journal, 153*, 1423–1431.

Rogers, E. M. (1995). The challenge: Lessons for guidelines from the diffusion of innovations. *Journal on Quality Improvement, 21*, 324–328.

Schulberg, H. C., Katon, W., Simon, G. E., & Rush, A. J. (1998). Treating major depression in primary care practice: An update of the Agency for Health Care Policy and Research Practice Guidelines. *Archives of General Psychiatry, 55*, 1121–1127.

Silverman, M., Bongar, B., Berman, A. L., Maris, R. W., Silverman, M. M., Harris, E. A., et al. (1997). *Risk management with suicidal patients*. New York: Guilford Press.

Springer, T., Lohr, N. E., Buchtel, H. A., & Silk, K. R. (1996). A preliminary report of short-term cognitive-behavioral group therapy for inpatients with personality disorders. *Journal of Psychotherapy Practice and Research, 5*(1), 57–71.

Swenson, C. R., Torrey, W. C., & Koerner, K. (2002). Implementing dialectical behavior therapy. *Psychiatric Services, 53*, 171–178.

Torrey, W. C., Drake, R. E., Dixon, L., Burns, B. J., Flynn, L., Rush, A. J., et al. (2001). Implementing evidence-based practices for persons with severe mental illness. *Psychiatric Services, 52*, 469–476.

Turner, R. M. (2000). Naturalistic evaluation of dialectical behavior therapy-oriented treatment for borderline personality disorder. *Cognitive and Behavioral Practice, 7*, 413–419.

Witterholt, S. (2006, November). *Certification*. Paper presented at the meeting of the International Society for the Implementation and Teaching of Dialectical Behavior Therapy, Chicago.

CHAPTER 3

Implementing Standard Dialectical Behavior Therapy in an Outpatient Setting

Katherine Anne Comtois, Cedar R. Koons, Soonie A. Kim, Sharon Y. Manning, Elisabeth Bellows, *and* Linda A. Dimeff

Dialectical behavior therapy (DBT) was originally developed and evaluated in an outpatient setting, so how does it make sense to include a chapter on outpatient DBT in a book devoted nearly exclusively to adaptations of standard DBT? The simple reason is this: While Linehan's manuals (1993a, 1993b) very clearly describe what is and isn't DBT, very little information is provided about *how* to develop, implement, and sustain a DBT program or to implement DBT. Additionally, since the publication of these seminal manuals, there have been considerable advances in DBT applied in the outpatient setting. These include further elaboration of how to structure the DBT treatment program to facilitate building a life worth living (e.g., graduating from the mental health system, seeking and retaining employment, getting off of psychiatric disability, successfully pursuing a life that is consistent with one's ultimate goals and values; see Comtois et al., 2006).

Our goals for this chapter are twofold: First, we provide the reader with the collective wisdom we have developed over the past decade in building our own DBT programs and consulting to many others applying DBT in an outpatient setting. By providing you with all we know, we hope to help you "fast-track" the effective development of your own DBT program. We discuss common misconceptions, obstacles, barriers, and errors in implementation, and we suggest DBT-adherent solutions to these problems. We provide step-by-step tips for developing your DBT program—from consideration of inclusion and exclusion criteria to strategies for insurance reimbursement. Second, we provide specific instructions for building a DBT advanced program aimed at transitioning patients into jobs, school, and other normative activities of a life worth living.

We make the following assumptions: First, that readers of this chapter are knowledgeable about DBT principles, assumptions, and strategies, as well as about the theories on which it is based (see Koerner & Dimeff, Chapter 1, this volume). Second, that the reader's intention is to build a comprehensive outpatient DBT program to fidelity (see Koerner, Dimeff, & Swenson, Chapter 2, this volume). Third, the individuals served by the reader's program are severely disordered, chronic, and multidiagnostic clients, including those with borderline personality disorder (BPD). Fourth, the reader intends to build or improve a Stage 1 DBT outpatient program for Level 1 clients (see Chapter 1 for definitions).

Swimming against the Currents: The Necessary Paradigm Shift

As you may already know, DBT often constitutes a radical departure from "treatment as usual" for clients with BPD—it is nothing short of a paradigm shift on many fronts for therapists, administrators, and clients alike (Kuhn, 1962). Recognizing and acknowledging the paradigm shift, as well as the differences between DBT and more traditional approaches, can be extremely helpful in anticipating, assessing, and solving implementation problems as they arise. We highlight several of these differences below:

• *The goal of DBT is a life worth living*, not *palliative care*. The intent of DBT is to help the client develop the capability and motivation to build a life that is indistinguishable from the authors' lives or the reader's life—one that includes solid and lasting relationships, employment at a living wage, and other aspects that provide meaning and relevance to life, as deemed by the individual him- or herself. Inherent to this goal is the assumption that the client will no longer require mental health services and/or psychiatric disability on an ongoing basis for BPD. (This is not to say that he or she would not seek out psychotherapy in the future, just as "ordinary" people do for assistance with "ordinary" problems.) Thus, it assumes that the diagnosis of BPD is *not* a life sentence—that people diagnosed with BPD can be fully and successfully treated with DBT, where they become "diagnosis-free."

It is not uncommon during the early phases of implementation to hold on to the core belief that the program's patients with BPD are "lifers" (i.e., that they will require mental health services forever) and to narrowly define a life worth living as the absence of self-destructive, impulsive behavior (e.g., suicide attempts, nonsuicidal self-injurious behaviors, substance abuse), despite the fact that the person is still dependent on the mental health system for his or her social and financial support. This is a mistake, as this outcome expectancy may ultimately create the reality it envisions. One alternative approach is presented at the end of this chapter: an advanced DBT program that systematically pushes for and reinforces the client and the therapist for their efforts in actively moving the client toward behaviors and activities consistent with building a life worth living.

• *Clients get more of what they want based on functional (vs. dysfunctional) behavior.* This basic principle courses throughout DBT and is a radical departure from the standard disease model approach of providing clients *more* when they are dysfunctional. The classic illustration is the 24-hour rule: In DBT clients are required to wait 24 hours before initiating telephone contact with their primary therapist after engaging in self-injurious behaviors, but they can contact their therapist for skills coaching whenever there is a need for such coaching as a means of averting dysfunctional behavior. Similarly, *more* treatment in DBT (following the initial treatment agreement) is provided contingent on tangible progress on treatment goals and not on the declining mental status of the client or his or her lack of change. In a nutshell, all good things (i.e., reinforcers) come to the client in the presence of *functional* behavior, while reinforcers are withheld from the client in the presence of his or her dysfunctional behavior.

The anti-DBT error of providing *more* reinforcers in the presence of dysfunctional behavior often shows in those new to DBT in the following contexts: (1) the therapist stays on the phone longer and is more soothing when the patient is more suicidal, dysfunctional, or noncollaborative; (2) the therapist allows the client to control the session and discuss whatever is on his or her mind despite the fact that the client had engaged in dysfunctional behavior during the past week; (3) the therapist offers the client additional months or years of treatment despite the fact that he or she has not demonstrated significant behavioral progress on treatment goals; and (4) the therapist increases session frequency and/or length when the client is engaging in dysfunctional behaviors.

• *DBT is a high-risk treatment.* There is no question about it: Compared to treatment as usual, DBT is high risk. Think about your own program: What is the protocol when a client becomes suicidal? At what point, if any, does the therapist move to hospitalization? What is your own comfort zone for risk?

In DBT, hospitalization is used minimally and generally as a last resort; considerable effort is exerted to keep the client out of the hospital. The rationale for this position in DBT is described thoroughly by Linehan (1993a). The bottom line is that for most patients with BPD, hospitalization does not reduce the risk of suicide and can instead have an iatrogenic effect on such patients (Paris, 2005; Krawitz et al., 2004; Lieb, Zanarini, Schmahl, Linehan, & Bohus, 2004; Linehan, 1993a). From a DBT perspective, it is imperative that the client find and use DBT skills to effectively manage whatever situation is precipitating the urge to kill him- or herself. There is no way to ultimately achieve a life worth living except by going through difficult situations, using skills, and getting to the other side of the situation without engaging in dysfunctional behavior.

Swimming against the current, while necessary to apply DBT, is both challenging and wearing for the therapist. This is particularly true early in the implementation process before there is clinic-specific evidence that DBT works at the local level. It can be still harder in public-sector systems serving psychiatrically disabled clients accustomed to receiving services "from cradle to grave." Given that DBT represents a paradigm shift for many, it can help to orient people (e.g., staff, administrators, clients, spouses, and parents) ahead of time to the message that *doing* DBT may mean doing things radically differently from the ways to which they are accustomed. Before embarking on building a DBT program (and certainly as new staff and clients join the program), we suggest getting an individual commitment from all of these individuals to *doing* DBT. As part of this commitment process, we suggest doing *pros and cons*. There are certainly easier approaches than DBT for treating BPD; they simply may not be as effective (see Koerner & Dimeff, Chapter 1, this volume).

Getting Started: Designing Your DBT Program and Taking the First Steps

Like building anything from the ground up, there are a number of foundational decisions that must be made before construction can begin. Take building a house, for example:

Where will it be built? How many bedrooms and baths will it have? Will it contain two (or more) levels, or be a one-story structure? Who is responsible for the design and construction? Relevant questions for the development of your DBT program include: Where will DBT be situated (e.g., within an existing program or agency, as a stand-alone service program)? What clients will be served by DBT (e.g., those with BPD and/or severely disordered problem behaviors)? Who will staff the different DBT treatment modes? What is the typical caseload size? Who and what factors will determine treatment duration? What does the treatment consist of? This section seeks to help generate an initial "blueprint" for DBT.

Who Will Receive DBT?: Defining Inclusion and Exclusion Criteria

Deciding on the types of clients to be served by your DBT program is an important first step as it often influences other decisions, including the staff you recruit, where you house the program, how you advertise for and recruit clients to the program, and how you assess a person's "fit" during the intake/assessment phase. The entrance criteria can range from relatively narrow (e.g., the person must meet criteria for BPD, have a history of multiple suicide attempts, *and* be among the system's highest utilizers of inpatient and emergency room services) to relatively broad (e.g., the person must have severe behavioral dyscontrol due to emotion dysregulation, whether or not he or she meets criteria for BPD). Recognizing the cost savings success of DBT for difficult-to-treat clients with BPD, some agencies have applied DBT to all difficult-to-treat, high-utilizer clients. Others have considered offering DBT to clients who have repeatedly "failed" with other approaches.

We recommend initially adhering as much as possible to the population DBT has been validated on: Level 1 patients with BPD, including those who are chronically suicidal and drug-addicted. If it is necessary to *widen* the criteria (e.g., there are too few Level 1 clients with BPD available to your clinic to justify a DBT program), consider inclusion of those non-BPD Level 1 clients for whom behavioral dyscontrol stems from emotion dysregulation. If it is necessary to *narrow* the criteria (e.g., there are *many* clients with BPD seeking referral), you may consider focusing on those patients with BPD who utilize the greatest number of services or are generating the most problems for your system. Demonstrating clinical success and cost savings with the most costly of clients is a very reliable way of receiving continued support for your DBT program, from colleagues and administrators, and from behavioral health organizations. Alternatively, practicalities may demand that the limiting factor is the client's ability to pay for services—either out of pocket or because his or her insurance covers it.

We encourage two simple rules of thumb as you proceed. First, start with an evidence-based therapy for the problem the client has. For example, the application of DBT for treatment of panic disorder would be ill-advised if the client does not have BPD and has not yet received panic control treatment (Barlow & Craske, 2006), a highly effective treatment for panic. Similarly, we would not recommend DBT for bulimia unless several attempts at the evidence-based therapies for bulimia (with different treatment providers) had failed *and* emotion dysregulation was a prominent clinical feature. However, we would recommend DBT as the frontline treatment, for clients with panic disorder or bulimia *and* BPD, as DBT is structured to treat multiple disorders, in addition to BPD. Or one might choose DBT because the client has many behaviors that interfere with the treatment process regardless of BPD diagnosis—this may be known from previous treatment failures or become apparent when the diagnostic treatment is tried. The second recommendation is to be parsimonious. All things being equal (i.e., two treatments have comparable outcomes), apply the simpler treatment first.

Choosing the Right Location for Building the DBT Program

Whether you are in private practice or in a public-sector system, chances are that you will face many different options for where to position your DBT program. These decisions will inform the extent to which a clinician's caseload involves providing DBT—ranging from some DBT to exclusively DBT—as well as a strategy for training clinicians to adherence in DBT. While some smaller agencies may require that all their clinicians know and be prepared to apply DBT when receiving a referral for a client with BPD, other agencies (often medium to large in size) will design a DBT specialty unit. In this latter approach, clinicians elect to be on the DBT team where they can dedicate themselves to treating the agency's clients with BPD with DBT. Similarly, in private practice, some clinicians dedicate themselves and their practice exclusively to providing DBT to patients with BPD (indeed, a number of DBT centers have emerged in the United States and abroad over the past several years). Other private practitioners limit their DBT practice to a handful of clients with BPD and may join other private practitioners (either in or outside their practice) to create a DBT program (e.g., three or more solo practitioners provide DBT individual therapy for their own clients and join together to offer a DBT skills training class and for peer/team consultation). Table 3.1 summarizes these different agencies and private practice models and highlights the pros and cons for each.

It is important to consider whether the DBT program will share staff with other agency teams. Having another job with different rewards and challenges and/or having fewer difficult-to-treat clients with BPD can reduce burnout. However, there is a risk that non-DBT clinic demands, including meetings, new training initiatives, and the like can interfere with building a strong, cohesive DBT program. There is a further challenge for the clinician who is expected to apply radically different treatment philosophies (paradigms) with similar clients depending on the team or clinic. When this is the case, it is important to consider changes, additions, or clarifications in policy to strengthen the DBT team's identity and freedom to adhere to the model. The weekly consultation team meeting of 60–120 minutes can play a central role here. If, on the other hand, it is the client who receives treatment from different teams or clinics, it is crucial to clarify the following:

1. Which team/clinician is ultimately responsible for the primary treatment plan?
2. Which team/clinician has clinical authority during a clinical crisis?

To be adherent to DBT, the ultimate responsibility for the patient with BPD in both cases resides with the DBT individual therapist.

Another way to address the latter issue is to consider whether DBT clients will work partially, primarily, or exclusively with the DBT team. A partial model indicates that part of the client's care is managed by the DBT team and part by another team; a primary model indicates primary responsibility for the client is with the DBT team but that other teams of providers interact with the client; an exclusive model has the client working primarily with DBT clinicians, although he or she may bave contact with ancillary treatment providers. Given the need in DBT for one primary therapist and team, it is rare that a partial model will work—especially one where crisis management resides outside of the DBT team. Conflicts can arise when clients are suicidal or making complaints that are hard to resolve when multiple treatment teams share responsibility. While the exclusive model is generally easiest from a management perspective, primary models can allow clients access to services not provided by the DBT team such as housing, financial, and vocational services. Note that conflicts in treatment perspective will still arise in a pri-

TABLE 3.1. DBT Program Structures

Type	Description	Pros	Cons
Private practice: Single group practice model	Group practice with one legal entity, business name, tax ID number. Typically one facility with standardized clinical and business policies and procedures.	• Easy to share clinical coverage. • Greater quality control with respect to adherence to DBT treatment manual and fidelity to DBT program structure. • Can negotiate a single contract with third party payers.	• Shared liability for clinical mistakes and debt. • Requires greater organization, commitment, and financial resources to establish and maintain. • Requires that all clinicians have interest in treating clients with BPD and applying DBT.
Private practice: multiple solo practitioners	Multiple solo practitioners from own independent practice join together for purpose of offering DBT. Each clinician is responsible for his or her own finances and administrative tasks. Services *may* be offered at multiple facilities.	• Relatively easy to form and dissolve. • Colleagues uniformly highly motivated to learn and apply DBT. • Fewer conflicts about day-to-day operations, policies, and procedures. • Each clinician can continue to determine scope of practice with respect to application of DBT, number of patients with BPD receiving services by practice, etc. • Greater individual autonomy.	• Relatively easy to form and dissolve. • Limited opportunities to see each other and develop collegial relationships outside of consultation team. • May be clinically liable for cases seen by consultation team members whom other team members have not met. • Unless teams have clear structural safeguards in place to ensure that team members apply DBT to adherence, as well as clear contingencies for failing to do so, teams of solo practitioners can drift out of adherence. • The independence of the solo practitioners and the voluntary nature of the team formation can complicate hiring and firing of team members. A strong team leader whose authority is accepted is essential to establish and maintain quality control. • Team leaders may find themselves spending a lot of unpaid time dealing with administrative issues. • Clinicians may not be aware of the extent of their shared liability.
Agency: specialty service	Agency referrals of some or all BPD clients go to dedicated treatment team specializing in DBT. Clinicians comprising this team work exclusively with DBT clients (for the portion of their time dedicated to DBT team).	• Shares the advantages of single group practice model described above. • Agency can direct its training resources to fewer staff, thus creating the potential for more thorough, comprehensive training in DBT. • Sustained focus applying DBT may increase DBT program effectiveness. • Staff cohesive and coordination has potential of being high.	• Potential for increased risk of burnout as clinicians are treating the agency's most severe and difficult-to-treat patients. • Other units within agency do not benefit from universal clinical strategies used in DBT to manage difficult-to-treat patients. • Greater risk for losing DBT service and expertise with staff transitions.

(continued)

TABLE 3.1. *(continued)*

Type	Description	Pros	Cons
Agency: integrated service	Each unit within agency has clinicians dedicated to providing DBT, but do not exclusively treat BPD or provide DBT. Many or all units within the agency provide each DBT mode.	• Clinical skill learned in DBT to treat patients with BPD can be applied, as needed, to treat other difficult-to-treat patients in caseload. • Caseload can include diversity of clients, balancing easier-to-treat with more complex cases to prevent burnout.	• Multiple agency initiatives to learn other evidence-based therapies make it difficult for a large number of clinicianst to fully develop DBT clinical skills/competence and to devote sustained effort to maintaining DBT program. • Difficult to maintain DBT program cohesion; risk of moving out of DBT adherence because DBT is not "front and center" in mind of clinician. • Risk of general DBT program diffusion. • Limited DBT program cohesion.

mary model that the client may have difficulty reconciling. A common example in community mental health might be a tacit message that a client is not capable of independent action. This message may come from, for instance, a housing team in the agency (e.g., validation of "mental patient" role) and will conflict with the DBT assumption of capability leading to the perception that DBT "expects too much" or that housing services are "enabling" the client. Finally, in partial and primary programs, it is important to assure that the multiple psychological as well as practical demands of each treatment do not overwhelm the client. While there is no single way to proceed, concerted discussion of these issues early in program development can prevent confusion in a crisis and bad feeling all around.

Selecting a Team Leader

In our experience, those programs that survive and thrive are ones with strong administrative support *and* a strong team leader. Ideally, the team leader has *natural authority* on the DBT team (e.g., has the most experience with DBT, is a supervisor, is a unit lead, is an experienced clinician), *time* to assume the additional responsibilities required, *talent* (e.g., he or she is organized, a clear communicator, follows through, is personable), and is *willing*. The DBT team leader should also be a clinician on the DBT team, serving either as a DBT primary therapist, a skills trainer, or both. (This generally means the DBT team leader cannot be the agency manager if that person does not do clinical work within the team.) The team leader need not be the individual who runs the DBT team meetings (this can rotate), but is ultimately in charge of the DBT team and program. In a nutshell, the function of the team leader is to ensure that the program achieves and maintains structural fidelity to DBT; that clinicians adhere to the DBT treatment manuals in their respective mode(s); and that clinicians continue to increase their core competencies, as well as to solve problems and overcome barriers that interfere with program fidelity and clinical adherence. A final function of the team leader is to ensure that the DBT team as a whole remains energized and motivated to continue providing DBT services to the highest standards possible. (It is expected that future certification in DBT will include a specific certification for DBT team leader and that all DBT-accredited programs will have a certified DBT team leader. Team leader certification is expected to require separate certification in DBT skills training and individual therapy, thus requiring that the team leader is proficient in these treatment modes.)

Staffing Your Program

One of DBT's basic tenets is that participation should be voluntary. *This is just as true for clinicians as it is for clients.* When participation is mandated, the clinicians may resist the initiative, slow the team's development, and ultimately significantly compromise the program's viability. We have seen this effect over and over, even when DBT teams have included other members who were highly motivated to do DBT, despite the mandate. The negative effect of even a single unwilling clinician on a DBT team of otherwise willing staff cannot be overstated.

So where does this leave administrators and program managers who wish to move forward with a DBT initiative with reluctant and/or uninterested staff? First, consider if you really have to include them. It is often easier, faster, and more effective to transfer motivated clinicians from other clinics or to hire DBT clinicians rather than convert those who are committed to another form of treatment. Second, the key to motivating those with reluctance is to remember that the carrot (i.e., reinforcers) is more powerful than the stick (i.e., punishment, coercion) and to know what the carrots and that sticks are for each clinician. Then the task is to apply the strategies of DBT to turn around the attitudes and willingness of even the most reluctant of staff. These strategies will include linking DBT to staff goals, using DBT commitment strategies, creating such a positive valence around the DBT initiative through effective marketing that a groundswell of interest follows, and structuring employment conditions that facilitate motivation (e.g., DBT clinicians have smaller caseloads; learning DBT and making a commitment to serve on the DBT team for 2 years results in a salary increase or upgrade in employment status resulting in a pay raise; coveted agency positions require knowledge and 2 years of experience applying DBT). Such structural incentives can be particularly helpful with highly reluctant and resistant staff during the early implementation phase before the natural reinforcers of doing the treatment take hold. Table 3.2 lists a variety of additional strategies to facilitate willingness and interest in applying DBT.

In most cases, however, recruiting staff from within and outside your agency to do DBT may not be as difficult as one might think. Indeed, in many instances, it is the frontline staff themselves (looking for effective strategies for their most challenging cases) that initiate and push for the development of a DBT program. Often graduate students, social work and psychology interns, and psychiatry residents from educational programs nearby are also highly motivated to seek out opportunities to join a DBT team in exchange for learning the treatment. Students are keenly aware of the value of this experience when they are on the job market, whether competing for clinical or academic positions. For recent graduates and other professionals, joining a DBT team, either at an agency or within a private practice group, can be highly motivating, as they are more able to get on insurance panels (i.e., approved clinicians for that company to whom the insurance company directs referrals), thereby inheriting a ready-made referral base and attendant income.

The more formidable challenge for many DBT programs is *maintaining* their highly trained and skilled DBT clinicians. Their experience and training in applying DBT make them extremely competitive on the market for lateral DBT positions or promotions to develop or oversee a DBT program. Some may decide instead to build their own private practice. The best way to promote staff retention is to develop and pursue a business plan in which staff can see the prospect of continuing professional and financial advancement. For example, newly recruited staff in a private practice can be asked to accept a certain number of low-fee cases during their initial training period (1 year perhaps) and are then

TABLE 3.2. Persuasion Techniques for Getting Others to Buy Into DBT

Strategy	Examples
1. If clinicians already have difficult clients in their caseload, show them how DBT will help them to become more clinically effective and less distressed/burned out.	• Adopt their hard clients and succeed. • Run "office hours" or a monthly "case consultation" to identify effective strategies, skills, and approaches for use with their difficult-to-treat clients. • Teach the clinicians the DBT skills—as helpful treatment strategy or as employee assistance/stress management.
2. Link acceptance and mastery of DBT to the colleague's own professional or personal goals.	• Make learning and applying DBT (or specific aspects of it) a work requirement that is (like other work requirements) reviewed during the employee's annual performance review. Link pay increases to successful completion of DBT tasks (as measured and evaluated on performance review). • Offer other reinforcers for learning and applying DBT (e.g., once 80% of unit can pass DBT skills knowledge test at 80% or better, supervisor throws a pizza party for team). • Have clinician do the part of DBT that is most tied to the clinician's favorite part of the job (e.g., group, individual, case management).
3. Elicit the clinician's pros and cons for promoting versus declining DBT.	• Do a group exercise where everyone does pros and cons of doing DBT and not doing DBT. • Do contingency clarification on the short- and long-term consequences of doing or not doing DBT in this job. • Assess for whether DBT is truly voluntary or involuntary for that clinician.
4. Validate and then validate again.	• Don't oversell—that is functionally invalidating. • Validate that learning evidence-based practice does imply that current treatment is inadequate but that clinician is not inadequate. • Validate the grief or frustration of doing something new or unwanted. Repeat this validation as needed (e.g., don't assume validating once is enough).
5. Positively reinforce and shape all use of DBT techniques in the clinicians' daily work and in their team participation.	• Evaluate the clinicians' reinforcers—Do they want attention or to be ignored? • Figure out all the DBT strategies the clinician already uses and reinforce those when they occur. • Be systematic—develop a shaping curve of desired clinician behaviors and stick with it. • Watch for satiation—easily reached for those feeling pushed into something.
6. Use any and all of the DBT commitment strategies including "freedom to choose and the absence of alternatives."	

allowed to charge higher fees if they stay on longer. The other critical ingredient is to make doing DBT personally rewarding, whether it is having loads of fun on the DBT team, witnessing the turnaround in clients with BPD whom many had previously given up on, or opportunities to do the modes of DBT the clinician most enjoys.

Determining Caseload Size

Several considerations are critical in determining caseload size, including whether the individual is providing DBT exclusively on a full-time basis or is shared with other teams. For our purposes here, we will assume a full-time caseload where the individual is exclusively providing Stage 1 DBT to severely disordered patients with Level 1 BPD. (Readers can then adjust the numbers accordingly for staff in their setting.) Generally speaking, it is expected that a full-time clinician assigned exclusively to a DBT outpatient team will have between 15 and 18 suicidal individual clients with BPD and will conduct or colead one to two 2-hour DBT skills training groups per week. This caseload size assumes sufficient time for phone consultation and/or *in vivo* skills coaching (e.g., an average of 20 minutes per client per week), weekly participation in a 60–120-minute consultation team, and completion of paperwork. Furthermore, this assumes productivity standards of 60–75% (which range based on degree of paperwork required, requirement for training and supervising other staff, etc.), as well as a client no-show rate of 30% (Comtois, Elwood, Holdcraft, Simpson, & Smith, in press; R. Wolbert, personal communication, January 5, 2006; Sayrs, personal communication, January 5, 2006; DuBose, personal communication, January 5, 2006).

Other factors that may influence standard caseload size include (1) experience in treating clients with BPD; (2) experience in applying DBT; (3) number of unusually complicated or severely suicidal clients already on the caseload; (4) number of new clients with BPD in first month or two of treatment; and (5) team size and referral demands. Less experienced clinicians or those with limited familiarity with DBT may start off with slightly fewer clients with BPD. Additionally, unusually extreme and severe clients may count as two clients given the amount of effort required to intervene outside scheduled sessions. Moreover, a DBT clinician's caseload may be reduced during a period when he or she starts off with several new clients, as it is expected that clients in the first 2 months of treatment require considerably more time.

Determining Length of Treatment

One of the primary topics discussed and agreed to in the initial DBT "commitment" session is the *length of treatment*, the period both parties (client and therapist) agree to remain engaged together in DBT. The agreement can be "renewed" or extended for another specified period of time as the treatment length is about to expire, should additional treatment be indicated (see below). It is imperative to determine treatment length prior to the initial meeting between the DBT individual therapist and a prospective client as the therapist will want to get an agreement from the client to participate in treatment for this specified duration.

The majority of DBT programs, including those at the University of Washington (where DBT was developed), begin with a year's commitment. To ensure that the client completes two 6-month rotations of DBT skills training group, the "year" is yoked to the start date of the DBT skills class, not to the initial meeting with the DBT therapist. Because the prospective client meets *first* with the DBT individual therapist *before start-*

ing the DBT skills training group, it may be that the actual treatment length ends up being 13–14 months for some clients as a consequence of when the start date falls for entering the DBT skills training group and the fact that the client may continue to see the clinician for a couple of weeks following group graduation. (DBT skills training groups typically are open for new clients for 3–4 weeks, then close for 4–5 weeks, then open again for another 3–4 weeks, then close for 4–5, and so on, so that clients enter during mindfulness training and the beginning of a module and not in the midst of a module.)

The most frequent mistake made by new DBT teams is to fail to define the length of treatment. Sometimes failing to define the length is a simple oversight as the clinicians are not accustomed to determining a specified length of treatment at the start of working with a new client. In other cases, the program considered doing so but opted, in the end, not to set a length. The logic provided is this: "Our clients are too severe to offer only a year of treatment" or "We work with public-sector, disabled clients; we are legally and ethically obligated to continue to provide mental health services to our consumers." *Both arguments represent a misunderstanding and misapplication of DBT.*

Several DBT principles apply to this situation. First, reinforcers (e.g., contact with therapist, progress in treatment) are used to strengthen clinical progress, not the status quo or greater behavioral dyscontrol. This may be particularly relevant for clients with BPD who have systematically been reinforced for dysfunctional behavior over the course of their lives. Second, contingencies create capability—in other words, clients will work harder and more quickly develop and use behavioral skills (vs. engage in dysfunctional behavior) if doing so means they can get more of what they want: typically ongoing connection with the DBT therapist, whether this contact is formal or informal. DBT leverages these reinforcers, including attachment to the DBT therapist, in the service of the client's treatment goals. (These principles are discussed thoroughly in Linehan's [1993a] *Cognitive-Behavioral Treatment for Borderline Personality Disorder.*) Therefore, *more treatment* beyond the initial treatment contract *should be contingent on significant clinical progress.*

As is highlighted in the description of the advanced DBT program below, the DBT primary therapist should begin discussing termination and "What next?" around the eighth or ninth month of treatment. It should not be automatically assumed that an additional 6 months or year will be needed at this time. However, if it is determined by the therapist (in consultation with the DBT team) and the client that additional therapy *may* be required/appropriate upon completion of the initial year, the DBT therapist should clearly communicate what is expected of the client between now and graduation. In cases where the client is working hard and making steady progress, the therapist might simply highlight this pattern and state that so long as he or she continues like this, the therapist will be more than happy to discuss extending work together, should it be needed. In cases where the client is stuck and shows little progress on Stage 1 primary target behaviors, the therapist might instead describe the behaviors that must change by the year's end in order to receive additional treatment.

What if a client refuses to change; communicates "I can't change; you're asking too much"; or wants to change, has worked hard to change, but has still fallen short, and graduation is around the corner? These are important and complicated clinical issues that should be carefully considered by the therapist in collaboration with the consultation team. Teams that are in their early stages of learning DBT may opt for consultation with an expert to ensure that the solution generated is optimal and fully adheres to DBT principles. Assuming that the therapist has clinically proceeded in a DBT-adherent fashion, treatment should be terminated at the contract's end and the patient transferred to another treatment that may be more effective for him or her or (if he or she chooses) to working things out on his or her own. By definition, this means losing his or her primary DBT therapist as well as the skills training group which, for many clients, will create the conditions to shape up while there is still time to do so rather than risk this terrible fate. For others, DBT may truly not be effective and the ethical course is to try something else. Regardless, clients should be told what would be expected of them in order to reapply to the DBT program (if they can) should they wish to do so in the future.

If Adapting, Adapt Well

As previously noted, adoption of comprehensive DBT "by the book" may become even more important once accreditation in DBT is established. As described in Chapter 2, there are occasions, however, where even outpatient programs must adapt the structure of DBT to their unique setting. Sometimes these adaptations may be temporary (as the DBT program gets established); other times, they are longer term. We recommend that before adapting, every effort is made to look for solutions and syntheses to the problem consistent with DBT fidelity and that veering from the standard course is only done as a last resort.

Within outpatient programs, the mode that is most challenging to implement is phone consultation. In some systems, union rules or a clinician's job classification may be the barrier. In other agencies, it is the DBT clinicians themselves who are simply unwilling to take after-hour phone calls. In some situations, clinicians are willing *in principle* to take calls, but become so fearful of their limits being crossed that they become exceedingly unwilling to actually take the calls, or even refuse altogether. In our experience, barriers, resistance, and reluctance can often be overcome and fidelity preserved if the *actual* concern or problem is carefully assessed and solutions are thoughtfully generated. For example, some apprehensive clinicians have been willing to provide phone consultation to a few clients with BPD initially as a "test" to see what it is *really* like (as with phobias, the anxiety and fear are often far greater than the reality). Others agree if they can be assured that they will have sufficient supervision to effectively respond to client calls that are past their limits. Union rules and requirements are designed to protect the worker and not be a barrier to service provision: Clinicians generally *can* provide after-hours services so long as they are *willing* to do so and are not forced or otherwise coerced by the employer.

There may be situations, however, when it is simply not possible for the DBT individual therapist to take any after-hours calls. What are some solutions when this proves to be the case? In some systems, this means rotating call duty between crisis intervention team members who are trained to be DBT skills coaches. Some states have implemented toll-free DBT hotlines that are staffed by skills coaches. Other systems require their mobile crisis team members to be trained in DBT skills coaching.

While addressing the function of telephone coaching, these solutions are imperfect. Elements not addressed by these solutions include (1) the relationship between the client and the individual therapist and the ability of each to decrease feelings of alienation and to repair rifts in the relationship outside of work hours; (2) the expertise by the telephone coach on what skills work best for a particular client; and (3) determining the focus of treatment at the time of the phone call. Effective strategies to compensate for some of the inherent shortcomings that arise when primary therapists are not taking all calls include very explicit crisis plans made by the primary therapist and the client; contingency management of crisis staff that reinforces adherence to the crisis plan; if crisis plans are found to be unworkable for crisis staff, crisis staff can request revision by therapist and client (but should not revise themselves); scheduled calls with the therapist during work hours;

and "consultation time" in the therapist's workday schedule when clients know to call. It should be noted that while these strategies may be helpful in compensating for some of what is lost therapeutically by not offering DBT phone consultation, they are nonetheless *partial solutions*. It is for this reason that many DBT experts would not deem a program without standard DBT phone consultation as comprehensive, standard DBT. It is anticipated that the DBT phone consultation mode will be a requirement for future accreditation.

Marketing Your DBT Program and Building a Referral Base

The popularity and reputation of DBT as an efficacious, cost-effective treatment for BPD has made it relatively easy to market over the past decade. Indeed, the popular demand for DBT has resulted in the proliferation of programs describing themselves as DBT even when they offer only one DBT treatment mode: DBT skills training or DBT individual therapy. With efforts underway to develop DBT program accreditation and DBT provider certification, it is quite likely that the future of marketing a DBT program and building a referral base will be tied to whether the program is DBT-accredited and the extent to which its clinical staff are certified in providing DBT. Presumably, those with certified staff and program accreditation will be in the best position to secure a strong referral base. It is all but certain that accreditation for outpatient programs will require all modes and functions of DBT—in other words, standard, comprehensive DBT. In the meantime, it can be helpful to highlight to potential referral sources that not all DBT programs are alike—some may represent themselves as DBT, but not actually offer a comprehensive DBT program, whereas your program *does*.

The first step in advertising and marketing your DBT program is to identify the most likely sources of referrals. These may include managed care representatives, primary care physicians, a local chapter of the National Association for the Mentally Ill, pharmacotherapists with large BPD caseloads, and so on. Once you have done so, plan a meeting with each source of referrals to discuss your DBT program. Ideally, contact the referral representative who has the greatest power or influence over referrals for each source. Personally telephone the potential referral to initiate the meeting. Request that anyone interested who is in a position to refer patients with BPD attend, including case managers, supervisors, and claims representatives. If your budget allows, plan the meeting as a lunch in-service meeting for all who can attend and provide the lunch. Some public-sector agencies without marketing budgets have instead provided freshly brewed coffee and homemade desserts to those in attendance. Structure the meeting to include a formal presentation about DBT and your DBT program. We recommend that this presentation be no longer than 20 minutes. This will provide ample opportunity for people to ask questions at a leisurely pace. During the formal presentation itself, provide a high-level overview of DBT, including a brief summary of the research findings on DBT (see Koerner & Dimeff, Chapter 1, this volume). Link your presentation to the values and goals that matter the most to your audience (e.g., clinical outcomes, cost savings, recovery focus; see Table 3.3). Before you conclude, provide explicit information about how those in attendance make the referral (e.g., provide name of person to contact, phone number) as well as explicit information about who to refer (i.e., your program's inclusion/exclusion criteria). Additionally, be sure to prepare and provide flyers, business cards, and brochures.

Possibly the most important data to "sell" your DBT program will be outcomes from your DBT program that answer the question: *We know that DBT works, but does it work in your setting?* We encourage the reader to carefully read and review Rizvi, Monroe-DeVita, and Dimeff (Chapter 12, this volume) for tips in evaluating your DBT

TABLE 3.3. Values Shared between DBT and Managed Care/Behavioral Health Organizations

Value	Description
1. Evidence-based therapy	• DBT is an efficacious treatment, with more rigorous randomized controlled trials supporting its effectiveness for multidiagnostic Level 1 patients with BPD than any other treatment. (See Chapter 1 for a description of outcomes from DBT RCTs.) • DBT is an empirically derived treatment. It is made up of strategies, components, structures, and behavioral skills, which themselves have empirical support.
2. Significant cost savings compared to treatment as usual	• In the seminal RCT of DBT, Linehan et al. found that DBT saved $9,000 per patient during the initial treatment year compared to treatment as usual ($8,610 vs. $17,609, respectively; Linehan & Heard, 1999; Linehan, Comtois, & Kanter, 1999). • Pre–post data for patients ($n = 14$) completing a year of DBT in a community treatment program showed significant decreases in psychiatric service utilization when compared to the prior year: 77% decrease in hospitalization days, 76% decrease in partial hospitalization days, 56% decrease in crisis beds, and 80% decrease in emergency room contacts were reported. Total service costs also fell dramatically—from $645,000 to $273,000 (American Psychiatric Association, 1998).
3. High rates of client retention and satisfaction	• DBT studies to date consistently demonstrate its effectiveness in retaining clients in treatment despite the relatively long (typically 12 months) length of treatment. • Client satisfaction, a factor in treatment retention, is high for DBT.
4. Strong recovery focus	• The goal of DBT is building a life worth living, not merely symptom relief or a decrease in expensive psychiatric services. By definition, a life worth living in DBT is attainment of ordinary happiness and unhappiness (Level 3; see Chapter 1)—where behavioral dyscontrol, emotion dysregulation, and mental health problems do not define or limit the individual's capacity to live a full, fulfilling, and (extra)ordinary life.
5. Clarity and precision emphasized throughout all aspects of the treatment	• Clearly defines behavioral targets. • Clearly specifies functions for each treatment mode. • Clearly specifies how other treatment providers (DBT and non-DBT) interact with each other, as well as role of primary treatment provider in planning treatment and coordinating other services in service of client's goals. • Specifies criteria for determining when to begin formal exposure for PTSD in a way that guards against iatrogenic effects.
6. Flexible, principle-based treatment for multidiagnostic patients	• DBT is a principle- (vs. protocol) driven treatment that is flexibly tailored to the specific needs of the patient within a standard, structured framework. • Structure of DBT allows for treatment of comorbid Axis I disorders, including substance use disorders.
7. Tracking clinical progress through continuous monitoring of specific behavioral targets throughout course of treatment	• DBT promotes the weekly monitoring of outcomes through use of the DBT diary card (for clients) and session notes for therapists. • Client progress (or lack thereof) is tracked by the DBT consultation team; DBT teams move to assist therapists with case conceptualization and treatment planning when DBT clients are showing little improvement or when a relapse has occurred. • DBT encourages DBT programs to collect program outcome data on the overall effectiveness at treating DBT target-relevant behaviors and building lives that are worth living (e.g., attaining jobs, working steadily, enrolling in college, getting off psychiatric disability). • If clients do not show significant improvement after standard course of DBT, alternatives, including termination, are found.

program. The key is to keep the effort simple. The most persuasive data is that which your program will automatically collect from weekly diary cards and session notes (e.g., number of suicide attempts, nonsuicidal self-injurious behavior, admissions to emergency room, psychiatric inpatient admissions, number of days hospitalized). The success of your former DBT clients, now graduates of your program, will also naturally sell your DBT program, as other non-DBT staff and/or the claims representative are likely to notice the dramatic change in former DBT clients. Some programs incorporate "testimonials" from DBT graduates to further sell their DBT program. Positive feedback about your program often naturally occurs as DBT graduates informally talk to others about their lives, experiences, and the role of DBT in helping them to achieve their goals.

Getting Reimbursed for DBT Services

Strategies for reimbursement vary according to whether your agency is or is *not* a part of the public sector. Strategies for both are described below. Several overarching strategies are important irrespective of the type of system. First, it is often imperative to orient the managed-care company or claims representative on how DBT is unique from many other treatments: It is a comprehensive treatment involving multiple treatment modalities and providers. Fidelity to DBT involves offering the comprehensive treatment package; fidelity is breached if DBT is offered in an "à la carte" fashion (based on what the client wants or the insurance provider is willing to pay). Additionally, while DBT initially begins with making an agreement to 1 year of treatment, it is not assumed that a year will be sufficient for all clients with BPD. A second year may be required and offered *contingent on progress* in the first year and medical necessity. Second, it is recommended that you complete reimbursement negotiations *before* accepting the client into your DBT program; you will have the greatest leverage at this point in the process and you have not yet assumed legal and ethical responsibility for a (presumably) high-risk client. Third, push for reimbursement of comprehensive DBT for the full year, with provisional approval of an additional year, should it be required. Finally, if an insurance provider is initially reluctant to reimburse as described above, strike a deal to treat (with full reimbursement and caveats above) and collect outcome data on two or three of their most problematic and/or expensive clients. (This is a less viable option when the DBT therapists are new to DBT.) Provide intermittent reports on their progress, and plan to return to a final decision about reimbursement for other clients following completion of their treatment. This strategy allows claims representatives to limit their risk as they evaluate for themselves the value of your DBT service.

In the private sector, the primary problem is that DBT requires a commitment of time and money that exceeds the limits set by most managed care and insurance plans. Typical benefit plans do not cover all modes of treatment that comprise standard outpatient DBT for an entire year. Those that do pay for DBT individual therapy and DBT skills training group may not necessarily pay for phone consultation. Still fewer will be likely to reimburse the consultation team at first blush. Whenever possible, we advise working to negotiate a flat or "bundled" weekly rate for DBT services that includes all modes of treatment. When a program bundles services, the insurance company is billed for a week of all DBT services and the billing is coded "DBT treatment," instead of billing for each treatment session separately. In some instances, DBT programs have successfully secured a flat reimbursement rate, even for weeks when the client "no shows" to treatment. This can be justified on the basis that the DBT therapist is expected to continue to treat the patient, independent of whether he or she attends the session (e.g., actively calling the client to assess/problem-solve those factors that are interfering with attending session, going to a client's home to mobilize the client back into treatment), and such weeks are balanced by weeks of managing crises or *in vivo* exposure that may involve multiple calls, sessions, or outreach that is also covered in the weekly charge. On occasion, it can be necessary to work with clients on an individual basis to devise creative solutions to reimbursement. Table 3.4 summarizes a number of such strategies.

In the public sector, the issues are often exactly the opposite. While public managed care is also designed to provide services more efficiently, there is little focus on number of sessions or duration of therapy, as the system expects that most clients who are suicidal or who have BPD will remain in care indefinitely. The primary reimbursement challenge faced in the public sector involves a move to reduce funding as soon as stabilization is achieved (e.g., once the client is no longer actively suicidal or in crisis); services for the BPD client who is no longer engaging in suicidal and nonsuicidal self-injurious behavior are discontinued before the client is fully prepared to "fly" on his or her own. A cutback in services at this time can result in decompensation or the client remaining a "chronic but quiet mental patient." An important strategy for maintaining payment is to highlight the number and types of supports provided to the individual to achieve stabilization including the amount of therapy provided, assessment of continued suicide risk, how close the client has been to being admitted to a hospital, the frequency of phone coaching to keep the client at home, and the range of treatment strategies used to manage the client during group and individual sessions. However, when the client is remaining stable with fewer supports, the state or county may not want to pay for the client to continue to improve. If this is the case, it helps to go back to the public mission statement where states and counties often use language of recovery, including client-driven treatment and employment supports, not just reducing risk or symptoms. You can then use their own words to highlight how DBT is a good fit for public insurance dollars. If all else fails, you may need to help the client find employment that offers a private insurance you can accept.

Some practitioners seek to supplement their income by contracting with referral sources or by offering special services. Especially for new practices, applying for contracts with state agencies, such as social services, vocational rehabilitation, labor and industries, or child and family services, is one means of building a practice while providing a treatment that would otherwise be unaffordable to clients. One may also want to provide individual therapy or groups for caregivers, partners, or dependents of DBT clients. DBT clients of all ages are often in relationships that experience high stress. Issues of caregiver burden and burnout are particularly salient during Stage 1 DBT treatment of both adoles-

---

TABLE 3.4. Strategies to Pay for DBT

1. Transfer inpatient benefits to outpatients benefits (alternative treatment plan).

2. Bill insurance for the most expensive service (i.e., individual treatment); client pays for less costly groups.

3. Submit insurance bills with their covered Axis I diagnosis (as opposed to BPD); use of a parity Axis I diagnosis often increases available benefits.

4. Consider alternate sources of funding: family, church, school, employer, community organizations.

5. If therapist is not on provider panel, making a single case agreement (or accommodation) allows client to use in-network benefits and might pay your full fee.

6. Refer to a therapist for a reduced fee (student, trainee, licensed therapist learning DBT).

7. Reduce fees for clients after they complete 6 months of treatment.

8. Run a training group for therapists that can be paid fee for service as supervision.

---

cents and adults. Caregivers are often eager to participate in groups that provide support and teach principles of validation and behavioral change. These groups can be provided on a self-pay basis, usually at an extremely reduced rate such as $15.00–$20.00 per session. If such caregivers groups are fee for service, they require no administrative support other than issuing payment receipts. Often caregivers' distress is significant enough to warrant therapy in its own right, regardless of whether the client is in DBT. These caregivers may have acceptable private pay or insurance funding and appreciate a therapist who understands what they are facing and can give advice for managing their family member and their own emotion distress.

Accepting Referrals and the Intake/Assessment Transition

Clients often enter DBT desperate for help with few effective strategies for managing their distress. Some arrive with a (non-DBT) therapist to whom they are very attached and are reluctant to "give up" in order to begin DBT. Others may be eager to begin *now* and are impatient with the preliminary clinic intake and assessment procedures. Responding to the various crises and preventing suicide attempts during this transitional intake/assessment period while keeping the client sufficiently motivated to continue moving through the process can be quite challenging. Several pointers may be helpful during this phase.

- *Orient the prospective client and his or her existing provider to the process and identify who is clinically responsible for the individual during the intake phase.* At the very first contact, the intake staff should explain how the intake process works, including the steps and timeline. It is important to clarify who is clinically responsible for the client during this time. If the client *has* a therapist, it is recommended that the existing therapist continue to assume clinical responsibility for the client and that the individual continue to follow the existing crisis plan established by the current provider. Should crises occur during the intake phase, the intake clinician should assist the individual by contacting the current provider and/or executing the already established plan. If, however, the individual does *not* have a current mental health provider, a primary care provider or crisis clinic can temporary assume this role. The basic idea is to not assume that the individual will meet the DBT program criteria or want to participate in DBT after learning about the program. Drawing a clear line in the sand between assessment and treatment helps to guard against getting clinically "stuck" with a client who is at high risk and who does not want or fit the criteria for your program. Clarify this plan with the referring clinician at the outset, and repeat the expectation throughout the intake process with all relevant individuals, including the prospective client and his or her family. Using the metaphor of specialty medical care is often helpful—while patients expect to be able to enroll in primary care quickly, specialty medical services such as surgery or rheumatology often requires a delay and specialty clinicians do not take clinical responsibility from the primary care clinician before treatment has begun. We recommend screening a prospective client for eligibility to your DBT program on the telephone before initiating a more extensive assessment or conducting a first session. This approach is helpful in identifying many clients who will not meet entry criteria so their hopes are not further established, should it not work out.
- *Helping clients transition from their existing (non-DBT) therapist.* Sometimes clients and/or their referring non-DBT clinicians are reluctant to give up therapy together; they prefer to add DBT to the total treatment package. Linehan (1993a) describes a thorough rationale for why this is ill-advised and problematic. The question is how to make the transition well. We recommend the following: First, make sure to clarify at the time of referral that transition is the expectation; should the individual be accepted into the DBT

program, he or she will need to discontinue treatment with the existing therapist. Second, help ease the transition. This can be done by framing the transition as "temporary"—once the client completes DBT, he or she can certainly return to his or her current therapist. Again, it can be helpful to draw a analogy to medicine: The existing clinician is like the generalist; the DBT treatment providers are the specialists. Once the specialized treatment is completed and the problem that was beyond the skills of the generalist is resolved, the client may resume with the generalist. It can also be helpful to offer alternative models for the role of an ex-therapist: Rather than disappearing altogether, the ex-therapist can remain connected to the former client. Like relationships with other important people or mentors in the client's life (e.g., rabbis, priests, teachers), the ex-therapist and client relationship could consist of occasional meetings (e.g., phone calls, walks, meetings for coffee or lunch), discussions, and correspondences. Ex-therapists, however, do not do therapy. Specifically, they do not respond to crisis calls, develop or impose treatment plans, or engage in other formal planning of therapeutic activities.

Maintaining High Standards for Excellence over the Long Haul

Perhaps because of the high-risk nature of the clients served and the profound suffering in the lives of people with BPD, DBT emphasizes clarity, precision, and compassion throughout the treatment. Furthermore, it is deeply committed to science and excellence. Whether striving for full fidelity to the treatment, evaluating a program's clinical outcomes, or adhering fully to the manual (Linehan, 1993a, 1993b), in each treatment mode and at all times DBT requires a number of competencies from providers and the team leader alike. This section details several strategies that are critical for maintaining the strength of the DBT team—both clinically and programmatically—over the long haul.

Measure Your Program's Outcomes

This point cannot be emphasized enough. Rizvi et al. (Chapter 12, this volume) provide simple, pragmatic instructions for collecting outcome data, which will be invaluable for maintaining referrals to your DBT program. For programs situated within larger community mental health agencies, outcome data can also be very helpful in persuading administrators to continue their support of the DBT initiative—from allocating resources and further training opportunities to continuing to its structural support of DBT. Data also demonstrates to the team its strengths and weaknesses, which guides quality improvement. As emphasized throughout Chapter 12, collection of outcome data need not be complex; the most important outcome data will naturally be collected from the diary card and session notes.

Watch For and Address Anti-DBT "Drift"

Despite significant efforts to maintain fidelity to DBT principles early in the program, drift can occur over time—often in response to clinic changes, a push for other training initiatives, changes in reimbursement rates or policies, or simply the popularity of the DBT program. The most frequent situation is one in which the agency generates solutions to a perceived problem or concern that are incompatible with DBT. For example, in response to a recent serious event, an administrator institutes a policy in which all clients who contact crisis services be given a next-day appointment. While this solution addresses a real problem, it becomes a DBT problem by providing the client with BPD greater access to his or her DBT primary therapist following (contingent on) dysfunctional behavior. In cases where the DBT primary therapist is a reinforcer, this programmatic policy may function to strengthen dysfunctional behavior.

When this occurs, the first thing to do is to *conduct a skillful assessment* of the problem the solution seeks to solve. It is only after understanding the problem that the team can both validate the agency director's concerns and offer alternative DBT-compatible solutions. For example, a thorough assessment of the problem that facilitated a change in clinic policy might reveal that the emergency room (ER) and crisis clinic have been complaining for a while that clients are overusing their services and yesterday there was a big problem case where a client came to the ER three times in a week but no outpatient clinician had seen the client during that time. Thus, the administrator generated the solution of next-day appointments. The DBT team is, of course, concerned that crisis behaviors may be reinforced with extra appointments or that, since they are part-time or work on scheduled appointments, fitting in next-day appointments is impractical.

After thoroughly understanding the problem the administrator is seeking to solve, *look for and propose DBT-compatible solutions and/or a synthesis.* In this example, a DBT solution might be that the client would have a scheduled phone contact with their therapist instead of a visit following an ER admission, and the DBT therapist would explicitly chart that overuse of crisis services was a targeted behavior. The therapist might also describe the reasons why it was not useful for the therapist to see the client immediately after use of crisis services both in the chart and at an inservice or staff meeting of that ER. It is typically the role of the DBT team leader to then work with the administrator on the team's concerns and possible solutions.

Apply DBT Principles and Strategies to Administrators and Other Colleagues

The example above illustrates another important ingredient: Whenever possible, apply the principles and strategies of DBT when working to address problems within the system. This strategy is particularly important in the interpersonal realm—when making requests of administrators, referring agencies, insurers, and employees. This strategy is critical because DBT often requires organizations to make exceptions to standard mental health protocols (as seen in the example above). Effective use of DBT skills can be extremely beneficial. Consider the mindfulness skill of effectiveness (i.e., doing what's needed in a situation), as well as DBT interpersonal effectiveness skills. For example, use the Factors to Consider in determining whether it is a good time to make a request/say no to a request/present an alternative solution; apply DEAR MAN GIVE FAST skills to how the request is made, and so on. Always remember to keep reciprocity on your side by jumping in to do what is needed quickly and volunteering help when appropriate. It can be useful to think of doing four times as many things as you request, as this is considered a good ratio of positive reinforcement to aversives (e.g., demands, criticism). Use the DBT consultation team to practice, provide feedback, coach, and reinforce team members in the process of interacting with administration, other clinicians, and so on.

Networking and Building Goodwill

DBT programs that succeed over time prioritize building and sustaining strong relationships with DBT stakeholders (e.g., advocates, social service agencies, insurers, legal aid, administrators, and other colleagues) and generating goodwill toward and positive attitudes about the DBT program. Possibly the most effective and enduring way to do this is by helping the clinic (administrators and clinicians alike) effectively treat its most challenging, difficult clients. Providing consultation and training to other staff within the agency can also be helpful and often results in interested participants asking things like, "Will you come and talk to my staff?" or "Why isn't this more available?" or "Can I refer this client to you?" Some DBT programs offer "office hours" or monthly lunch meetings to discuss difficult non-DBT cases. Part training and part peer-to-peer consultation, these brown bags provide an invaluable opportunity for non-DBT colleagues to get assistance with difficult cases by applying the tools of DBT.

Keeping It Going

As the DBT team and program mature over time, old struggles and concerns soon fade and new ones emerge. These include attending to staff motivation, structuring ongoing training, preventing burnout, and dealing with staff leaving. This section is devoted to sharing successful strategies that help to sustain your DBT program.

The Changing Team

One of the stresses for the team is that its membership changes over time. Occasionally, there is someone whose departure is welcome, but this is rare among groups of clinicians who have developed their team together. In addition to the team's experience of grief and loss, there is often pressure to recruit and hire new staff, or to absorb clients into already full caseloads. This focus on filling the position can interfere with processing the loss of a valued team member, which can subsequently interfere with fully welcoming the new member.

Adding new members to a consultation team is a moment for dialectical thinking if there ever was one. On the one hand, it is important to socialize the new person to the dynamics of the existing team. On the other hand, trying to keep the "old team" with new members is probably impossible. Thus, the dialectical skill of allowing natural change comes to the fore. Watch for the moment when orienting begins to feel more like controlling and realize that the time has arrived to elicit and accord respect to the input of new members. During such transitions, it can help to acknowledge the new dynamics by discussing the team goals for the clinic or to engage in mindfulness exercises focusing on appreciation of all members' strengths.

A different approach may be required when trainees regularly rotate in and out of the team. Trainees are generally present to learn DBT. This is fortunate because it obviates the necessity of shaping the team too much toward them. In fact, changing to accommodate trainees can "lower the bar" of adherence and competency of the team which is not desirable for anyone. Instead, it can be very useful to inoculate trainees against outsider feelings by emphasizing that their primary job is to learn DBT thoroughly by participating in a well-functioning team. Individual supervision of the trainee can be a place for further discussion of the trainee's observations and questions about the treatment. It is important to note that only those trainees who actually treat patients on the DBT team should attend the consultation team (all trainees can attend didactic/training sessions). Trainees should be assigned to a mode that they can be expected to complete during their rotation (e.g., serving as a coleader for 6 months of DBT skills or picking up an individual client should they be able to make a long enough commitment to the DBT team).

Enhancing Therapist Capabilities through the Consultation Team

The most challenging problem for many successful DBT teams is the large size of the team and the considerable number of clients it serves. For such a DBT team, too many therapists means that some will seldom receive case consultation and few will receive in-depth consultation on cases. There are several ways to manage this situation. One method is to start the meeting with a "team review" of life-threatening behaviors; therapy-interfering behaviors including important issues such as staff burnout and client at risk of missing four sessions in a row before the next meeting; and positives or good news since the last meeting. When done mindfully, this can be accomplished quickly and with the addition of business items can be the basis of the meeting's agenda. Then in-depth time can be spent on a few (e.g., maximum of two or three) therapists. Another strategy is to use internal e-mail or voicemail systems to give updates on group attendance, group homework, therapists' out-of-town dates (to arrange clinical coverage), as well as other announcements that do not require discussion.

While effective in some circumstances, these strategies may not be effective in situations where there are a number of highly lethal, suicidal clients new to the DBT team. When this is the case, it may be necessary to divide the consultation team into multiple teams, either temporarily or permanently. Some teams have developed a model, for example, of a monthly lottery to one of two teams (Team A or Team B) that meet at the same time. Each month, each member has an equal (but random) chance of ending up on Team A as on Team B (members pull their assignment from a hat). This method allows for the members to split into two smaller teams, but preserves the cohesiveness of the larger group.

Another way to improve consultation is to review videotapes or audiotapes of therapy sessions. When clinicians play a tape that demonstrates the problem they need help with, assessment can begin with a minimum of narration. The target for consultation is shown rather than described and other problems, such as secondary targets, often become clear during the session review. Viewing session tapes during team meetings is one of the most effective ways to improve DBT adherence in individual therapy. Clients must consent to being videotaped and therapists usually have to overcome some anxieties about their perceived competence. As long as the team does not punish showing tape, therapist anxiety will diminish over time.

Continuing Training in DBT

One question that often arises is how to meet the different training needs of experienced and beginning clinicians—especially if they are working on the same team. Beginning clinicians often have a steep learning curve and can benefit from studying the treatment manual, conducting individual or group DBT, and experiencing the modeling provided by colleagues in the clinic. However, more focused training can speed the process along. One intervention many clinics have found useful is running a skills training group for clinicians. This has been done as a teaching format per se, but has also been conducted as stress management under the auspices of human resources or employee assistance programs. When conducting such a group, all participants choose behavioral goals they would like to achieve but have not been able to previously (e.g., reducing lateness, on-time paperwork, more effective observation of personal limits, reduced irritability with clients, regular exercise.) The DBT skills are taught to assist the clinicians to accomplish these goals. Progress is tracked weekly on a clinician diary card. Such a group accomplishes many things simultaneously: defining problems behaviorally, teaching DBT skills, understanding the difficulty of completing diary cards consistently, experience with the effectiveness of self-monitoring, empathy for the difficulty of changing long-standing behaviors, and practice blocking avoidance strategies that arise in the face of the task.

Another efficient strategy is to have newer therapists act as cotherapists in DBT skills training groups. This is excellent training and also serves to fill clinic staffing needs. However, there are a number of common pitfalls. The most frequent problem is that the trainee falls into the student role and stops acting as cotherapist. This often occurs because the trainee is fascinated by the skills, which are very helpful in his or her own stressful life, and acts like a client learning rather than like a therapist teaching. Alternatively, the trainee has not sufficiently studied the material ahead of time to play an active role as coleader. It can also occur when the primary therapist is less confident of his or her trainee and does not allow the trainee to function as a cotherapist. Other approaches include having the trainee observe the DBT skills teaching class, participate in individual or small-group supervision, and teach a DBT skill to the supervisor each week (or prior to the DBT skills training group, if they are coleading).

For the more senior staff, training may occur in a separated, dedicated meeting or retreat focused on a particular topic area of interest, or may include one-on-one (as-needed) peer supervision. For those in private practice, such supervision is not only not reimbursed time, but may represent a loss of income for hours devoted to supervision. Thus, the supervision needs to be sufficiently reinforcing. In agencies, provision of training can be used as an incentive or reinforcement for past hard work. If outside training is not possible, it may be critical to keep the consultation team meeting to the level of the more experienced staff and limit trainee participation unless there is available supervision to get trainees quickly to advanced levels. That decision is best related to the mission of the team (e.g., training vs. standard program) and whether the majority of team members are new or experienced. A summary of training activities that experienced teams have found particularly effective is presented in Table 3.5.

Enhancing Therapist Motivation and Preventing Burnout

One way to enhance therapist motivation is to prevent burnout—the main reason (other than more money) that clinicians leave a team or have a slump in their work. Part of burnout is being emotionally overextended and exhausted by one's work. This is often best addressed by matching DBT tasks to therapist preferences. For instance, a list of all team tasks (individual therapy, skills training, crisis coaching, teaching, providing supervision, being supervised, providing case management, providing medication management) can be ranked on a scale from 1 (e.g., "I hate this and couldn't take it for long") to 5 (e.g., "The opportunity to do this is critical to my job satisfaction"). While it is never possible to completely match therapist preferences to tasks, new information is often uncovered that was not apparent in therapist behaviors. Better matching of tasks means more reinforcement for therapists and less burnout.

Even favored tasks can burn out a DBT therapist when therapists (1) do the same thing day in and day out, (2) do a lot of tasks that are not compensated, (3) don't see clients progress, (4) work with the highest risk clients or those who are angry or critical, and (5) work with clients who overuse phone consultation. These burnout factors need to be balanced by positive factors in the DBT team such as being your own boss, ability to see non-DBT or non-BPD cases if this is reinforcing, support from team members, fun

TABLE 3.5. Training Exercises for Enhancing DBT Therapist Capability

Strategy	Potential problems	Troubleshooting strategies
Review audiotapes or videotapes of sessions	• Buying equipment • Access to equipment • Time to review tapes • Time to give feedback • Clients' reluctance to be taped • HIPAA concerns	• Cameras now inexpensive • If the review and feedback is consistent and reinforcing, therapist works hard to tape • Assure reinforcement for tape watching (which is not favorite activity) or put on set schedule to prevent avoidance • Do behavioral and solution analysis for not taping or watching • Make feedback written • Shape frequency of taping and watching • Start with tapes therapist thinks are terrible so not defensive • Reinforcing ratio is 4 positive to 1 negative feedback • Orient clients that taping is just like phone company "recording call to assure service quality" • Tapes have been treated by HIPAA officers as "process notes" following those rules
Rate sessions for DBT adherence	• Not trained in DBT adherence scale • No ability to tape sessions	• Photocopy tables from Linehan text into handout that is good proxy for adherence • If can't videotape, audiotape • If can't tape at all, self-rate immediately after session.
Use DBT strategies to help clinicians solve their problems of doing therapy	• Therapists resist therapy strategies used on them • Worry about too much team time and not enough time to review clients	• Do orientation and commitment to this approach in team before starting • Remember team meeting for enhancing therapist skills and motivation not talking about clients
Use DBT skills on each other: teach skills, try new skills, validate, use chain analysis	See above	See above
Give a didactic presentation of a journal article or summarize a teaching seminar	• Time to prepare	• Make funds for outside training of team member contingent on teaching the team about what they learned afterward • Use articles team members already found and liked anyway instead of making new task • Don't have everyone read ahead
Engage in role plays or behavioral rehearsal instead of "talking through" your suggestions and recommendations	• Avoidance of role playing	• Schedule someone each week to prepare to role-play • Commit to one role play per team meeting so someone has to do it • Have frustrated therapist be his/her difficult client and someone else role-play (reinforcing to see someone else struggle and helps generate phenomenological empathy for client)

(continued)

TABLE 3.5. (continued)

Strategy	Potential problems	Troubleshooting strategies
Case presenters do their homework: describe behavior, identify questions for consultation, have recent chain analysis and a videotape ready to share	• Time to prepare • Team gets mindless and forgets to stick to plan	• Everyone takes responsibility not to give suggestions until asked what therapist wants help with • Make very simple set of prep questions (e.g. client's overarching goal, target you are working on, help that you want) that becomes habit • Put plan on "table tents" as reminder • Schedule previous week for someone to bring tape (so no diffusion of responsibility)
Practice irreverent or reciprocal communication styles during team discussions	• Forgetting • Lack of awareness of whether doing it	• Make one meeting a month "irreverence day" and everyone try and say one irreverent thing at that meeting • Ring bell when someone does "strategy of day"

(parties, evening events), and celebrating successful interventions and not just successful cases.

Another problem of burnout is the therapist feels or acts with increasing emotional distance to clients or team members. If this happens, a lot of validation from team members for the difficulty of the task is needed as well as observation of whether the therapist is moving outside his or her limits. Skills to maintain limits and metaphors or other dialectical strategies to help find balance in the stress are needed. The team needs to assure that the therapist has the skills needed for clients to improve and to help the therapist to target hopeless and helpless thoughts. The key is often finding ways for therapist to evaluate the effectiveness of his or her interventions apart from positive reinforcement from the client or client improvement; this could be checking DBT adherence, highlighting extinction bursts as indicators of success, and team reinforcement for desired therapist behaviors. Reminders and lots of attention on the occasional stellar success experiences do not hurt either.

Burnout can also be reduced by sharing the treatment tasks for very difficult clients. For instance, family members, social service providers, insurers, or apartment managers may be desperate for the client's behavior to change and make demanding phone calls to the therapist. Meanwhile, the client him- or herself is already very demanding of the therapist's time and energy. It can be helpful in these cases to ensure that the therapist can defer complaints and demands from individuals other than the client to a clinic director, supervisor, or another clinician. This deflection helps prevent the therapist from being punished by the client *and* everyone else for slow treatment progress. It also helps to maintain the treatment alliance between the primary therapist and the client. Occasionally, a therapist needs a break after a run of high-risk suicide calls or serious occasions of crossing of the therapist's limits; at the same time, the client may continue to need an active coach closely involved. A couple of coaching sessions with another clinician or a week of another clinician taking phone calls often helps to return the primary therapist's interest in and commitment to the client.

Lack of personal accomplishment or lack of feelings of competence and successful achievement in one's work can also lead to burnout. The previous strategies apply here too, but more importantly, the therapist needs to be using the skills for which he or she was trained and finding opportunities to stretch further. This can often be accomplished by taking on a client with difficulties that match the area in which the therapist wants to learn or by choosing a specific focus for peer supervision. Targeting therapist therapy-interfering behavior in a routine way during team meetings puts therapists' learning goals on the table and provides opportunities for help, contingencies to try harder, and reinforcement for success. Another intervention is to regularly present data collected on individual client progress or teamwide summaries at consultation team meetings to remind clinicians of successes and to identify areas that need improvement.

Another strategy to prevent burnout is to make burnout an explicit part of the regular consultation team agenda (i.e., have each team member rate burnout at beginning of meeting from 0–10). This serves two purposes. First, it provides a cue for therapists to consider their burnout level, and thus identifies burnout much earlier than if the team waited for the therapist to initiate. Second, it normalizes burnout as an expected result of working with challenging clients. This allows the therapist to be less defensive and actively work to reduce burnout and the team to help without anxiety that the person is about to quit. However, burnout is a challenging therapist problem to treat as it makes one very sensitive to invalidation. A team trying to intervene quickly without sufficient assessment of the problem, validation, and time to discuss it can make the situation worse rather than better. Substantial team time may be required to assist the individual to address the problem and it may take several weeks to resolve so the team and individual need both patience and persistence.

Adhering to the team consultation agreements provides an atmosphere of respect and warmth that is essential to mastering DBT and targeting burnout. A strong team reduces therapist burnout by providing support, encouragement, humor, and community for the therapists. A team becomes most effective when all members are consistently dialectical, radically genuine, ready to address problems, willing to make repairs, and mindful of the overarching goals. If the team drifts off course, spending team time on strategies to improve the team pays off like spending time on client therapy-interfering behavior does—that is, taking time to fix the "tool" of therapy instead of continuing with a broken tool is often a lot faster way to get to a goal.

Legal and Ethical Issues

Good risk management is an essential part of any mental health practice. For DBT teams, liability issues related to suicidal clients are usually the most salient. The most common bases for malpractice lawsuits related to client suicidal behavior are wrongful involuntary commitment, wrongful release, and failure to take precautions against suicide (Roswell, 1988). As long as DBT is the most evidence-based, efficacious treatment for BPD, the best risk management strategy to reduce legal and ethical exposure is simply to follow the DBT treatment manual (Linehan,1993a), doing DBT by the book and documenting that you have done so and how you have done so. While DBT may fail to prevent death for some cases, it is far more effective than most alternative approaches and is substantiated by rigorous (and now numerous) research trials.

Awareness of suicide risk is likely to be high among DBT therapists. Appropriate protocols are well documented in Linehan (1993a). However, periodic training (e.g., a "suicide summit") on suicide and risk management is important to continue to be considered an expert in the area. New material can be divided between consult team members and then taught to each other to minimize nonbillable time. Most clinicians are well aware of the importance of documentation and consultation with qualified professionals in risk management. The remainder of this section is devoted to specifics with respect to documentation and consultation in DBT.

DBT Suicide Crisis Plans

DBT suicide crisis plans are an efficient means of documentation as well as communication. Important items for a DBT crisis plan include the client's physical address and all phone numbers, names and phone numbers of friends and family, DSM diagnoses, date of birth, medications, body weight in pounds and kilograms, a description of the client's car and its license plate number, as well as a few "best" skills or important phrases that can be applied by a backup therapist who may not be as familiar with the patient as his or her primary treatment provider. It can include a brief description of client's behavior both at baseline and in crisis, as well as effective skills or strategies to use in a crisis situation. If this crisis plan is available at all times to the therapist and anyone providing clinical backup, it maximizes as well as organizes treatment. In addition, referral to a crisis plan in a chart note prevents cumbersome repetition of documentation (e.g., "Continuing to follow DBT suicide protocol as described in crisis plan of xx/xx/xx"). Crisis plans are strongest if they are developed with the client. Fully orienting the client to the therapist's legal and ethical obligation to take action and to breach confidentiality in the event of an impending suicide crisis will increase the likelihood that the client will effectively collaborate on the plan and stick with it during a crisis. Whenever possible, the therapist, the client, and relevant family members can meet together to discuss what *each* can do in the event of a suicide crisis. These discussions are then incorporated into the plan, further decreasing the chance that it will be ignored during a crisis or challenged later.

Peer Consultation

Individuals who consult together on psychotherapy cases share, to some extent, liability for those cases. Team members should be fully insured, not only for their own private practice, but also for the work they do in collaboration with others, including attending team and coleading groups. To document consultation, a chart note can be written for each client discussed in the team meeting including the proposed treatment plan or strategies and who attended team that day. A copy can then be placed in the client's chart, strengthening the position of the individual therapist by adding the weight of the team's opinion. The fact that a member is consulting weekly with a group of other professionals on a difficult case will almost always be an advantage in the case of a lawsuit.

For those working in a larger agency, review of suicide risk management with the larger agency is imperative in preventing last-minute overruling of crisis plans, warmer and clearer support after a suicide or serious attempt, and better handling of complaints from clients or family regarding management of suicide crisis. (Private practice teams might also want to have these discussions among themselves.) These discussions are best handled before a crisis occurs. The following topics can be helpful to discuss: when to hospitalize a client, when to call 911, what to do if client injures him- or herself in the facility, what if a client is violent or threatening, what consultation is needed in high-risk situations, what counts as a high-risk situation, how documentation will be done in high-risk situations, how consultation will be documented, and the appropriate procedure for grievances by staff, clients, family, or outside agencies. While the interaction needs to include enough discussion so that everyone is comfortable with the plan, bringing in a first draft of a DBT protocol for each of these topics to start from saves time and prevents administrators from suggesting plans that they then have to be talked out of.

In spite of all of these efforts, with such a high-risk population, it is nearly inevitable that your DBT team will lose a patient to suicide at some point in your careers. "Postvention" is a word coined by suicidologists for the needed processing or debriefing after a suicide. There are several postvention options, as well as monographs for family and friends effectively surviving a suicide available through suicide prevention websites (e.g., *www.suicidology.org*, *www.afsp.org*, and *www.sprc.org*). It is the role of the team to support the therapist and to help him or her to effectively interact with other clients, family, and friends affected by the suicide in the most effective ways. Based on clinical experience, it is strongly recommended that the individual therapists speak to their respective clients separately *before* group leaders discuss the suicide in the DBT skills group. It is hard to predict how group members will respond. If members come late, it can result in retelling about the suicide and processing too much at first. It is also important to check on HIPAA standards in your agency regarding telling other clients about the deceased. As with risk management (discussed above), it can help to discuss ahead of time how the team wants to handle managing and communicating about a suicide should it occur.

Helping Clients Transition Out of the System

One of the biggest challenges faced by individuals with BPD is radically discarding the identity of a "mental patient" and moving out of the mental health treatment system and fully into an "ordinary" existence (e.g., facing ordinary problems of living). This may be particularly challenging for those individuals with extensive histories of severe behavioral dyscontrol, mental health treatment, numerous inpatient psychiatric admissions, and years on psychiatric disability public assistance. When constructing a blueprint for your DBT program, it is important to give consideration to how (programmatically) to assist your patients with BPD move "out" of the mental health care system and into a life that is not defined or limited by a previous history of BPD. This section offers several models for helping patients transition out of the system. The first two are intended for Level 1 patients with BPD following the initial Stage 1 course of DBT. The third was designed specifically for Level 3 individuals and builds on skills and strategies learned years earlier while in the first year(s) of DBT. All three models are in the initial phases of evaluation and, as a result, lack data from rigorous randomized controlled trials. However, all three are built on the basic tenets of DBT; preliminary pre-/postdata from all three are very encouraging.

DBT Accepting the Challenges of Exiting the System

Developed by Comtois and her colleagues (Comtois et al., 2006), in close collaboration with Marsha M. Linehan, DBT Accepting the Challenges of Exiting the System (DBT-ACES) is an innovative 2-year DBT program focused on systematically building a life worth living outside the public mental health system. DBT-ACES focuses on skills training and self-sufficiency, gradually adding such skills as goal setting, problem solving, trouble shooting, dialectics, and reinforcement. Furthermore, the program includes contingencies for working or attending college to compete with the multitude of systemic contingencies, including psychiatric disability, that function to reinforce dysfunctional behavior (Comtois et al., 2006). Specifically, receipt of a second year of DBT is contingent on successful completion of the first year and willingness to get a job and/or go to school in the second year. These programmatic contingencies focus and reinforce the therapist and client to "cross the divide between *wanting to work* and *working*" (Comtois et al., 2006, emphasis added). Preliminary pre–post and anecdotal data indicates that DBT-

ACES is a promising new approach to aiding patients with BPD transition out of the system into jobs and school.

Structure Used in DBT-ACES

The structure of the initial year is identical to standard outpatient DBT. Clients are encouraged to get active during the initial year—"doing something that is *normative* (i.e., you act as if you don't have emotional problems around people who act as if they don't have emotional problems) and *productive* (i.e., structured, active, goal-oriented and rewarding) outside the mental health system" (Comtois, Elwood, Holdcraft, Simpson, & Smith, in press). Programmatic goals are specified for number of structured hours per week (which can include volunteer and paid work but also going to a gym, socializing, or other activities that weren't already in the client's repertoire). Hours increase incrementally throughout the course of the year (see Figure 3.1). By the year's end, clients are expected to engage in 20 hours of structured activities per week.

The admissions process for the second and final year of DBT begins approximately 4 months before graduating from the initial year (approximately the eighth month of treatment). Those wishing to pursue a second, advanced year of DBT must meet the following criteria: (1) relative stability (e.g., no recent suicidal and/or other dangerous behavior, attends and complies with treatment, continues progress on normative, productive goals), (2) an extensive application that details how DBT-ACES will help him or her achieve living wage employment, (3) 75% or better score on a DBT skills test as a demonstration of his or her knowledge and fluency in DBT skills, and (4) willingness to obtain paid work and/or matriculate at a college, university, or vocational school during the second year (Comtois et al., in press). Those who wish to continue but are not immediately accepted for the advanced year are informed of the explicit criteria required for entry into the advanced DBT program and are encouraged to apply whenever they meet those criteria. All clients who complete the standard first year of DBT graduate whether they continue to advanced DBT or not.

Primary targets for the second year are the same as for standard DBT. Additional behaviors are subsumed under quality-of-life-interfering behaviors in DBT-ACES. These targets include (1) attaining normative/productive active requirements leading to living wage employment, (2) self-sufficiency, and (3) the development of a normative social network outside community mental health (Comtois et al., 2006). Clients continue to attend weekly DBT individual psychotherapy and one advanced skills training group per week that emphasizes problem solving, decreasing depression, anxiety, and other mental health issues that disrupt quality, as well as issues pertaining to leaving the mental health system. As-needed phone consultation is provided, as is the consultation team for DBT clinicians. It is expected that clients will have secured competitive employment (no less than 10 hours per week) or will have matriculated in a school program no later than the 16th month of treatment (see Figure 3.1). Clients who do not meet the incrementally advancing hours for structured activities and work are placed on a vacation from therapy until the program criteria are met. By the conclusion of treatment, clients are expected to be engaged in competitive employment or to be enrolled in school no less than 20 hours per week for 4 months.

Findings from DBT-ACES and Analysis

Results (*n* = 21) from the initial pre–post evaluation (*n* = 21) by Comtois and colleagues (2006) are promising. The combined program (standard DBT during Year 1 and DBT-

Treatment Month	# Hours Normative and Productive Structured Activity	# Hours Working/Attending School
0 to 4 months	• Start getting active	
4 to 8 months	• Stay active 10 hours week	
8 to 12 months	• Stay active 15 hours/week	
12 to 16 months	• Stay active 20 hours/week (paid work and school included)	• Start/prepare for 10 hours paid work or matriculation
16 to 20 months	• Stay active 20 hours/week (paid work and school included)	• Engage in paid work or school 10 hours per week and work up to paid work or matriculated school 20 hours/week
20 to 24 months	• Stick with paid work or matriculated school 20 hours/week for all 4 months	

FIGURE 3.1. DBT-ACES schedule for structured activity and work/school.

ACES in Year 2) among a sample of psychiatrically disabled, severely disordered, chronic BPD clients in a routine community mental health setting was associated with increased productivity, employment, and quality of life, as well as standard outcomes that parallel outcomes from randomized controlled trials of standard DBT: reduced suicide attempts, inpatient admissions, ER services, and treatment retention (Comtois et al., 2006). At the end of the second year, over 80% of the clients were in paid employment or matriculated at a college, university, or vocational school. Median hours worked weekly (for those employed) was 25 and increased during the 12-month follow-up period. By the end of the follow-up period, only 40% of the original sample was still receiving public mental health services. While further research is critical to determine that DBT-ACES is more effective than an active control group, this data demonstrates that such outcomes are feasible, which many clinicians do not realize.

DBT Adapted for Vocational Rehabilitation with Very Significantly Disabled Patients with Personality Disorders

Koons and her colleagues (2006) developed an adaptation of standard outpatient DBT for high-utilizing, psychiatrically disabled individuals who had used, on average, over $10,000 in department of vocational rehabilitation services without ever attaining 90 days of continuous employment. Like DBT-ACES, the goal of treatment was to successfully help clients transition off of psychiatric disability and into the workforce. Actively suicidal clients and those who had been hospitalized in the previous 6 months were excluded from participating in the clinical trial.

Comprehensive DBT was provided for 6 months in a group format. Two groups were provided weekly: a 2-hour standard DBT skills training class (covering all skills and thus allowing for only one full cycle of skills training) and a 90-minute skills generalization group, consisting of review of the diary card, chain analysis, and behavioral rehearsal. Specific behavioral targets for obtaining and sustaining employment were tracked on a weekly basis. Behaviors analyzed using the chain analysis procedure in group included those most noted to interfere with getting or keeping a job: substance use, nonattendance to DBT and non-DBT therapy appointments, isolating, ruminating, interpersonal conflicts, and neglect of physical health needs. In addition to DBT, all clients had a number of non-DBT ancillary treatment providers, including a non-DBT individual therapist, DVR counselors, psychiatrists, and job coaches (Koons et al., 2006). Ancillary treatment providers received a half-day of training on DBT and were invited to attend the DBT consultation team once monthly to discuss client progress.

Results from a small ($n = 12$) pre–post trial of this adaptation are encouraging. Eight individuals (66%) completed the treatment (Koons et al., 2006). Treatment completers made significant improvements across a number of mental health outcomes, including depression, hopelessness, and experience of anger at posttest and at the 6-month follow-up compared to baseline. Perhaps most notably, treatment completers had a significant increase in total number of hours worked weekly at the 6-month follow-up.

DBT Mindful Living Process Group

Developed by Betts, Koons, and their colleagues in 2004, this DBT group was constructed as a Stage 3 treatment for graduates of DBT programs (see Koerner & Dimeff, Chapter 1, this volume for a definition of levels and stages of treatment; C. Koons, personal communication, January 5, 2007). The group was initially designed and developed for DBT graduates with ongoing interpersonal skills deficits and a high degree of interpersonal sensitivity. While structured in a fashion to address problems of living, mindfulness-based acceptance strategies are strongly emphasized; furthermore, members are encouraged to practice "in the moment" mindfulness as they listen to and interact with other group members.

Group Structure

The group meets for 2 hours and is cotaught by two DBT group coleaders. The first half is evenly divided between mindfulness practice and didactic presentation. Mindfulness typically includes a 10–20-minute practice followed by a brief debriefing of the practice by group members. The didactic portion (approximately 30 minutes) is taught by one of the two DBT group leaders on a topic of relevance to group members (e.g., operant conditioning, stimulus control, dialectics, validation, radical acceptance and mindfulness, behavioral analysis, and other problem-solving-based strategies). The emphasis of the second hour shifts to process-based discussion of members' problems in living. Members share the time to discuss specific goals they are working toward and steps taken to achieve these goals; time can also be used to discuss specific problems members have encountered or anticipate encountering in the weeks to come as a means of receiving helpful feedback and tips from the group. The group concludes with a mindfulness-based wind-down practice.

Group Process

As members discuss problems in living during the second hour of group, emphasis is placed on practicing mindfulness and interpersonal effectiveness skills when receiving feedback from others and when providing feedback to others. For example, is the member judgmental, overly tentative, or not behaviorally specific in the feedback provided? Do change-based suggestions include sufficient validation? Using the group as a fertile ground for *in vivo* practice (often avoided in Stage 1 groups), members receive coaching and feedback from the leaders and group members in how they make and receive comments in the moment (e.g., "The essence of what you're saying to Joey is great—it makes sense and you're being very clear about what Joey needs to do to change. The problem is that your tone of voice sounds pretty judgmental which makes it difficult to actually *hear* what you are saying"; "Sarah, I'm not sure you're aware of it, but you are looking really angry as Chiza is providing you feedback. What about practicing half-smile and maybe opposite action? Maybe uncross your arms, sit back in your chain, take a few calming breaths, and half smile?").

Group Member Inclusion Criteria and Group Length

Participation is voluntary, based on readiness for a Stage 3 treatment (i.e., no suicidal and nonsuicidal self-injurious or other severely disordered behaviors for at least 4 months before applying to group; graduated from Stage 1 DBT program; completed Stage 2 exposure treatment, as indicated) and a recommendation from the individual's DBT primary therapist.

This open-enrollment group does not specify a specific length of treatment for a member's participation in it. Because the group is viewed as a means of helping patients transition into ordinary lives, the expectation (conveyed at every turn throughout the group) is that members will leave the group after achieving the group goals: improved interpersonal skills and diminished interpersonal sensitivity. The average length for the group is approximately 11 months.

Conclusions

Creating a comprehensive outpatient DBT program is a considerable challenge, particularly at the beginning stages of implementation. DBT often requires a radical paradigm shift for the many stakeholders involved, from agency administrators to frontline clinicians, clients, and their family members alike. The requirements are more than philosophical: implementation of a comprehensive DBT program, done in a way that preserves fidelity to the treatment, frequently requires revising clinic policies and procedures to ensure that they are consistent with DBT for those served by DBT. Furthermore, because of their risk for suicide, the severity of behavioral dyscontrol across many behavioral domains (including interpersonal), and their multitude of other Axis I and often Axis II problems, clients with BPD are among the hardest and most stressful to treat. As a direct result of this fact, DBT is a complex and, for many, difficult-to-learn and difficulty-to-apply treatment. Indeed, DBT is a comprehensive, multimodal and multifaceted treatment; clinical mastery of the treatment requires that the clinician know DBT inside and out, as well as numerous other evidence-based treatment manuals for the client's other Axis I problems.

Given the personal stresses and strains in treating clients with BPD, some are tempted to ask, "Why do it?" When translated, this often means, "Why work with clients with BPD when there are so many other clients who are so much easier and simpler?" or "Why *do* DBT all the way?" After having learned DBT and built our DBT programs, it is now easy to say, "We wouldn't have it any other way." The benefits and rewards, despite the struggles we faced particularly early on, are plentiful, both professionally and personally (i.e., the skills we teach our clients "cross over" into our own lives and relationships). Many discover that the behavioral skills and strategies in DBT are useful with other clients. For others, answering the "why do it" has all to do with the deep satisfaction and fulfillment they experience in helping someone move from a miserable life to a full and rich life worth living. For still others, DBT has provided their agency a specialty in the community that has served all stakeholders (from clients to top administrators) well.

Our intent in writing this chapter was to provide the reader with the benefits of foresight *and* hindsight by instilling here all we have learned over the years in developing our own DBT programs and consulting to many others. We attempted to address all the commonly asked questions as well as the common barriers in implementing DBT across a range of diverse outpatient settings, from private practice to public-sector community mental health agencies. We focused on topics sequentially, beginning with those required during the early stages of implementation of an outpatient program (e.g., therapist selection, caseload size) to issues that typically arise later. We conclude by describing several DBT models aimed at incrementally moving psychiatrically disabled patients to paid employment with living wages and/or enrolled in college, university, or vocational programs, and ultimately to a life that is lived congruently with their greatest values, goals, and aspirations.

REFERENCES

American Psychiatric Association. (1998). Integrating dialectical behavior therapy into a community mental health program: The Mental Health Center of Greater Manchester, New Hampshire. *Psychiatric Services, 49,* 1338–1340.

Barlow, D. H., & Craske, M. G. (2006). *Mastery of your anxiety and panic: Therapist guide* (4th ed.). New York: Oxford University Press.

Comtois, K. A., Elwood, L. M., Holdcraft, L. C., Simpson, T. L., & Smith, T. R. (in press). Effectiveness of dialectical behavior therapy in a community mental health center. *Cognitive and Behavioral Practice.*

Comtois, K. A., Huus, K., Hoiness, M., Marsden, J., Mullen, C., Elwood, L., et al. (2006). *Dialectical behavior therapy: Accepting the Challenges of Exiting the System (ACES) manual.* Unpublished manuscript.

Koons, C. R., Chapman, A. L., Betts, B. B., O'Rourke, B., Morse, N., & Robins, C. J. (2006). Dialectical behavior therapy adapted for the vocational rehabilitation of significantly disabled mentally ill adults. *Cognitive and Behavioral Practice, 13*(2), 146–156.

Krawitz, R., Jackson, W., Allen, R., Connell, A., Argyle, N., Bensemann, C., et al. (2004). Professionally indicated short-term risk-taking in the treatment of borderline personality disorder. *Australasian Psychiatry, 12*(1), 11–17.

Kuhn, T. (1962). *The structure of scientific revolutions.* Chicago: University of Chicago Press.

Lieb, K., Zanarini, M. C., Schmahl, C., Linehan, M. M., & Bohus, M. (2004). Borderline personality disorder. *Lancet, 364,* 453–461.

Linehan, M. M. (1993a). *Cognitive behavioral treatment of borderline personality disorder.* New York: Guilford Press.

Linehan, M. M. (1993b). *Skills training manual for borderline personality disorder.* New York: Guilford Press.

Paris, J. (2005). Understanding self-mutilation in borderline personality disorder. *Harvard Review of Psychiatry, 13*(3), 179–185.

Roswell, V. A. (1988). Professional liability: Issues for behavior therapists in the 1980s and 1990s. *The Behavior Therapist, 11*(8), 163–171.

CHAPTER 4

Dialectical Behavior Therapy on Inpatient Units

Charles R. Swenson, Suzanne Witterholt, *and* Martin Bohus

Introduction and Rationale for Inpatient Dialectical Behavior Therapy

Dialectical behavior therapy (DBT) was developed as an outpatient cognitive-behavioral treatment approach for individuals with borderline personality disorder (BPD). Eight randomized controlled research trials and many more quasi-experimental studies of DBT converge on similar outcomes: reduction in self-harming behaviors, improvement in treatment retention, and reduction in hospitalization (Dimeff, Monroe-DeVita, & Paves, 2006; Robins & Chapman, 2004). The standard DBT team helps DBT clients to build community-based lives that feel worthwhile and fulfilling, in the process eliminating the raison d'être for suicidal and other dysfunctional behaviors in their repertoires. Because of the considerable potential of inpatient hospitalization to inadvertently reinforce suicidal and other severely dysfunctional behavior, in combination with an evidence base demonstrating that hospitalization for patients with BPD is not efficacious, the DBT team is biased against hospitalizing their clients for suicidal episodes unless absolutely necessary.

While DBT was developed for *outpatient* treatment, many *inpatient* programs have used it to address individuals with BPD. Constraints have become apparent. First, even though skills can be acquired and problems solved during inpatient admissions, it is far less obvious or likely that these skills and solutions will effectively generalize to where they are needed in outpatient life. Second, if hospitalization becomes a strategy of choice for coping with distress, it can stand in the way of exercising and strengthening other more adaptive strategies for surviving crises and building a life. Sometimes "saving" the client's life in the moment actually weakens his or her capacity to endure in the long run. Third, admission can interrupt outpatient treatment relationships and other supports that might actually be strengthened if brought to bear on that crisis. Fourth, inpatient units often bring the patient into contact with an overload of stressors that have nothing to do with his or her care, and with multiple examples of dysfunctional coping behaviors that can be "contagious." Fifth, because a crisis admission can bring immediate relief to a client, a therapist, a team, or a family, it can actually reinforce the very behavioral patterns that prompted the admission. The impression that an individual's hospitalization has prevented his or her suicide can paradoxically increase the likelihood of his or her future suicidal behaviors that prompt hospitalization. For certain individuals, suicidal behavior and hospitalization can become a way of life that is difficult to change.

On the other hand, a well-timed hospital treatment can (1) save a life, (2) interrupt a spiraling crisis, (3) remotivate a beleaguered patient, (4) provide a breather and time for consultation for a weary outpatient clinician or team, (5) bring a new perspective to diagnosis and treatment, (6) allow for a difficult family intervention, or (7) make a medication trial possible. A DBT inpatient program can allow for:

1. A clear and compassionate orientation for the client regarding his or her disorder.
2. An unusually detailed behavioral chain analysis leading to an expanded case formulation and new solutions.
3. An intense review and practice of selected DBT skills.
4. Safe processing of emerging trauma memories that lead to dangerous dissociative episodes.
5. Review, repair, and remoralization of a strained outpatient therapy.

We have learned that the clear specification of goals and targets in DBT can define a realistic and finite hospital intervention, and that the pragmatic and concrete solutions in DBT fit well with inpatient nursing philosophy and the current emphasis on efficient, outcomes-oriented approaches.

Those who have implemented DBT on inpatient units have had to address the fact that typical features of DBT are a mismatch with typical features of inpatient settings (Swenson, Sanderson, Dulit, & Linehan, 2001). DBT thrives on a collaborative relationship between equals, but the hospital setting structures a one-up, one-down relationship between staff and clients. DBT is based on a nonpejorative understanding of behaviors that comprise the diagnosis of BPD, while inpatient units seem to be fertile soil for judgmental and stigmatizing attitudes toward individuals with BPD. In DBT, therapists consult to patients regarding how to interact with other professionals; in hospital treatment, staff members typically join together in managing the patient and trying to minimize inpatient "splitting." DBT therapists encourage active emotional expression and assertiveness; hospital milieus tend to reinforce compliant and passive problem-solving styles that do not disrupt the community.

All three authors have developed and maintained comprehensive inpatient DBT programs. In the course of their training and consultation, they have become familiar with dozens of inpatient DBT programs located in Canada, Europe, New Zealand, Australia, and throughout the United States. These include acute inpatient units where patients stay from 2 days to 2 weeks, intermediate units where patients stay between 2 weeks and 3 months, and long-term units where patients stay beyond—sometimes well beyond—3 months. This chapter applies most directly to acute and intermediate settings, but where relevant we do indicate modifications relevant to the long-term program.

Some inpatient DBT programs have primarily targeted individuals with BPD and related conditions (e.g., substance abuse, eating disorder, dissociative disorders, posttraumatic stress disorder [PTSD], antisocial disorders), while others have modified DBT to address a broader diagnostic range. For instance, there are inpatient general psychiatry programs that offer a subset of DBT skills to all patients, skills that are then prompted and reinforced by nursing staff members throughout the day. Others have used DBT-based diary cards for patients to monitor their behavior and progress, behavioral chain analyses integral to standard DBT as assessment tools, and some of DBT's contingency management strategies to shape adaptive behaviors. In this chapter we describe a comprehensive and systematic implementation of standard DBT on inpatient units, based on a narrow body of inpatient DBT research and considerable clinical consensus among those who have established comprehensive inpatient DBT. While the use of DBT in inpatient psychiatry overlaps considerably with similar work in forensic inpatient settings (McCann, Ball, & Ivanoff, 2000; also see McCann, Ivanoff, Schmidt, & Beach, Chapter 5, this volume) and partial hospital programs (Simpson et al., 1998), the focus of this chapter is on the psychiatric inpatient program.

Research on Inpatient DBT

At least five studies have been conducted to evaluate the effectiveness of DBT inpatient treatment. Barley and colleagues (1993) describe an inpatient program with a stay of several months, dedicated to individuals diagnosed with BPD, where several features of DBT were adapted: a DBT orientation upon admission, a prioritized treatment target list, individual DBT therapy, group skills training, self-monitoring with diary cards, unitwide incorporation of contingency management strategies, an emphasis on validation and compassion, and behavioral chain analysis. The investigators used a quasi-experimental design to compare the frequency of parasuicidal acts for three time periods: at pretreatment for 19 months prior to introducing DBT on an inpatient unit, during the 10 months when DBT was being introduced, and over the 14 months while DBT was in full operation. Rates of self-harm behaviors were significantly lower during the third time period than during the other two periods, and similar rates did not change throughout the entire 43 months on a traditional general psychiatric unit in the same hospital.

On an acute unit with a 12.3-day average length of stay, Springer, Lohr, Buchtel, and Silk (1996) compared outcomes between those patients assigned to a creative coping (CC) group that incorporated DBT skills versus others assigned to a wellness and lifestyles discussion group. Patients in each group attended an average of six sessions. While those exposed to DBT skills in the CC group were more likely to believe that their skills would help them after discharge, they "acted out" on the unit more than the patients in the other group. The way in which the CC group was conducted, where patients were encouraged to share details of their self-harm behaviors, varied considerably from the cardinal principles that inform the way that in the conduct of DBT skills groups are conducted, where such sharing is prohibited. While it is interesting that the two groups showed differences in the measured outcomes, the differences can hardly be attributed to DBT.

Bohus et al. (2000) published the pre–post data of 24 female patients who had finished a 3-month inpatient DBT treatment. The treatment incorporated behavioral analysis of the targeted behavior, orientation to the basics of DBT and BPD, skills training with a focus on skills to prevent future hospitalizations, and contingency management of reinforcers following self-injurious behaviors. Comparing the patients in the month prior to hospitalization to the patients in the month after discharge, the authors found significant improvements in ratings of depression, dissociation, anxiety, and global stress, as well as a highly significant decrease in the number of self-mutilating acts.

In another study from the same group, Bohus et al. (2004) compared individuals in their 3-month length of stay inpatient program to individuals assigned to a waiting list. Clinical outcomes, including changes on measures of psychopathology and frequency of self-mutilating acts, were assessed for 50 female patients meeting criteria for BPD. Thirty-one patients had participated in the DBT inpatient program; 19 patients had been placed on a waiting list and received treatment as usual in the community. Posttesting was conducted 4 months after the initial assessment (i.e., 4 weeks after discharge for the DBT group). Pre–post comparison showed significant changes for the DBT group on 10 of 11 psychopathological variables and significant reductions in self-injurious behavior. The waiting list group did not show any significant changes at the 4-month point. The DBT group improved significantly more than did participants on the waiting list on seven of the nine variables analyzed, including depression, anxiety, interpersonal functioning, social adjustment, global psychopathology, and self-mutilation. Forty-two percent of those receiving DBT were clinically recovered on a general measure of psychopathology. The data suggest that 3 months of inpatient DBT treatment is significantly superior to nonspecific outpatient treatment, with relatively fast improvement across a broad range of psychopathological features.

In a fifth study, Katz, Cox, Gunasekara, and Miller (2004) present pretreatment and posttreatment outcome data on 62 suicidal adolescents, comparing two different inpatient units using two different treatment models addressing suicidal adolescent populations. One of the units employed a comprehensive application of DBT and the other used a traditional, psychodynamically oriented crisis assessment and treatment model. The mean length of stay was 18 days for both groups. The DBT unit offered daily skills training sessions conducted according to a manual; twice-per-week individual DBT psychotherapy utilizing diary cards, behavioral analyses, and cognitive-behavioral solutions; and a DBT milieu where the staff was trained to facilitate skills generalization. The DBT treatment team, including the full-time nursing staff, met regularly. DBT significantly reduced behavioral incidents during admission when compared with the other unit. Both groups demonstrated highly significant reductions in self-harm behavior, depressive symptoms, and suicidal ideation at 1 year. This pilot study concluded that DBT can be effectively implemented in acute-care child and adolescent psychiatric inpatient units.

In summary, research demonstrates that DBT can be successfully adapted and implemented on inpatient units, a significant finding given that DBT was developed as an outpatient model. Furthermore, it suggests that self-harm behaviors and other associated behaviors may be reduced. Insufficient standardization of the inpatient application of DBT, inadequate control groups, and lack of randomization limit the power and generalizability of these findings. Further research on inpatient DBT may benefit from the further definition of the treatment approach provided in this chapter.

Foundations of Inpatient DBT

DBT stripped to its foundations is a synthesis of three paradigms—behaviorism, mindfulness, and dialectics—for the purpose of reducing dysfunctional behaviors, increasing skillful behaviors, and building a life worth living. An understanding of inpatient DBT begins here. Consistent with DBT's foundation as a cognitive-behavioral treatment, the hospital staff collaborates with each patient to specify those behaviors to be targeted during the admission, uses behavioral analysis to analyze the factors maintaining these behaviors, uses cognitive-behavioral procedures including skills training as solutions, and uses diary cards as a means to monitor progress on the identified targets. The approach is straightforward, transparent, pragmatic, at times directive, always active, and always oriented toward change.

For this approach to be effective with individuals with BPD, it is balanced with a second approach based on mindfulness and with an emphasis on nonjudgmental awareness and radical acceptance of things as they are. There is considerable pain associated with having BPD, there is additional pain associated with trying to change old behavioral patterns, and there is another layer of difficulty in living on an inpatient unit. The DBT inpatient staff work to validate all this pain and to find the wisdom in each patient's behavior, even as they insistently push for behavioral change.

The skillful and fluid synthesis of these two poles, insistent change and radical acceptance, is the primary example of the third paradigm of DBT, dialectics. A staff member moves from truly validating a patient's suffering one moment to firmly requesting that he or she change his or her behavior the next. In community meetings, staff meetings, and group therapy meetings, there is a search for the validity of each position and the synthesis among them rather than for the "right" or "correct" position. Within practical limits, the staff works to find creative ways to resolve tensions without premature closure. DBT individual therapy has been likened to the shifting movements of two individuals at opposite ends of a seesaw, trying to find balance while moving closer to each other at the middle. A more fitting metaphor for inpatient treatment is that of a large group of individuals, many of them strangers to each other, riding through whitewater on a large inflatable raft on the Colorado River. To succeed, the raft needs to follow established rules for whitewater rafting, will be neither too rigid nor too flexible, will realize the interdependency between the group and each individual, and will seek balance at every turn.

DBT's theory for explaining the development and maintenance of BPD behavioral patterns is a dialectical one, and more specifically a transactional one. The biosocial theory holds that the dysfunctional patterns typical to BPD arise out of the transaction between an emotionally vulnerable individual and the pervasively invalidating environment in which he or she lives (Linehan, 1993a). The theory is an active presence in DBT inpatient treatment in several ways. For one thing, it is used to orient staff, patients, and families to the nature of the problem and the rationale for its treatment. Correctly understood, it provides a compassionate and sympathetic way to understand the behaviors of these patients, who are often demonized by frustrated providers and others in their social network. Second, while it is sympathetic, it is also a call to action, to address the patients' dysregulated emotions and their accompanying behaviors. The theory is brought up time and again in team meetings as therapists formulate the problem behaviors of their patients in a manner both compassionate and effective. Perhaps the most powerful application of this theory in hospital care is its use by the staff as a lens to clarify troubling transactions between the staff and the patients on the unit. The staff may find themselves again and again in the role of the invalidating environment trying to control the emotionally dysregulated patient, who then responds with greater dyscontrol, and so on. This is the genesis of some of the most painful scenarios of inpatient work. Aware of the transaction, the staff may be able to identify it as it happens and then find a way to step out of the spiraling process. Finally, the biosocial theory suggests that what the patient needs is a validating (enough) environment in which he or she is taught to regulate his or her emotions, deal with interpersonal conflict, tolerate distress, and find balance amid the storms. In a nutshell, this is the goal of inpatient DBT.

Goals, Targets, and Phases in Inpatient DBT

The treatment team works with the patient to define a prioritized list of targets to be accomplished during his or her stay in the program. The target list should be specific, behaviorally defined, prioritized, and realistic in scope. A well-designed target list sets the stage for a crisp and effective treatment plan. The team and the patient work their way from the top to the bottom of the list from admission to discharge, revising the list as needed. The therapist or other designated staff member develops a diary card as the vehicle with which to monitor progress on the targets. Some units have simply used DBT's original standard outpatient diary card (Linehan, 1993b; see Appendix 4.1), making revisions to suit each patient on the unit. It is completed once or more per day by the patient and is reviewed by the therapist or other staff member. The card may be revised during the admission—that is, some target behaviors could be added and others deleted as the patient progresses toward his or her goals. A collaboratively derived target list with an associated diary card focuses the staff and each patient on a step-by-step road map from admission to a successful discharge. (See Appendix 4.2 for a standard inpatient diary card and Appendix 4.3 for examples of completed diary cards across different phases of inpatient DBT treatment.)

Because the scope of problems and problem behaviors is at times huge for this patient population, it is especially important to focus the patient and the staff shortly after admission on those targets best accomplished *during* the hospitalization, saving everything else for outpatient life *later*. For instance, for a patient with chronic suicidal ideation and long-standing interpersonal difficulties who is then hospitalized due to a suicide attempt, the target list should focus on the factors leading to *this* suicide attempt and to *this* hospitalization, not on resolution of the patients' chronic patterns. This distinction between *current* inpatient and *future* outpatient targets helps to challenge the natural reflex of both patient and staff to begin addressing whatever problems seem to come up, which blurs and lengthens the task of inpatient treatment. The goal of most inpatient DBT programs of a short-term or intermediate nature is to decrease the likelihood of future hospital admissions, essentially to eliminate themselves as functional solutions in the patient's lives. The long-term inpatient DBT program is an exception. There, the target list is more extensive and more closely matches the one in outpatient DBT, and may include the processing of PTSD responses after initial stabilization. In the program established by Bohus and colleagues (2000, 2004), the goals and targets reflect its special nature as a 12-week introduction to a long-term outpatient DBT treatment.

The following three-phase approach is proposed for the majority of acute and intermediate inpatient DBT programs, where a chief aim is to reduce reliance on hospitalization and strengthen the capacity to stay out of the hospital. We describe the three phases as sequential and nonoverlapping to help with conceptual and strategic clarity, but in practice the phases overlap and some patients will move back and forth among them before moving to discharge. The phases, and the behaviors targeted in each phase, are listed in Table 4.1.

TABLE 4.1. Phases for Inpatient DBT Programs

Phase	Goal	Target behaviors
Phase 1: getting in	Develop and get commitment to inpatient treatment plan	1. Increase collaborative behaviors 2. Increase commitment to the inpatient treatment plan

Phase 2: getting in control	Reduce behavioral dyscontrol requiring hospital care	1. Decrease life-threatening behaviors that *prompt or prolong* the hospital stay
		  a. Suicidal or homicidal behaviors
		  b. Near-lethal behaviors without suicidal or homicidal intent
		2. Decrease treatment-destroying behaviors that prompt or prolong the hospital stay
		  a. Outpatient behaviors, by patient and/or providers, that prompt or prolong the hospital stay
		  b. Inpatient patient or staff behaviors that destroy treatment and therefore prolong the hospital stay
		3. Decrease egregious, suicidal, and nonsuicidal self-injurious behaviors in the hospital that prolong the hospital stay
		4. Increase skills for behavioral control
		  a. Distress tolerance skills
		  b. Mindfulness, emotion regulation, interpersonal skills

Phase 3: getting out	Develop and successfully execute discharge plan	1. Increase troubleshooting skills for getting out and staying out of the hospital
		2. Increase DBT skills for getting out and staying out of the hospital
		  a. Interpersonal effectiveness skills
		  b. Distress tolerance, emotion regulation, mindfulness, and self-management skills

Phase 1: Getting In

The entry phase comprises four main processes, usually overlapping one another: *orientation* of the patient to the program, *assessment* of the patient, coming to *agreement* on the inpatient plan, and getting a *commitment* to that plan that is as strong as possible. Orienting the patient to the unit is an enormous opportunity that we often miss for many reasons: unpredictable admission times, inadequate staffing, the pressured flow of inpatient life, and absence of a clear protocol for orientation. If we are ready, we can welcome the patient respectfully and sensitively, validating his or her distress and clarifying the nature and role of the inpatient unit in his or her overall care. We can convey real acceptance of the patient's plight while offering a realistic step-by-step plan to change his or her behavior. We can teach the patient about his or her disorder and about the inpatient treatment, prepare him or her for the possibilities and disappointments of his or her stay, and immediately get him or her started on a behavioral chain analysis of the events leading to this particular hospitalization. To standardize the orientation and to ensure that a meaningful orientation takes place on the day of or the day after admission (in the case of late-night/early-morning admission), some DBT units have created orientation videotapes, lasting 20 minutes or so. A videotape can introduce the patient to the unit; outline its purpose, rules, and organization; lay out the main goals of a typical hospitalization; present an overview of the skills package to be taught on the unit; and perhaps provide some tips for making the best use of hospitalization. After watching the video, the patient can sit down with a staff member who further orients him or her and answers questions.

Standard inpatient assessments are performed that are routine for that unit, leading to a diagnosis, a medication plan, a nursing care plan, and a prioritized list of goals and targets to be accomplished during the stay. While this list is based on the template presented above, it is individualized in each case. The more the patient has collaborated in the process of assessment, especially around the behavioral chain analysis, and in identifying the targets, the more one can expect him or her to "own" the target list. The initial chain analysis is a preadmission "story," reconstructed step by step, beginning with the patient's vulnerabilities, identifying major prompting events that set a chain of events in motion (e.g., actions, feelings, thoughts, other events) leading up to the problem behaviors for which the patient was admitted. Consequences of being hospitalized are identified, with special emphasis on those consequences that seem to be candidates as reinforcers for future admissions. (In fact, whether a particular consequence serves as a reinforcer for getting admitted to the hospital can only be determined by analyzing several admissions.) An inpatient chain analysis of this type will search for all the factors supporting the problem behavior, but especially for those factors that favored hospital admission as a "solution." We want to lay the groundwork so that in the future, even if the patient were to proceed down the same chain of events toward problem behaviors, it could be managed in an effective outpatient treatment.

Having identified factors that prompted admission and other factors that may prolong the admission, and perhaps making an initial listing of what will be required to get out and stay out of the hospital, the results are turned into the inpatient treatment plan. If this is done in a focused, task-oriented manner, and in a timely manner even if the patient him- or herself is still dysregulated emotionally, momentum can sometimes be established as a counterpoint to the despair and hopelessness that often accompany the patient entering the hospital. One wants the initial assessment to conclude with a clear, written plan, consisting of goals, approximate time frames, specific targets, and a listing of the methods for accomplishing the targets. Some programs have made it part of the entry process to begin filling out a discharge planning form, which helps to orient the patient to the finite nature of the inpatient stay. The diary card is created at this point, although it evolves during the patient's hospitalization, as previously mentioned. For example, in an acute-care setting, a diary card for a patient with a preadmission suicide attempt might begin by tracking suicidal behaviors and urges, use of distress tolerance skills and mindfulness skills, scheduled and unscheduled check-ins with nursing staff members, and progress on the chain analysis. Soon, after the patient gains better behavioral control and moves beyond the entry phase, the card may be shifted to track the use of emotion regulation skills and interpersonal skills in dealing with individuals on and off the unit, the contacts made in the process of discharge planning, and the emotions associated with discharge efforts.

Having come to an agreement with the patient on a target list, several questions might serve as a point of review. Do the goals make sense? Do the targets and proposed treatment methods make sense in light of the goals? Does the diary card capture the essential targets to be monitored day by day? Is the approximate time frame reasonable? What factors are most likely to interfere with progress on the plan? What can the staff do to help the patient move forward on this plan? Who should be involved from the outpatient treatment world and from the family? The readiness to adopt the plan might be formally noted by a "moment of agreement" of some kind, a "handshake" either literal or metaphorical. This might be the second formal "moment" of this kind, the first having been the moment of orientation. Marking these steps deliberately, even with a ritual, can help to strengthen the treatment relationship and a sense of forward momentum.

Having oriented and assessed the patient, created a plan and some agreement on the plan, the DBT team moves onto the final step in the entry phase: commitment. The fact that some patients are legally "committed" to the hospital, or may feel that they have no choice but to be there, creates a problem for a treatment approach that emphasizes making a voluntary choice to enter into it. Ideally, there is a "program in a program," in which the patient can choose the DBT program or track, or choose not to be in it. Then, even the involuntarily committed patient on the unit can truly choose DBT or not. The stage is then set for a therapist or other staff member to work with the patient on making a commitment to the treatment plan, using the six commitment strategies available in standard DBT. The therapist can highlight the freedom to choose, while at the same time describing the consequences of making that choice. The unit can be structured so that the consequences of choosing to engage in DBT are reinforced. On one comprehensive DBT unit, newly admitted patients begin in a commitment group with other new patients. In the group, commitment to the targets and agreements of treatment is the total focus. Patients who develop a strong commitment graduate from the group, and as a consequence are awarded increased freedom, more flexibility in scheduling, more on-grounds pass time, and more choice in off-grounds passes. These rewards serve as powerful reinforcers for commitment behaviors.

The therapist or designate also helps the patient weigh the pros and cons of making a commitment, to make as large a commitment as possible and then try to add to that (the foot-in-the-door strategy), to recall former difficult steps in their lives to which they had committed (the eliciting-prior-commitments strategy), and take every opportunity to reinforce small indicators of commitment (the shaping strategy). Testimonials from patients soon to graduate from the program, citing the difficulty of getting started but the sense of accomplishment at the end, can inspire the wary or willful new patient. At times commitment can be enhanced by teaching a highly distressed new patient some concrete crisis-survival strategies. Whether there is a commitment group or not, marking the patient's commitment with some kind of graduation ritual or congratulatory community meeting announcement can serve as another boost.

Phase 2: Getting in Control

The goal of the second phase is to establish better behavioral control at a level that would be consistent with a resumption of outpatient life. The highest priority is the reduction of life-threatening behaviors toward self or others, especially those that interfere with outpatient life. These may include suicide attempts, self-harm behaviors of sufficient severity to prompt or prolong hospitalization, assaults, or serious credible threats of harm to others. Some of these life-threatening behaviors are those that occurred prior to admission; others may occur during the hospital stay. The second highest priority in this phase is the reduction of those preadmission behavioral patterns that disrupted or seriously threatened the viability of the outpatient treatment enough to contribute to hospitalization. For example, these may be behaviors of the patient that seriously cross the personal limits of the outpatient therapist and result in therapist burnout or termination. Conversely, they could be behaviors of an outpatient therapist or other treatment provider that violate professional or ethical guidelines, resulting in traumatization of the patient. The range of behaviors that destroy outpatient treatment for these highly emotionally vulnerable and reactive patients is wide, and should be identified in the assessment.

Next in priority are those behaviors on the current inpatient unit by either the patient or the staff that damage the treatment environment and necessitate a prolonged stay. An example is the patient who may have no life-threatening behaviors remaining, but who may be distributing phone numbers of drug dealers to other patients. Or a staff member might violate ethical and professional guidelines by having sexual contact with a patient. Other egregious behaviors are those that are not life-threatening and not imminently destructive to the unit environment, but are nevertheless seriously dysfunctional behaviors in that context—for example, the patient with anorexia who is secretly and intentionally vomiting, or the sexually promiscuous patient who is offering sexual favors to anyone who will be kind, or the patient who impulsively disrobes and runs through the unit.

Finally, the treatment plan during Phase 2 emphasizes the acquisition and practice of skills for accepting reality as it is in the moment, for getting in control of behavior. Distress tolerance skills are especially relevant here, as patients need concrete ways to weather intense emotions without making things worse. The targets to be negotiated in Phase 2 vary considerably from patient to patient. They need to be identified during the evaluation in Phase 1 so that efforts can be devoted in Phase 2 to the particular behaviors that prompt and prolong hospitalizations for that individual.

Phase 3: Getting Out

The third phase is focused on getting out and staying out of the hospital. With a therapist or staff member helping, the patient outlines and pursues a discharge plan that includes living circumstances and outpatient treatment. These steps can themselves set off emotional dysregulation, which can again set off behavioral dyscontrol. This back-and-forth work between steps toward discharge, emotional and behavioral dysregulation, strengthening a commitment, getting in better control, and so on, is typical. Having outlined and worked toward a discharge plan, the patient is helped to use troubleshooting skills to anticipate the factors that will foil the plan, which are then targeted. The skills curriculum on the unit offers distress-tolerance skills to help the patient tolerate anxieties about getting out, interpersonal skills to help the patient negotiate for objectives and relationships in the process of getting out, and emotion-regulation skills that enable the patient to develop more resilient emotional responses. Some DBT units at this level have used transition groups or discharge groups in which patients approaching discharge can work on their concrete plans, anticipate interpersonal and emotional challenges, and strengthen DBT skills that will help them navigate those challenges. In the attempt to bridge the often frightening gap between inpatient and outpatient life, some programs have allowed patients to attend the transition group for another 1–2 weeks after discharge. Former patients of the unit who have successfully negotiated the transition to outpatient life can be invited to the group on occasion to share their experiences and suggestions. As the patient who has completed all three phases gets ready to leave the unit, a graduation ceremony of some sort can be very important, for it allows everyone on the unit a chance to see and to hear from a patient who has gone all the way. He or she is a model for patients in the first two phases of treatment and he or she can receive encouragement from the patient population in facing life after discharge.

Functions, Modes, and Strategies in Inpatient DBT

Any comprehensive DBT treatment provides five functions that are effectively coordinated with one another. *Modes* are the treatment modalities or vehicles through which a function is realized and delivered. For instance, enhancing capabilities is a function; an outpatient weekly skills training group is a mode that serves that function for the patient.

Generalizing capabilities to the patient's natural environment is a function; telephone calls to the outpatient therapist is a mode through which the therapist realizes the function by coaching the patient to be skillful then and there. While the modes for delivering the five functions in standard outpatient DBT are well established (see Comtois et al., Chapter 3, this volume, where these are discussed in depth), the inpatient context is vastly different than the outpatient clinic and requires creative development of modes to serve each of the five functions. We next present each of the five functions with their corresponding inpatient modes, highlighting DBT strategies typically used in these modes. A more detailed discussion of DBT's entire armamentarium of strategies can be found in Koerner and Dimeff (Chapter 1, this volume).

Function 1: Structuring the Environment

In outpatient DBT, a director or team leader is charged with structuring the *treatment environment*, working to provide the patients with a clear, coherent, well-organized approach that incorporates all DBT modes and therapists. In structuring the inpatient environment, the inpatient unit chief (IUC) or the designated inpatient DBT program director is concerned with structuring the treatment program itself and with structuring the relationship between the inpatient unit and each patient's outpatient treatment program. This stands in contrast to the role of the DBT individual treatment provider who is in charge of defining and directing the implementation of DBT for a particular patient, or tailoring the general environment established by the IUC to the specific needs of that patient and tailoring that patient's relationship to the outpatient treatment network.

Operationally defined, "structuring the patient's inpatient environment" involves establishing unit rules or policies, daily and weekly schedules, the use of physical space, the organization of relationships and roles among the staff, DBT-based assumptions about patients and about staff, and three sets of DBT-based agreements (patient agreements, staff agreements, and team agreements) that govern interaction among staff members.

Unit Rules and Policies

For purposes of facilitating DBT on the unit, what is important about the rules and policies is that they are as *few*, as *clear*, as *transparent*, and as *consistently observed and enforced* as possible. The rules and policies should be consistent with DBT principles. Some inpatient DBT programs are compromised from the outset by policies and procedures that are incompatible with DBT—for instance, those that narrowly limit staff responses to promote what appears to be consistency among them in order to minimize "splitting" by the patients. Staff should know, and patients should learn, the important rules. In a sense, the rules and policies are the *limits* of the program, and more personally are an expression of the limits of the program director. They represent a synthesis of overall hospital policies and mandates and of all policies and procedures of other governing bodies (e.g., Joint Commission on the Accreditation of Hospitals) that affect the unit, the philosophy and primary tasks of that unit as defined by the director, the staffing patterns and other resources available for treatment, and the state of the unit over a given period. These rules and policies can shift over time as things change, and they can be more or less flexibly applied in the moment. For the person structuring the DBT inpatient environment, the important thing is to make them clear, consistent, coherent, and public. Ambiguity and confusion in the control and definition of resources and rules will invariably become a treatment-interfering or therapy-destroying behavior by the unit leadership, and certain patients' treatments will be adversely affected.

Unit Schedule

A DBT inpatient program, or a DBT track within a general unit, typically begins the day with some meeting in which patients identify their concrete goals for the day. This may be a community meeting or a small-group meeting. Staff members orient everyone to the schedule of the day, help patients define their goals for the day, and always look for opportunities to encourage and to positively reinforce adaptive behaviors. For a Phase 1 patient, the goals for the day may be to work on the initial behavioral chain analysis, to view the orientation videotape, to fill out the first draft of the discharge planning form, and to attend a class for learning some crisis survival strategies to use while trying not to act on urges to self-harm. For a Phase 2 patient, the goals for the day might be to practice observing and describing emotions, to "act opposite" to the urge to withdraw into his or her room for the day, to sit in on a transition group for the first time, to use mindfulness skills and crisis survival strategies whenever he or she senses the onset of a dissociative episode that day, to set up a meeting with someone from the residential program he or she hopes to return to, and to get help doing a behavioral chain analysis of his or her urge to assault a fellow patient. For a Phase 3 patient, daily goals will typically be focused on the contacts, the plans, and the skills necessary for getting out of the hospital.

The goals meeting or community meeting will typically begin with a brief practice of the skill of mindfulness. This provides an opportunity to practice that skill that is central to all other skills in DBT, that of bringing attention voluntarily, in the present moment, and without judgment, to some chosen focus. Staff members can describe the skill, let everyone practice it, and give feedback and coaching. Other opportunities to practice core mindfulness skills, formally taught in the skills curriculum on the unit, punctuate the day at other transition points (e.g., meals, other meeting times, time for getting medications from the nursing staff).

The daily schedule will typically incorporate skills training sessions, psychotherapy sessions, pharmacotherapy sessions, check-in meetings with nursing staff, and perhaps a commitment group (in Phase 1) or a transition group (in Phase 3). Some programs develop specialized applications of DBT skills tailored to the needs of their patient populations: mindful eating skills for the patients with eating disorders, skills for generating compassion and empathy for those with antisocial features, skills for grounding for those with dissociative disorders, and skills for reducing anger for those prone to angry outbursts. All of these groups of skills are found in the total DBT skills package, but can be emphasized and adapted to specialized comorbid populations. Figure 4.1 provides a schedule from one comprehensive DBT inpatient program.

The Use of Physical Space

The physical space should be pleasant and functional, with a visible emphasis on DBT and the work to be done, but not so comfortable as to reinforce patients for coming to the hospital. Bulletin boards and wall posters can illustrate sets of skills or DBT principles, offer inspiring pictures and quotations, and present anything else that might inform or encourage. The schedule, the unit rules, and the DBT-based agreements and assumptions can all be posted. A table with handouts about DBT, related topics (e.g., trauma, BPD, biology of emotions, substance abuse), and worksheets for the application of DBT

Time	Activity
9:00 A.M.	Mindfulness skill of the day and mindfulness practice
9:30 A.M.	Community meeting
10:00 A.M.	Break
10:15 A.M.	Daily goal setting and homework review
11:00 A.M.	Break
11:15 A.M.	DBT skills training group and homework assignment
12:00 P.M.	Lunch (including a mindful eating practice for those with eating disorders)
1–4 P.M.	Individualized meetings with psychotherapists, milieu staff, pharmacotherapists, and other ancillary professionals, and specialized skills application groups
4:00 P.M.	Afternoon check-ins with milieu staff (possibly including diary card reviews)
4:45 P.M.	Break
5:00 P.M.	Evening exercise (stretching, calisthenics, yoga, etc.)
5:30 P.M.	Evening meal, free time
7:30 P.M.	Evening wind-down with mindfulness practice and time to complete diary cards

FIGURE 4.1. Sample schedule from a comprehensive DBT inpatient program.

skills is useful. Ideally, the unit will have a special location reserved for the practice of mindfulness and/or calming down. An organizational chart showing the various staff roles and team structure should help patients to understand the unit makeup and indicate whom to go to for what.

Relationships and Staff Roles

The role-related and informal relationships among the staff are an important part of the inpatient environment. Two features are desired on a DBT inpatient unit. First, the task roles among the staff should be clear. On a unit with considerable emotional intensity and frequent dysregulation, where rules and policies are challenged and crises are part of the expected work, each staff member should know his or her role, what to do, what not to do, and what the protocol is for crisis situations. When confusion arises, it presents a good opportunity for clarification in staff meetings and supervisions. Second, staff members should look for opportunities, publicly and privately, to validate one another and to comment on the use of DBT skills and strategies. The atmosphere of mutual validation and positive reinforcement among the staff will enhance staff resiliency and motivation and will provide opportunities to model skillful behaviors for the patients.

Unit leadership decides whether to have a primary therapist for each DBT patient. On units where a primary DBT therapist plays a central role, he or she orients and assesses the patient; reviews the agreements and gets the patient's commitment to treatment and target behaviors; creates the prioritized target list and the associated diary card with the patient; reviews the diary card daily; does behavioral chain analysis with the patient; implements indicated problem-solving, validation, and dialectical strategies; gives homework assignments; monitors progress; and consults to the patient in the discharge-planning process. He or she has a key role in the DBT team meetings on the unit, and is centrally involved in the daily decision making regarding the unit or the patient. In other words, in a comprehensive inpatient DBT program, the individual therapist plays a role similar to that of the standard outpatient DBT primary therapist, serving as the "quarterback" of the treatment team. Due to resource limitations, however, some inpatient programs have tried to incorporate individual therapy strategies into other modes. For instance, and this may be especially true of acute units, these treatment functions may be taken on by a nursing staff member assigned as the primary nurse, or by a clinician who helps the patient with concrete planning (in this latter case, the clinician acts more as a diary card coach and planner than as an individual primary therapist). Some programs have established therapy groups in which a group therapist helps patients to determine their targets, work on commitment to the treatment plan, review diary cards, analyze chains of behavior, and generate and practice skillful solutions. There is no evidence, even on an outpatient basis, that these arrangements are effective, but they represent creative attempts to adhere to the principles of DBT. At the very least, for each patient there should be a staff member who works collaboratively with the patient to help him or her get oriented to treatment on the inpatient unit, develop and express commitment to a treatment plan, monitor progress toward achieving his or her inpatient goals, and ensure his or her use of DBT principles and strategies toward a successful outcome. Designation of this role and assignment of tasks by role are all part of structuring the environment and must be clear and coordinated.

Assumptions about Patients and Treatment

Inpatient DBT adapts the list of assumptions that are used in standard outpatient DBT to help therapists maintain attitudes about patients and treatment that promote compassion and effectiveness. Some of the inpatient assumptions are exactly the same; others are based on the standard assumptions but modified for use in an inpatient setting. Certain assumptions are *unique to inpatient* DBT. Table 4.2 summarizes the DBT assumptions about patients in an inpatient unit.

The first four of these assumptions, borrowed directly from standard DBT, promote a compassionate viewpoint. Staff members need to review, and even argue about, these assumptions, since patients at any given moment may appear to be doing less than the best that they can, or look like they do not want to improve, or even seem not to be suffering at all. It is understandable that staff members who work on the front lines day after day in a setting marked by episodes of behavioral dyscontrol may develop attitudes or assumptions that run counter to the assumptions about maintaining a compassionate

---

TABLE 4.2. Assumptions about Patients

1. Patients are doing the best they can.
2. Patients want to improve.
3. Patients cannot fail in DBT.
4. The lives of suicidal individuals with BPD are unbearable as they are currently being lived.
5.[a] Patients must learn new behaviors in all relevant contexts on and off the unit: in meetings, in the milieu, and ultimately in natural life contexts outside the hospital.
6. Patients may not have caused all of their own problems, but they have to solve them anyway.
7. Patients need to do better, try harder, and/or be more motivated to change.
8.[b] The inpatient environment is powerful and hierarchical, often rigid and invalidating, and may contribute to patients' emotional dysregulation; nevertheless, patients must work toward their goals on the unit.

---

[a] Based on the standard assumptions of outpatient DBT but modified for use in an inpatient setting.
[b] Assumption unique to inpatient DBT.

viewpoint. That is why these assumptions are so important in the inpatient setting. Similarly, assumptions about treatment in inpatient DBT are adapted from assumptions about treatment in standard outpatient DBT. Assumptions are described in Table 4.3.

Inpatient Agreements: Patient, Staff, and Team Agreements

As with assumptions, we have modified the patient, staff, and team agreements for use in the inpatient settings, while retaining the original agreements detailed by Linehan (1993a) for use in a comprehensive outpatient setting. One aims to have as few agreements as needed to establish clarity and consistency. These agreements are listed in Table 4.4.

Relationship between Inpatient and Outpatient Treatment Contexts

The unit director defines the overall relationship between the inpatient unit and outpatient providers, to be tailored in each case by the inpatient therapist. Obviously, the outpatient providers have important information to share regarding the patient's preadmission history and postdischarge resources, and usually have opinions about the goals of hospitalization. Contact during Phase 1 is therefore indicated. All such contact should conform, to the highest degree possible, to the consultation-to-the-patient agreement. In other words, the patient should be centrally involved in getting and sharing that information, and all inpatient-to-outpatient provider contact should include the patient to the highest degree possible.

Beyond this sharing of information toward assessment and goal setting, the inpatient DBT team will want to minimize contact between the patient and outpatient providers until the patient approaches discharge. Inpatients often want to phone their outpatient therapists during their episodes of emotional dysregulation on the unit. While this would be the correct DBT protocol on an outpatient basis, the ready availability of the outpatient providers in addition to the inpatient supports can reinforce behaviors that prolong hospitalization. Conversely, the suspension of contact, and the anticipation of the "reunion," can serve to reinforce progress toward discharge.

Inpatient DBT's emphasis on the patient's central role in gathering and sharing information during Phase 1 and on the suspension of contact with outpatient providers during the better part of the hospital stay deviate from standard practice. Therefore, the patient and the outpatient providers need to be oriented to these policies and their rationale during Phase 1.

TABLE 4.3. Assumptions about Inpatient DBT Treatment

1.[a] The most caring thing the staff can do is to help the patients change in ways that make a life without hospitalizations a possibility.
2. Clarity, precision, and compassion are of the utmost importance in the conduct of DBT.
3. The relationship between staff and patients is a real relationship between equals.
4.[b] Because of the hospital hierarchy, staff automatically have considerable power over the patients, and that power must be used compassionately and in a manner that is consistent with Assumption #3.
5.[b] The DBT staff can fail to apply the treatment effectively.
6. Even when applied effectively, inpatient DBT can fail to achieve the desired outcome.
7.[a] The staff that is treating individuals with BPD need support, and this is especially true of frontline nursing staff.

---

[a] Based on the standard assumptions of outpatient DBT but modified for use in an inpatient setting.
[b] Assumption unique to inpatient DBT.

TABLE 4.4. Inpatient Agreements for Patients, Staff, and Team

Group	Agreement
Patients	1. Agreement to work on reducing behaviors that require hospitalization. 2. Agreement to work on getting out and staying out of the hospital. 3. Agreement to abide by the unit's rules and policies. 4. Agreement to attend required unit meetings (e.g., community meeting, skills training groups).
Staff	1. Agreement to offer effective and compassionate treatment. 2. Agreement to keep patient information confidential unless transmitted with patient consent. 3. Agreement to abide by professional and ethical guidelines. 4. Agreement to seek consultation as part of treatment. 5. Agreement to observe unit rules and policies.
Team	1. *Dialectical Agreement*: No one individual or viewpoint is the "right" one, everyone's viewpoint has validity, and the truth is arrived at by synthesis of differing, even opposing, points of view. 2. *Phenomenological Empathy/Nonpejorative Agreement*: Staff members will seek out the most empathic interpretation of the clients' and their colleagues' behavior, being guided by the empirical evidence. 3. *Consistency Agreement*: While different staff members should be consistent in focusing on each patient's targets, on observing unit rules and policies, and on implementing DBT principles and guidelines, they need not be consistent in matters of style or approach. 4. *Observing Limits Agreement*: Different staff members should honor their own natural personal limits on the unit. These limits will, of course, be different from one staff member to the next and may differ within staff across time (as long as all staff members are also observing unitwide limits as articulated in rules, policies, and leadership decisions). 5. *Fallibility Agreement*: All staff members are fallible, make mistakes, and therefore need not be defensive about this; we agree to use these moments as opportunities to better learn the treatment. 6. *Consultation-to-the-Patient Agreement*: All staff members will consult to the patient in managing his or her relationships with other professionals, including those professionals on the unit, rather than trying to manage those things for the patient.

There are, of course, exceptions to this baseline position. Each exception is warranted by the primary goal of the hospital stay: to strengthen the patient's capabilities in outpatient life and reduce the likelihood of future hospitalizations. The patient might request to take passes from the unit to attend the outpatient skills training group. This should be encouraged within the bounds of safety. If the patient's relationship to the outpatient therapist is new and is still rather weak, contact may be indicated to strengthen that relationship and to reduce the likelihood of future hospitalizations. If the outpatient therapy relationship is a troubled one, the inpatient team might offer consultation to that relationship, which could include face-to-face meetings with the patient and therapist. Finally, as discharge approaches and the patient enters Phase 3, the patient needs to set up meetings with outpatient providers as part of the discharge process.

Function 2: Enhancing the Patient's Capabilities

DBT primarily enhances patient's capabilities with skills training, psychoeducation, and psychopharmacology. Pharmacotherapy is a way of enhancing capabilities through neurochemical intervention. It is compatible with a DBT treatment. However, if medications and skills were equally effective in enhancing capabilities, the preference in DBT would be for skills. While there are ways to practice pharmacotherapy as a mode of DBT, using DBT principles, targets, and strategies, that is not our subject here. Psychoeducation and skills training are ideal as a curriculum for an inpatient setting, and they are the aspects of DBT most easily and commonly added on to non-DBT-based inpatient programs. But, as is the case with studies in outpatient DBT, there is as yet no data to support the effectiveness of this add-on strategy.

DBT's entire skills package (Linehan, 1993b) consists of four modules, each of which requires six 2½-hour sessions over the course of 6 months in outpatient DBT. Long-term units can teach the entire set of skills, but acute and intermediate units must select smaller subsets of skills suitable for their time frames. In standard outpatient DBT, the entire skill set is taught twice through, therefore requiring 1 year of treatment. Accordingly, in inpatient DBT, we suggest that the chosen set of skills be taught twice. If a given unit has an average length of stay of 2 weeks, this requires a 7-day skills curriculum, so that on average each patient is exposed twice to each skill. In the extreme, a unit with an average length of stay of 2 days perhaps should teach one skill over and over again.

The inpatient program is not limited to a weekly skills session. In fact, the consensus among DBT experts supports daily teaching. Depending on the expertise of the weekend staff, skills teaching could continue during the weekends, or the weekend could be a time for skills review and application. Whatever the skills curriculum includes, all staff members should learn and practice those skills themselves, and they should also learn how to coach patients in using them.

The outpatient skills group session typically moves through five steps: (1) a brief mindfulness practice, (2) a review of the previous week's homework, a (3) 15-minute break, (4) the teaching of a new skill and the assignment of a homework practice of that skill, and (5) a warm-down exercise intended to help with emotion regulation before the group ends. The inpatient context, with daily skills sessions and other opportunities in the day to promote skills, allows for variations on this theme. For instance, a new skill could be taught on Monday and combined with a homework practice, the homework practice could be reviewed on Tuesday, a new skill could be taught on Wednesday, the new skill could be reviewed on Thursday, and a skills review and practice session could take place on Friday. Alternatively, a new skill could be taught every day, with practices of that skill prescribed for the coming 24 hours, when the practice is reviewed and a new skill is taught. On one comprehensive long-term DBT unit, patients met each day in small groups for careful review of the practice of yesterday's new skill. After a break, they convened in larger groups where the new skill of the day was taught to all patients. On that unit, a nursing staff member provided a review of that skill during the evening for those who needed it. The variations are endless. Possible variations allow for maximal tailoring to the unit and the patient population. The goal is to teach each skill clearly, to allow time for practice, to allow more time for practice, review, and feedback, and to create an atmosphere supporting the use of skillful behaviors throughout the day.

For an inpatient unit where the length of stay prohibits teaching the entire skills manual, which skills should be prioritized in the curriculum? No research suggests an answer to this question, but the consensus of inpatient DBT experts suggests the following guidelines. The core skills, those that are prerequisites for the practice of all other DBT skills, are the core mindfulness skills. Learning the skills of observing, describing, participating, nonjudgmentally, one-mindfully, and effectively, in the service of generating Wise Mind, should be taught again and again, and formally practiced at designated times several times per day. The next priority, given the patients' high levels of distress and the unit's goal of helping to reduce problematic behaviors in the context of distress, is the teaching of distress tolerance skills. That module includes the teaching of radical acceptance of reality. This teaching is perfect for the person on the inpatient unit who has many difficult realities to accept. In conjunction with radical acceptance of unpalatable realities, this module offers concrete skills to help weather crises without making things worse. These should be prioritized. Core mindfulness and distress tolerance skills should be amply represented in any inpatient curriculum. On an acute unit, they might comprise up to 75% of the total curriculum. Skills should be selected from the other two modules, emotion regulation training and interpersonal effectiveness training, that offer means to change one's emotional responses and relationships. From the former, the skills of observing and describing emotions, reducing vulnerability to negative emotions, reducing suffering through mindfulness of one's current emotion, and acting opposite one's emotion are particularly useful. From the interpersonal effectiveness module the unit should prioritize the teaching of three priorities in relationships, the five factors interfering with effectiveness, and the guidelines spelled out in DEAR MAN, GIVE, and FAST. Table 4.5 suggests those skills within the acute and intermediate inpatient programs.

Each unit must develop its own DBT skills curriculum with the right focus and fit for the length of stay and the targeted patient population. In addition to the skills handouts themselves (Linehan, 1993b), the inpatient team can develop apt homework assignments, additional handouts, and other supporting materials. Some programs have created flash cards or decks of cards with the skills listed on one side and the description of the skills on the other. Some programs maintain a library of DBT skills training videos created for clients by Linehan (Linehan, 2003a, 2003b, 2003c, 2003d; Linehan, Dimeff, Waltz, & Koerner, 2000). A very distressed patient who has just observed another patient's episode of angry dyscontrol can be assigned to sit down at the television, practice mindful breath-

TABLE 4.5. DBT Skills for Intermediate and Acute Inpatient Units

Modules	Intermediate unit	Acute unit
Core Mindfulness Skills	Wise Mind Observe, Describe, Participate Nonjudgmentally, One-mindfully, Effectively	Wise Mind Observe, Describe, Participate Nonjudgmentally, One-mindfully, Effectively

Distress Tolerance Skills	Radical Acceptance, Turn the
	   Mind, Willingness, Willfulness
	Distract, Self-soothe, IMPROVE
	   the Moment, Pros and Cons
		Radical Acceptance, Turn the Mind
		Distract, Self-soothe, IMPROVE
		   the Moment, Pros and Cons

Emotion Regulation Skills	Observe and Describe Emotions
	DBT's Model of Emotions
	Reduce Vulnerability to Negative
	   Emotions
	Increase Positive Emotions
	Reduce Suffering by Mindfulness to
	   Current Emotion
	Act Opposite the Current Emotion
		Observe and Describe Emotions
		Reduce Vulnerability to Negative
		   Emotions
		Act Opposite the Current Emotion

Interpersonal Effectiveness Skills	Three Priorities in Interpersonal
	   Encounters
	Five Factors That Interfere with
	   Effectiveness
	DEAR MAN, GIVE, FAST Skills
		DEAR MAN, GIVE, FAST Skills

ing, and watch the skills video that covers radical acceptance of things you can't control and crisis-survival strategies.

A crucial aspect to inpatient DBT is that the staff must master the skills over time and become expert coaches in the milieu. This helps to avoid situations in which staff members actually have less exposure to and experience with the skills than the patients, leading them to feel less confident and to be less effective in the milieu. A well-defined skills package can engage and empower an entire staff as they come to see what valuable tools they can bring to the patients every day. One wants an intensive skills workshop atmosphere, with the language and concepts of the skills fully permeating the environment.

Function 3: Generalizing the Skills to the Inpatient Milieu and the Outpatient Environment

We have already mentioned generalization of skills as one of the important elements of inpatient DBT. Indeed, the milieu environment, offering full immersion into DBT skills acquisition, strengthening, and generalization "24/7," may indeed be one of the primary benefits of DBT offered in an inpatient environment. It is a primary task of the nursing staff members who interact with the patients day in and day out. Nearly every minute is an opportunity to suggest the use of skills or to reinforce active skill use that patients may or may not be aware they are doing. While striving to create an atmosphere filled with positive reinforcement, each staff member is asked to think about skillful, even slightly skillful, patient behaviors that they can reinforce. One wants to catch a patient in the act of a skillful behavior and right then note it in a reinforcing manner. Staff members can comment publicly on each other's use of skills.

Throughout the inpatient stay, staff should make connections between the skills being taught and the use of them after discharge. Patients can identify situations that may benefit from the skills as part of homework assignments, or in a transition group focused on discharge. Staff can help the patient locate avenues for continuing skills learning and practice outside the hospital.

Many patients, especially while still emotionally dysregulated shortly after admission, may be uncommitted, even opposed, to learning the skills. This is to be expected. For some, this indifference or opposition will remain true throughout their stay. The staff's spirit should be one of offering, offering, offering the skills, but accepting when certain patients are not ready to put their mind to that cause. The goal is to make the skills part of the curriculum and a pervasive part of inpatient life, to find ways to make the learning interesting and compelling, to reinforce the skills everywhere, and not to get discouraged or defensive if certain patients or groups of patients find the skills unhelpful or objectionable. Our experience has been that if the staff as a whole become familiar with the skills and find them useful in their own lives, they will act in a manner that reinforces patient interest and commitment to skills training.

As discussed above, the patient is taught the skills on the unit in several contexts: via formal teaching in skills training groups, in one-to-one sessions with a skills tutor or coach, by studying the skills manual and practicing on their own, by watching skills on videotape, and through the modeling of the skills that the staff does day in and day out. After he or she learns a particular skill, the patient is encouraged to generalize the skill to the various environments that make up inpatient life and then to the outpatient environment during passes and after discharge. This transfer of skills from one setting to another cannot be taken for granted; it must be attended to over and over again. To aid with generalization within the unit, the staff uses DBT skills worksheets and visual prompts around the unit, coaching on the fly, coaching in check-ins, self-monitoring cards with listing of skills, modeling of skills throughout the day, skills videotapes, and scheduled and ad hoc skills application groups. There is no end to the number of ways that skills transfer can be encouraged by a creative inpatient team. One of the very first inpatient programs to apply DBT skills taught "turtling" (an application of "vacation," a DBT crisis survival strategy). Turtling involves "pulling yourself into your shell" for awhile until things change internally or externally. Ceramic turtles, stuffed turtles, photographs of turtles, and actual turtles were to be found all over the unit. Another DBT inpatient program developed a game of "frog" to strengthen the skill of nonjudgmental stance: Each time a patient or a staff member made a judgmental statement, the patients would gently throw a frog bean bag at the individual to catch. As already mentioned, patients can carry their manuals, flash cards, or "cheat sheets" listing all the skills with them. During Phase 3 patients can try in advance to identify emotionally difficult situations they will face after discharge and develop specific action plans, including use of skills, for those situations. When a patient goes on a pass into the community, he or she can enact a deliberate plan for using the skills. While a patient works on the practical steps toward discharge, and reexposure to some stressful situations, he or she has an opportunity for skills strengthening and generalization.

Certain skills worksheets from the DBT skills manual (Linehan, 1993b) have proven to be invaluable on inpatient units. These should be abundantly available at the nursing station. From the interpersonal skills module, the worksheet on preparing for a stressful interpersonal encounter is ideal for a wide range of inpatient situations. The patient who is having a conflict with a roommate, with a new patient on the unit, with a particular staff member, or with a visitor who is coming that afternoon can prepare for the next encounter by completing that worksheet. By doing so, the patient has an unusual opportunity to consciously rehearse, perhaps including a role play with a staff member, such an encounter before it takes place. It can then be reviewed afterward with a staff member with a focus on what skills were used and how they worked. The patient who is emotionally dysregulated by any of the thousands of stressors of inpatient life can use the "Observing and Describing Emotions Worksheet" to step back and establish a stance from which to observe and describe the current emotions, and in that way learn the power of observing and describing without acting upon emotions and associated urges.

To help the inpatient who is emotionally dysregulated and is progressing down the path toward dysfunctional behavior, some units have developed "safety protocols" to help that patient change direction and to use DBT skills. The steps of a typical safety protocol will include:

1. It becomes apparent to the patient or to a staff member that the patient is on a path toward problem behavior.
2. The patient acknowledges that her or she is on such a path and asks to enter onto the safety protocol (or a staff member may make this suggestion).
3. If possible, the patient removes him- or herself from whatever circumstances are setting off or promoting the problem chain (e.g., remain distant from a certain individual, or retire to one's room).
4. The patient creates and/or reviews a list of skills that might help him or her shift to a more adaptive chain of events.
5. The patient chooses one of those skills and tries it.
6. If necessary, the patient tries another one, and another one, and so on.
7. The patient meets with a staff member to get support and further suggestions.

Certain resources can facilitate the safety protocols. Worksheets from the distress tolerance skills module can be used to identify a distressing situation, rate the level of distress, consider the various crisis survival strategies, choose and apply one of them, and rate the level of distress before and after using the skill. Similarly, other worksheets can prompt the use of radical acceptance, breathing and body awareness, half smile, and the use of willingness. If there is a particular place on the unit that is slightly removed; is soothing; has visual prompts, readings, metaphors, and sayings; and has worksheets associated with mindfulness practice, patients can choose to visit that place in order to regain a sense of balance and calm. Too often, individuals resort to self-harm and other dysfunctional behaviors simply because at that moment they can imagine nothing else that could end their free-fall into the chasm of suffering. The unit equipped with safety protocols, skills training, and associated resources can help break the fall.

"Coaching on the fly" and check-ins with nursing staff are powerful modes for generalization of skills to the inpatient environment. Coaching on the fly should primarily rely on in-the-moment reminders of the use of skills, and most of all on the use of positive reinforcement at the moment a patient uses a skill. It is one of these unique advantages of inpatient DBT that staff is there to comment reinforcingly the very moment that a staff member sees a patient, struggling with an urge to self-injure or to strike out angrily in response to a cue, act opposite to that urge, radically accept that situation in that moment, and use a distress tolerance skill. It is a powerful moment when a patient's quiet heroic act in his or her battle to become stable and skillful—the kind of act that is almost never recognized by another human being—can be noticed and reinforced by another person. In one inpatient DBT program, staff members are asked repeatedly as part of their orientation, training, and ongoing work on the unit to think about skillful patient behaviors to reinforce that day and to constantly look for opportunities to reinforce them. To balance contingency management procedures on the inpatient unit, which can so naturally become a setting focused on maladaptive behaviors and their management, and therefore become an aversive setting for almost any patient and many staff members, one wants to go as far as possible to bring skillful behaviors to light, both on the fly and in all kinds of meetings.

Check-ins between nursing staff members and patients are a hallmark of inpatient care. These are often extremely important to patients as well as to staff members, providing those formal moments of extended contact (usually 5–15 minutes) where problems can be addressed, wounds can be soothed, supportive relationships can be fostered, and confrontations can be delivered as skillfully as possible. On inpatient units guided by a psychodynamic philosophy, those check-ins can readily become minipsychotherapy sessions. Unless the staff is extremely well trained, this is more often a problem than a solution, as the patient ends up with a half-dozen therapists. A skills training model provides a better match for nursing check-ins. In order of priority, the behavioral targets of such meetings should be (1) reducing behaviors (on that day) that are destroying the inpatient environment as a therapeutic setting, behaviors that are damaging to other patients' treatments, and behaviors that prolong the hospitalization; (2) increasing generalization of the patient's skills to the milieu; and (3) strengthening the relationship between that patient and that staff member. Functionally, the focus is on acquiring and strengthening skills for gaining control, for interacting on the milieu, and for getting out and staying out of the hospital—a perfect fit with the overall inpatient goal. The staff member is equipped with the skills and the check-in becomes an effective, time-limited, target-oriented mode. Sometimes a 10-minute check-in done in this manner in the heat of a distressing moment can be the single most important 10 minutes of the hospital stay. The frontline staff member then feels effective, identified with the overall unit mission, and very much part of the treatment team. This is one of the best antidotes to low morale and feelings of disenfranchisement in a nursing staff.

Diary cards have been discussed as vehicles for self-monitoring and for communication between the patient and the staff. Additionally, they can serve as portable reminders of the skills taught on the unit. The skills in the curriculum should be listed on the card in a way that allows the patient to indicate when he or she has used one. Checking off a skill on the diary card can teach patients to reinforce themselves for adaptive behaviors, much as someone may put stars on a calendar for each day of exercise. For some programs, especially some child and adolescent units, the card can additionally serve as a way to keep track of skillful behaviors. By using skills, the patient earns points, and those points then influence decisions about levels of status or privileges. In these cases, there are sometimes places on the diary card where staff members too can record observations of problem behaviors and skillful behaviors. Thus the card becomes a central means of keeping track of the balance of such behaviors and a powerful means of generalizing skills throughout the program.

The stance "Do as I say, not as I do" is widely known to be problematic. The DBT version of this can be "Why don't you use your skills (even though I don't know much about them)?" The concept of an intensive skills training workshop can only become a reality if staff members themselves learn and use the skills. We hope that staff members will actually find them to be useful in their own lives and their lives on the unit. They will usually use the skills without mention, but now and then it can strengthen the program if they point out publicly that they have used a DBT skill then and there, and that it has been helpful to them. That staff member thereby becomes a model and a reminder that the skills are for everyone and for a wide range of situations. For instance, in a community meeting charged with tension during the discussion of some violation of program limits, a staff member might say, "I am finding that in order to stay focused and balanced while we discuss this intense situation, sometimes I have to just realize that my emotions are rising and falling like waves and that I can just slightly step back from them and notice them going through me and then bring my attention back to the discussion."

Some units have developed DBT skills application groups to supplement the more standard skills training sessions. This is another mode for generalization of skills to the natural environment—in this case, the unit environment. In these meetings, skills that are being taught in skills training sessions are brought to bear to solve problems in daily life on the unit or beyond the unit. One program called their skills application group the "DBT Patient Consultation Meeting." In this setting, the unit psychologist met in a scheduled hour in a group room on the unit, consulting to any and all patients who chose, completely voluntarily, to come. Sometimes one patient attended, at other times every patient on the unit attended. Patients could put a problem on the agenda, with the understanding that DBT skills would be brought to bear as solutions. A patient might bring up a problem of dealing with a nurse on the evening shift, or dealing with her psychiatrist who seemed not to hear her concerns about side effects, or struggling to manage his urges to self-injure every day, or simply ask a question about how to apply a particular skill. The leader of the meeting tried to formulate the problem, often in a way that included a brief behavioral analysis, and worked with the group to identify what skills could be used in that situation. Whenever possible, the leader would have the group members practice that skill in the meeting, and encourage the patient to report back to the group members on how the skill worked in the situation where it was needed. One such meeting was attended by almost all the patients on the unit after a difficult incident in a community meeting. The unit chief, frustrated after several episodes in which furniture had been damaged by cigarettes (back in the days when smoking was allowed on inpatient units), suddenly made a rule that there would be no more smoking on the unit without any planning for how everyone would then cope with that addiction. The patients went to the consultation meeting where the psychologist helped them to articulate the problem(s) and to begin to identify skillful solutions. She had each patient in the room do a brief role play with her in which she was the unit chief and they were using skills to get him to modify his position. After lots of episodes of practice, which became rather lively, the psychologist called a special meeting of the group later in the day to which the unit chief was invited. Serving as the patients' coach, she helped each patient skillfully address the unit chief about the problem. This marked a huge step toward finding a less drastic solution, and more importantly it provided an extraordinary opportunity for a group of emotionally dysregulated individuals to learn and to practice effectively addressing an authority figure about an emotionally charged matter.

Function 4: Improving Patient Motivation

Accomplishing the goals of inpatient DBT requires structuring the program effectively, enhancing the patient's capabilities, and generalizing those capabilities to relevant inpatient and outpatient contexts. All this comes to naught unless the patient is sufficiently motivated to make use of the capabilities in his or her repertoire when they are needed. In standard outpatient DBT, the treatment mode that is focused on motivation is individual psychotherapy. Certainly, motivation is not ignored by the skills trainer or by any other DBT provider, but it is the special focus of the individual therapist. To increase motivation, in behavioral terms, is to increase those behaviors (public and private) that make an individual more likely to achieve an identified goal. Much of the work of increasing motivation involves decreasing those behaviors that interfere with goal attainment.

Modes for Improving Patient Motivation

The brevity and interpersonal complexity of the usual inpatient unit conspire against centering the function of improving patient motivation in any one mode or individual. The inpatient team takes the stance that, on any given day, or, for that matter, on any given shift, the best clinician to enhance a patient's motivation is the one on the team who is most effective at motivating the patient to behave in ways that bring him or her closer to his or her goals. "Staff," in this sense, of course, does not distinguish between disciplines. It refers to the psychiatrist as much as it does to the psychiatric aide. After discharge, it is not unusual for patients to report that they were most affected and motivated by one or another nursing staff member, a vocational counselor, a fellow patient, perhaps even the unit clerk. It simply is not possible to count on the individual psychotherapist, if there is one, to be the most salient reinforcement for the patient on the unit. On the other hand, the individual therapist may be the prime motivator if the unit is a long-term one and the therapy takes place off the unit two or three times per week; and/or when the therapist is the leader of the team that makes decisions about the patient's inpatient status and treatment plan; and/or because the patient happens to bestow special value on the therapist or feels most understood by him or her.

Even if the individual therapist is not the person for whom the patient is willing to work, he or she still can be the one who systematically defines the target list, works to get a commitment, uses in-depth behavioral chain analysis, plans the discharge, and tailors the patient's treatment structure. He or she may still be in the best position to understand what motivates the patient and what interferes with the patients' motivation, and to make use of this understanding to shift the approach to what works for that patient. The therapist then puts a primacy on being the teacher/consultant to the team member or members who are the most motivating for the patient. The inpatient psychotherapist must avoid becoming attached to a preconceived notion of his or her value to the patient, and remain observant enough to see who and what really matters to the patient. The ideal position for the individual therapist is that he or she is connected enough to the unit and to the team so as to be up to date on what is happening on the unit, but to be distant enough to be a consultant to the patient about how to handle what is going on there. The therapist's role is different if he or she is also a decision-making member, even the leader, of the patient's treatment team. This role may increase his or her value as a reinforcer for the patient, but may interfere with his or her role as a consultant.

In many inpatient programs, especially those with shorter lengths of stay, assignment of individual therapists can be too costly or too inefficient. Instead, the work of orienting the patient, getting a commitment, designating the targets, assigning and reviewing the diary cards, undertaking behavioral chain analyses, proposing and implementing solutions, monitoring progress, and so on—the usual tasks of individual psychotherapy and the building blocks of improving the patient's motivation—will be taken on in other modes and by other staff members. A nursing staff member, for instance, might serve as the patient's skills coach, as his or her diary card reviewer, and as the person who does the in-depth behavioral chain analyses with the patient. Sometimes the deficiency in basic psychotherapy training is compensated for by that staff member's daily availability, up-to-date knowledge of the system, support, and natural skill. She or he can be "all over" the case. While a complex role, in some settings it is a better match for the job to be done. That staff member needs to be supported in supervision and/or as part of a DBT consultation team.

Some settings have used group therapy, two to three times per week, as the centerpiece of improving motivation. One inpatient adaptation of a comprehensive DBT program assigned six DBT patients to a therapist. That therapist met with the six patients in a group, three times per week, supplemented by an occasional individual check-in with each patient. In the group patients worked on orientation, agreement about goals and targets, commitment, review of diary cards, behavioral chain analyses, finding and implementing solutions, some generalization of skills, and discharge planning. Whereas problem behaviors and their antecedents can be described and discussed in detail in individual therapy, such detail in a group setting can have contagion effects, triggering urges and actions in other group members. Modifications are necessary. The more restrictive approach is to prohibit the detailed description of target behaviors, referring instead to "target behavior" at that point in the chain. Detailed descriptions can be saved for one on one meetings with staff. The less restrictive approach allows for group members to fully describe their problem behavior chains (omitting unnecessarily graphic references), while the therapists are alert to the potential triggering effect on each member. The patient who experiences urges to engage in the same behavior that has been described can be prompted and reinforced for using skills to tolerate and reduce those urges. The well-managed group has proven powerful in harnessing considerable peer support and improving motivation in each patient, although limitations are inevitable on the amount of detail in behavioral chain analysis.

Finally, of course, the milieu staff as a whole plays an important part in improving motivation. This mode, the daily informal communication network on the unit, has perhaps the greatest potential for improving motivation and yet is the most unwieldy to characterize or define. Optimally, staff members will be familiar with, or have quick access to, each patient's specific targets, will be very familiar with the skills, and will be trained in contingency management strategies and learning principles. The relentless focus throughout the program should be on positive reinforcement of skillful behaviors. But this is easier said than done in a setting where there can be considerable emotional and behavioral dysregulation on the part of both patient and staff, and repeated interventions to maintain programmatic limits.

Strategies for Improving Patient Motivation

Whether the function of improving motivation is delivered through individual therapy, group therapy, individual relationships with designated staff, or with the milieu staff as a whole, the work relies on the same groups of DBT strategies (see Linehan, 1993a). Below we highlight those that are especially important in the inpatient context. Some have been discussed already (e.g., commitment strategies, behavioral analysis). The rest will be discussed in three groups: problem-solving strategies, validation strategies, and dialectical strategies.

DBT's problem-solving strategies are those of cognitive-behavioral therapy. By beginning the hospitalization with an assessment that includes a behavioral chain analysis and leads to identification of target behaviors, problem solving is underway. Then again, when presented with problem behaviors that have the potential of prolonging hospitalization (e.g., life-threatening and other unsafe behaviors), a staff member does another behavioral chain analysis with the patient. The unit should be well stocked with worksheets for carrying out chain analysis and the whole staff should be familiar with the procedure. This assessment/treatment technique becomes central to the unit's work. In fact, some programs have formally taught behavioral chain analysis as a skill for patients to learn.

The outcomes of these analyses, seen in the context of the patient's recent history, begin to illustrate patterns of behavior, that is, sequences that seem characteristic. These insights may lead to possible solutions that are considered by the team and the patient. For one patient it may involve recognition that the hospitalizations take place shortly after the therapist goes away for vacations or conferences, in spite of the fact that the patient may have seen the connection before. This leads to a discussion with the therapist and has implications for future planning. For another patient the chain analysis may evidence the patient's profound deficit in observing his own emotions, which precedes incidents of self-harm. Treatment then includes a focus on observing and describing emotions. In another case, a careful chain analysis reveals that the patient's presentation in the emergency room after an incident of self-cutting, where she completely withdraws from interpersonal contact and rocks back and forth, sufficiently frightens the emergency room staff that admission to the hospital becomes the necessary plan. In this case, the patient can be involved in working with her outside therapist and the emergency room personnel, in advance, to come up with a more effective way to assess her.

The behavioral chain analysis sets the level for the ensuing work. For instance, a patient in the hospital may have a strained and tenuous relationship with staff members in the residential program where she has lived for a year. In fact, admission to the hospital came about in part due to a further breakdown in that relationship. Because the only viable discharge plan is to return to that residence, it is seen by the inpatient team and the patient as a high priority to repair that relationship. But the patient finds that in any encounter, real or imagined, with those staff members, she feels too hurt, resentful, and angry to have a reparative conversation. Once the team recognizes that the woman's overwhelming emotions interfere with her skillful movement toward her goal, the team can work with the patient in finding a solution. A psychotherapist or skills coach, using a diary card, might zero in on strengthening those skills needed to have an effective negotiation when feeling very strong emotions. Role playing with the patient offers a chance to combine exposure to the cues and practicing of the needed emotion regulation and interpersonal effectiveness skills.

A more detailed example may be useful in demonstrating the kind of data that can come from a behavioral chain analysis upon admission to a unit. Clarissa, a 32-year-old single woman, well known to the community public health system, had been living in a group home for individuals with chronic mental illness. She was admitted to the hospital after carving the words "Die You Bitch" into her abdomen. She required sutures and she was kept overnight in the surgical intensive care unit to be observed and assessed for any perforation of the peritoneal cavity. In her group home, she had few friends and was generally hostile to the staff and fellow residents. She complained bitterly of being misunderstood when having flashbacks or dissociating. She asked to be called by a series of different names based on which altered identity was presenting in any given situation. Occasionally well groomed, she was more often unkempt, having neglected to bathe, with tangled hair and wearing old, used clothing much too large for her smallish frame. Her eating habits were poor; she rarely ate more than one scheduled meal a day. In addition to telling staff she "forgets" rules and directives they have reviewed with her before, she vexes them with her tendency to leave her personal space cluttered ("It's a health hazard!"), with dirty laundry, unwashed bed linens and potato chip bags and candy wrappers from her weekly binging and purging episodes. She had great difficulty falling asleep, and her rest was constantly interrupted by nightmares. She drank up to 10 caffeinated soft drinks per day. She had intrusive memories of past abuse at the hands of her father, who was arrested and jailed for child molestation when she was 12 years old.

The attending physician and admitting nurse met with Clarissa after her transfer to the inpatient psychiatric ward. As part of the assessment, they conducted a detailed chain analysis of Clarissa's self-injury that led to the hospitalization. They discovered a series of links related to her severe emotional vulnerability, interpersonal difficulties, intrusive recollections of past events, and dissociation. She told them she "can't remember" how she came to cut herself because she had "dissociated." They oriented her to telling them everything she could remember up to the time she dissociated and prompted her throughout the interview with questions designed to elicit the series of emotions and cognitions. When they were done with the assessment, Clarissa told them that what she "really wishes for, but I almost don't dare to because I know it is impossible" is to be less prone to emotional reactivity, less ashamed of herself, and not have to be "so alone."

Upon admission Clarissa is oriented to the procedure of behavioral chain analysis and with some staff assistance she fills out the worksheet. The following steps, beginning with a prompting event in her residence and ending with the hospitalization, are identified.

1. The day before these events, Clarissa had many nightmares, poor sleep, and was left feeling tired and stressed.
2. Peers are watching television in the common room. It is a "true crime" show.
3. Clarissa walks in and says she became "indignant."
4. She thinks "They know about my abuse, they know I can't watch this!"

5. She shuts off the television with no discussion.
6. Peers express anger at Clarissa.
7. Staff intervene and ultimately turn the television on again.
8. Clarissa goes to her room and shuts the door.
9. Clarissa is very angry but also starts to feel anxious.
10. She lies down and tries to sleep.
11. She remembers her family yelling at her. She "hears" her mother's voice, "inside my head" telling her, "You ugly bitch! It's your fault Dad went to prison."
12. Anxiety and a painful sense of loneliness build.
13. Not knowing what else to do, Clarissa takes an X-acto retractable knife from her cosmetic kit and carves the words "Die You Bitch" on her abdomen.
14. She feels "numb" and somewhat calmer.
15. She asks staff to call 911.
16. Clarissa notes a slight sense of excitement as she hears the sirens of the ambulance approaching the residence.

Behavioral chain analysis reveals dysfunctional links that will need to be addressed to reduce behaviors that prompt hospitalization or behaviors to get out of the hospital. In standard DBT there are four groups of possible solutions to address the problems: skills training, cognitive modification, exposure procedures, and contingency management. We have already discussed skills training above. *Cognitive modification* is done routinely by noting beliefs and assumptions that interfere with effective problem solving. Clarissa's thought, for example, that her peers at the residence were deliberately exposing her to a television program that she should not see is a dysfunctional thought that could be subject to challenge. If a patient has the idea that all staff members must be very consistent with one another, or else she cannot stand it, this thought can lead her to a helpless and desperate state. *Exposure procedures* involve the formal exposure of the patient to cues that prompt overwhelming emotional responses, working toward desensitization to those cues. While exposure to painful emotions goes on routinely, unavoidably, in inpatient DBT, it is usually not used as a deliberate procedure on the short-term unit except as a framework for the practice of skills. In long-term comprehensive DBT programs, or in short-term programs that specialize in trauma treatment, exposure procedures using standard exposure-based behavioral treatments (Foa & Rothbaum, 1998) will play a central role.

The final of the four groups of problem-solving strategies, *contingency management*, deserves more discussion. Most behaviors of interest are at least partly under the control of consequences. That is, a patient is more likely to use a given skill if it works to reduce suffering or to bring about a desired change. A patient's decision about whether to self-injure is influenced by the calculation, much of it outside of immediate awareness, that the desired consequences (e.g., reduction of tension and distress) outweigh the undesired consequences (e.g., a public review of that behavior in a group meeting). Similarly, a staff member is more likely to use positive reinforcement of patients' skillful behaviors if doing so brings him or her closer to his or her goal of helping patients or of getting positive recognition from other staff. If a patient notices that one of her peers gets considerable one-to-one contact with staff members as a result of an episode of angry dyscontrol, and if she wants that kind of contact, she may be more likely to lose control too. At every moment, consequences of behaviors on the unit are affecting everyone's behavior, mostly outside of their awareness. Staff's attention to consequences, known as "contingency management," is therefore one of the most powerful problem-solving interventions available. We highlight three levels of contingency management here: the informal use of contingencies, day in and day out, in all unit contexts; the formal structuring of the program in such a way as to reinforce skillful behaviors and to weaken dysfunctional ones; and the use of a formal protocol to decrease the likelihood of the most egregious behaviors on the unit.

As has been noted, the staff engages in a constant effort to recognize and reinforce skillful behaviors all across the program. Such constant engagement requires training and practice, and must be reinforced by unit leaders. It is difficult to maintain because the natural tendency is to direct attention to the troubling and problematic behaviors on the unit, easily overlooking all the adaptive behaviors going on at the same time. Natural reinforcers should be emphasized: enthusiastic praise, a high-five, a quiet word of approval, a knowing glance, or even an absence of any response. Any one of these may be the best natural reinforcer for a given person; staff members themselves have to notice what works best for each patient. What is aversive and punishing for some may be reinforcing for others; overt criticism, imposition of restrictions, even physical restraints can work this way. The point is that staff members must be able to step back, individually and collectively, and consider what is actually being reinforced on the unit. It might be quite different than what is intended.

While strengthening adaptive behaviors with reinforcement, the staff attempts to weaken dysfunctional behaviors with extinction and at times with punishment. To "extinguish a behavior" is to weaken it by removing or withholding reinforcers that maintain it. For example, a staff member might consistently not respond in a group meeting to mildly dysfunctional communication behaviors, putting them on an extinction schedule, while selectively and obviously responding to adaptive communications. The patient who pounds on the nursing station door to get someone's attention might get no response, but he does get a response when he asks politely to talk with someone. Knowledge of the patient's specific inpatient targets will influence what is attended to with positive reinforcement and what is subjected to extinction. Every staff member should be familiar with, or have ready access to, each patient's target list.

Some problem behaviors do not remit even if they are targeted for extinction, even if adaptive alternatives are reinforced. If those behaviors are high-priority target behaviors for that individual (e.g., life-threatening behaviors or behaviors that will clearly prolong hospitalization), or if they are serious violations of program limits or of a staff member's personal limits, they may then be met with aversive consequences. The informal version of aversive consequences takes place between a staff member and a patient. The most common and natural aversive consequence will be disapproval. The staff member may respond to the patient who begins to bang her head on the wall, and for whom that behavior is a pattern that is not interrupted by validation, soothing conversation, or extinction, with clear and firm disapproval, followed perhaps by insisting that the patient fill out a behavioral analysis worksheet to identify the chain of events that led to it. The rule is that aversive consequences should be used when (1) the behavior is of a high priority and (2) reinforcement and extinction are insufficient. When used, it should be done firmly, consistently, and with good follow-through. The use of punishment as a problem-solving procedure is best done in a thoughtful, compassionate context. It is less helpful and ultimately counterproductive in a punitive atmosphere, and can, in fact, destroy the possibility of promoting motivational relationships between staff and patient. Such a side effect of "punishment done punitively" is the most toxic risk of relying too heavily on contingencies to reduce a behavior as opposed to orchestrating contingencies so as to reinforce new, skillful ones that are incompatible with the dysfunctional ones. On the other hand, inpatient programs require program limits and rules to maintain order and safety, so the uses of aversive consequences occur more routinely than in standard outpatient DBT.

Many DBT programs have benefited by using a well-defined protocol to address life-threatening and other egregious behaviors on the unit (see Swenson et al., 2001) (see Appendix 4.4). Self-injurious behaviors, suicide attempts, violent outbursts and threats, and some other particularly egregious behaviors trigger the protocol. The protocol usually includes three steps. Patients are oriented to the protocol upon admission. It is explained that the behaviors covered by the protocol are the very highest priority of treatment when they occur because they threaten life, the safety and well-being of individuals, or the program itself. All other activities and privileges for that patient are suspended during work on the protocol and are reinstated only upon its completion. The protocol defines a clear series of steps with accompanying worksheets. Those programs that have implemented protocols, if done consistently and with staffwide support, have found that they reduce the number of incidents and bring consistency and order to the response to these behaviors that can otherwise disrupt a program over and over again. The following example is typical, but details need to be adapted to a given unit environment.

- *Step 1: Behavioral chain analysis.* The patient is given a chain analysis worksheet to complete. The worksheet helps the patient identify the steps in the chain to the problem behavior and the consequences that followed it. Those steps include the thoughts, actions, feelings, and events that led up to the behavior, and are a search for problematic links that could be handled differently in the future. The patient is asked for skillful behaviors that may make the difference in the future. The worksheet is to be completed independently, by the patient him- or herself, as soon as possible following the egregious behavior. Initially, the patient is to work on it as independently as possible and as thoroughly as he or she can. Patients with behavioral dyscontrol are helped first to regain control and then begin the chain analysis. Patients with cognitive deficits that interfere with understanding or doing the analysis are given assistance by staff. Illiterate patients may be asked to tape-record and/or to draw the chain of events. One wants to avoid unnecessary assistance and contact at this level, as this kind of one-to-one contact with staff may actually reinforce such problem episodes.
- *Step 2: Review and feedback.* When the patient completes the worksheet, he or she gives it to a staff member, who then reviews it with the patient. That staff member assesses whether it was done well enough to move forward, or whether it needs to be redone. He or she reinforces the good work that was done, points out the links that were found, and tries to help the patient expand on it with more detail and with other ideas for skillful solutions. In some comprehensive DBT programs, or those with a DBT "track" on the unit where peers are familiar enough with one another, the chain analysis might then be presented to the peer group for additional feedback. For those programs that do this, this step is the most aversive one for most patients and yet is also the step where patients may get the most important feedback from others who understand the chain from within. It is important that care be taken to prevent a contagion effect by discouraging the patient from providing explicit details of dysfunctional behavior to his or her peers. The patient should instead refer to behaviors as "target-relevant." At the end of Step 2 the patient has a meaningful chain analysis with one or two rounds of feedback, and will be expected to take this chain into a therapy session or a meeting with a staff member to build upon it.

• *Step 3: Repair.* At this step the patient meets with a staff member to briefly review what he or she has learned from the process, to get support for how difficult it has been, to be reinforced for the good work he or she has done, and to consider whether a repair of some kind is warranted. If the behavior in question was disturbing to a given patient or staff member, it may be that an apology or some kind of repair is in order. If the behavior was disturbing to the community as a whole, some act of repair might be made to the whole. The repair may consist of an apology in a community meeting accompanied by some kind of offer that pleases people in the milieu. The staff member helps the patient to plan a repair. When it has been completed, the patient is off the protocol. The patient is oriented to the nature of "repair" as something that "rights" the wrong, that is, an apology may not correct the situation and can sometimes be interpreted as a "less than" adequate effort. For example, if I dent a friend's car by accidentally hitting it in a parking lot, say, "Gee, I'm really sorry," and leave it at that, the dent still remains, and the damage has not really been addressed. If I apologize and then make arrangements to have the dent removed and to pay for the services, then I have really "repaired." This same spirit is brought into the repair work needed after an egregious behavior occurs in the hospital ward. For example, patient X "trashes the day room," overturning trash cans and throwing pop at the walls and all over the carpet. She repairs by helping the housekeeper clean up the room, making a poster of the mindfulness "how" skills to hang on the day room wall, making a nice card to apologize to and thank the housekeeper for his assistance in cleaning up the mess, and then apologizing for the disruption to her peers at the next community meeting.

Within the realm of contingency management is a DBT procedure known as "observing personal limits." Using it is important in the prevention of staff burnout. Staff members are to learn that each individual has different personal limits, different thresholds of tolerance, different sensitivities. It is the responsibility of each one to know those limits and to do what is possible to see that they are preserved. One staff member may be disturbed by swearing, and therefore may ask a patient to use other words to express feelings. The patient is asked if he or she would please respect those limits so that the staff member can be a more effective listener and support, not because there is something "wrong" with what the patient has done. Staff members may have limits as to how much personal information they share with patients, how much tolerance they have for repeated contact, even how close they can be to someone standing near them. Observing limits places the emphasis on the limits needed *by the staff member* to function optimally, not the limits placed upon the patient for his or her own good. As is the case in standard DBT, it may be necessary sometimes for staff to temporarily broaden their limits when it is in the client's best interest that they do so. The consultation team may be needed to assist the individual to expand his or her limits when doing so is extraordinarily hard.

Balancing the emphasis on an organized and persistent way of solving problems represented in the target list is the emphasis on *validation* of the patients for the pain they suffer in their lives, the particular pain they feel now for being inpatients, and the difficulty they have in participating wholeheartedly in treatment. It is the essence of DBT to convey deep sympathy, compassion, and acceptance while it also pushes patients toward behavioral change. The staff, who also practice validation of one another, look for the nugget of gold in the dysfunctional behavioral sequence. Within an episode of self-cutting, which one does not want to reinforce with validation of that behavior itself, one can find the validity of the patient's painful emotions and even the patient's urges to cut.

While insisting to the still-in-bed patient that she get up in the morning in time to get to her first meeting, the staff member can also validate how hard it is to get up when you are feeling tired, or when you have had a hard night, or when you are generally feeling hopeless about your life. Staff members sometimes need help to understand that the ideal position in DBT is to be compassionate and 100% validating in one moment, and then to be 100% insistent on behavioral change the next moment. This kind of agility and wholehearted involvement can be difficult, such that staff tend to move toward a compromise position in the middle that neither insists on change nor radically accepts the patient's difficult plight.

Dialectical thinking and *dialectical strategies* are DBT's answer to polarized and rigid positions, black-and-white thinking, and impasses in treatment. There is an emphasis on spelling out the polarized positions in a given tense conflict or impasse and then moving toward synthesis of the wise part of each position. Dialectics emphasizes "both–and" thinking rather than "either–or" thinking. It emphasizes speed, movement, and flow rather than stasis. While it would be too much to review the dialectical strategies of DBT in this context (Linehan, 1993a), these include the attempt to make "lemonade out of lemons" (i.e., turn a crisis into an opportunity) and to find metaphors for capturing tense and conflictual situations. The staff is dialectical in their style of communication in DBT, balancing a warm and responsive tone (i.e., a reciprocal communication style), especially when the patient is "going down the right track" working toward his or her goals, with a more confrontational and challenging style (i.e., irreverent communication), especially when the patient might benefit from "jumping tracks." These strategy groups are discussed in detail in Linehan (1993a).

As has been noted, the bias in DBT, when it comes to the relationship between a therapist, a patient, and everyone else in the world "out there," is to consult to the patient about how to solve problems in that world "out there." Addressing this bias can be challenging but also powerful in an inpatient setting, and it requires that the staff be well oriented to the concept. For instance, when a patient complains to Nurse A about Nurse B's behavior, Nurse A might consult with the patient about how to address problems with Nurse B. Nurse A might not even mention his conservation with the patient to Nurse B. In DBT, it is not Nurse A's job to defend Nurse B. It is this situation that many inpatient staff call "splitting," with the implication usually being that the patient is doing something pathological, setting up one staff member against another. In DBT the point of view is that it will be natural for staff members to differ in their style and content, and natural that a patient will have difficulties with one staff person more than with another staff person. That is reality. The best thing to do is to help the patient deal effectively with all the others. Staff members need to be helped to see the value of this stance, and they need consultation teams (discussed in the next section) where they can work together within a DBT framework and support this type of work.

Based on the same bias in DBT to strengthen patients in dealing with the environment rather than managing the environment for the patient is the emphasis, to the degree possible, on having the patient as the architect of his or her own treatment. Wherever possible, patients should be in the meetings where their treatment is discussed and planned, and in the center of other communications about them. He or she should be making all of the phone calls for discharge planning except those where he or she could not effectively accomplish what is needed (e.g., when an agency needs to hear from a staff member or a psychiatrist), and even then he or she should be included to the degree possible, such as assisting the staff by finding the phone number and dialing the phone, followed by remaining in the office with the staff member while the communication is completed. Staff should "do for" the patient only what is required by hospital policy and unit policy, or when it is the only thing that can accomplish an important outcome (e.g., get housing for the patient).

Function 5: Enhancing the Capabilities and Improving the Motivation of the Staff

Many think that this function, in which the providers of DBT are helped to develop their own skills and to stay motivated, is the key to DBT's success. The mode for this function in outpatient DBT is a weekly consultation team meeting, where DBT therapists provide therapy to one another in the service of enhancing motivation and strengthening their capabilities to treat their patients with BPD. The weekly consultation team meeting is often not feasible for "line staff" on an inpatient unit due to the nature of their shifting schedules. A more traditional, 90-minute consultation time will work for the professional/nonshift employees but other modalities must be employed for line staff. The crucial point here is that *all* staff, "frontline" and "professional," need to have regular meetings that attend to the staffs' needs in the service of the patients. These meetings are defined as "practitioner-centered" as opposed to "client-centered." Most "team meetings," "treatment planning meetings," "ward rounds," and the like are client-centered, so the need to build in these staff-centered meetings cannot be overemphasized.

Therapists might be able to attend such meetings faithfully, but nursing staff, with shifting schedules and unpredictable schedule impingements of many kinds, and sometimes with staffing patterns that do not permit meeting attendance, often cannot. This dilemma has to be solved because the frontline nursing staff are those who need the team the most, exposed as they are for so many hours, and usually with the least clinical training. Each staff member needs a chance to review difficult encounters with patients, learn more about how to apply the treatment, and receive validation and support from fellow staff and leadership. Otherwise—as is typical in inpatient care—staff end up burned out by the emotional demands of their jobs. As they deplete their personal resources, they become more detached, or mechanistic, or rigid and punitive. One can hardly judge them for merely being human. Frontline staff are to be forgiven much when one sees the emotional strains of their jobs and the typical lack of meaningful supervision and support they endure. In a DBT program this fifth function must be built in.

For instance, one unit provided two different clinician-centered consultation teams, one for therapists and one for nursing staff and recreational staff. The therapists met weekly in a more typical consultation team. For the nursing staff, the DBT program leader conducted miniconsultation team meetings, which came to be known as "chalk talks." During a lull in activity during a daytime or evening shift, he would bring together those nursing staff members who could be spared for 10–15 minutes, take them to the room behind the nursing station, and ask them to bring up encounters with patients in the prior few hours that they wanted to review. Once a trusting atmosphere was developed, with considerable validation and positive reinforcement, staff members looked forward to the meetings and became more forthcoming. The meetings were brief, focused on encounters with patients, and filled with practical ideas of what to do. Role playing became common and staff were given "minihomework" assignments for the next encounter with a given patient, where the staff members could practice. These chalk talks supplemented a training curriculum for nursing staff that was delivered in in-service meetings during which therapists on the unit helped to cover for nursing staff functions.

Another unit expanded on these chalk talks by assigning not only the program leader but also all senior DBT clinicians to be mentors for two or three line staff. Supported by the nursing supervisor, staff members and their mentor would meet for "30 Minute Hits" once a week. The didactic portion of these meetings, usually lasting 10–15 minutes, was based on a curriculum of DBT principles followed by role plays of patient encounters and assignments as noted above. The mentoring relationship expanded naturally to "shoulder-to-shoulder," *in vivo* modeling by mentors and students as they saw patients together throughout the week. Finally, in much the same fashion that outpatient DBT therapists are available for phone coaching to their patients between sessions, mentors made themselves available by pager to their "staff" for in-the-moment consultation regarding DBT strategies when staff were managing difficult patient encounters.

It has been our observation that the nursing staff has the toughest time of it on inpatient programs (excepting patients), and that when they are meaningfully appreciated and brought into a DBT-oriented approach, they can find themselves rejuvenated, remembering what brought them into mental health work in the first place. This, of course, translates into better care for the patients.

The staff should undergo an orientation and training curriculum when they join the program. In-service trainings should be conducted regularly to keep everyone's knowledge and skills at a fine edge. Among the topics most important to cover in any training curriculum would be those covered in this chapter:

1. Understanding the rationale for DBT on the unit.
2. Getting oriented to the foundations of DBT and its biosocial theory.
3. Using goals and specific prioritized targets to frame each patient's hospitalization.
4. Using diary cards to monitor progress.
5. Understanding and conducting behavioral chain analyses.
6. Using commitment strategies.
7. Learning, practicing, and coaching skills.
8. Using role playing with patients.
9. Applying reinforcement, shaping, extinction, and punishment.
10. Effectively administering egregious behavior protocols.
11. Observing personal limits and program limits.
12. Validating the patients and each other.
13. Using dialectical thinking and strategies.

Conclusions

Drawing from an extensive and diverse array of inpatient applications of DBT in the world, but with insufficient research evidence that recommends any particular type of implementation, we have presented a way of understanding and proceeding to practice DBT on the inpatient unit. Some of the inpatient modifications of DBT have enjoyed widespread use: emphasis on an orientation to DBT shortly after admission, the use of targets to frame the inpatient agenda, the use of behavioral chain analysis to identify and address the controlling variables for problem behaviors including those related to patients' hospitalizations, the teaching of skills in groups and their reinforcement through coaching in the milieu, and the use of the egregious behavior protocol as an organizing and educational response to serious problem behaviors in the IPU environment. Evidence to date suggests that applying DBT to a unit may reduce the incidents of dyscontrol. Bohus et al. (2000, 2004) provides evidence that a 12-week inpatient introduction to DBT may lay the groundwork for a more successful outpatient treatment than the usual alternative. While there has been some consensus in the overlap among programs in what has been reported as useful, we will benefit from further research on the process and outcomes of various forms of inpatient DBT.

REFERENCES

Barley, W. D., Buie, S. E., Peterson, E. W., Hollingsworth, A. S., Griva, M., Hickerson, S. C., et al. (1993). Development of an inpatient cognitive-behavioral Treatment program for borderline personality disorder. *Journal of Personality Disorders*, 7(3), 232–240.

Bohus, M., Haaf, B., Simms, T., Limberger, M. F., Schmahl, C., Unckel, C., et al. (2004). Effectiveness of inpatient dialectical behavioral therapy for borderline personality disorder: A controlled trial. *Behavior Research and Therapy*, 42(5), 487–499.

Bohus, M., Haaf, B., Stiglmayr, C., Pohl, U., Bohme, R., & Linehan, M. (2000). Evaluation of inpatient dialectical behavior therapy for borderline personality disorder: A prospective study. *Behaviour Research and Therapy*, 38, 875–879.

Dimeff, L. A., Monroe-DeVita, M. B., & Paves, A. P. (2006). *Summary of published and unpublished uncontrolled studies*. Unpublished manuscript.

Foa, E. B., & Rothbaum, B. O. (1998). *Treating the trauma of rape: Cognitive-behavioral therapy for PTSD*. New York: Guilford Press.

Hanh, T. N. (1999). *The miracle of mindfulness*. Boston: Beacon Press.

Katz, L. Y., Cox, B. J., Gunasekara, S., & Miller, A. L. (2004). Feasibility of dialectical behavior therapy for suicidal adolescent inpatients. *Journal of the American Academy of Child and Adolescent Psychiatry*, 43(3), 276–282.

Linehan, M. M. (1993a). *Cognitive-behavioral treatment of borderline personality disorder*. New York: Guilford Press.

Linehan, M. M. (1993b). *Skills training manual for treating borderline personality disorder*. New York: Guilford Press.

Linehan, M. M. (2003a). *Crisis survival skills, part one: Distracting and self-soothing*. Seattle: Behavioral Technology Transfer Group.

Linehan, M. M. (2003b). *Crisis survival skills, part two: Improving the moment and pros & cons*. Seattle, WA: Behavioral Technology Transfer Group.

Linehan, M. M. (2003c). *Practicing reality acceptance*. Seattle, WA: Behavioral Technology Transfer Group.

Linehan, M. M. (2003d). *This one moment: Skills for everyday mindfulness*. Seattle, WA: Behavioral Technology Transfer Group.

Linehan, M. M., Dimeff, L. A., Waltz, J., & Koerner, K. (2000). *DBT skills training video manual: Opposite action*. Seattle: The Behavioral Technology Transfer Group.

Linehan, M. M., Schmidt, H. I., Dimeff, L. A., Craft, J. C., Kanter, J., & Comtois, K. A. (1999). Dialectical behavior therapy for patients with borderline personality disorder and drug-dependence. *American Journal on Addictions*, 8, 279–292.

Linehan, M. M., Tutek, D., Heard, H. L., & Armstrong, H. E. (1994). Interpersonal outcome of cognitive-behavioral treatment for chronically suicidal borderline patients. *American Journal of Psychiatry*, 51, 1771–1776.

Lynch, T. R., Morse, J. Q., Mendelson, T., & Robins, C. J. (2003). Dialectical behavior therapy for depressed older adults: A randomized pilot study. *American Journal of Geriatric Psychiatry*, 11, 33–45.

McCann, R. A., Ball, E. M., & Ivanoff, A. (2000). DBT with a forensic inpatient population: The CMHIP forensic model. *Cognitive and Behavioral Practice, 7*, 447–456.

Robins, C. J., & Chapman, A. L. (2004). Dialectical behavior therapy: Current status, recent developments, and future directions. *Journal of Personality Disorders, 18*(1), 73–89.

Scheel, K. R. (2000). The empirical basis of dialectical behavior therapy: Summary, critique, and implications. *Clinical Psychology: Science and Practice, 7*, 68–86.

Simpson, E. B., Pistorello, J., Begin, A., Costello, E., Levinson, J., Mulberry, S., et al. (1998). Use of dialectical behavior therapy in a partial hospital program for women with borderline personality disorder. *Psychiatric Services, 49*, 669–573.

Springer, T., Lohr, N. E., Buchtel, H. A., & Silk, K. R. (1996). A preliminary report of short-term cognitive-behavioral group therapy for inpatients with personality disorders. *Journal of Psychotherapy Practice and Research, 5*, 57–71.

Swenson, C. R., Sanderson, C., Dulit, R. A., & Linehan, M. M. (2001). The application of dialectical behavior therapy for patients with borderline personality disorder on inpatient units. *Psychiatric Quarterly, 72*(4), 307–324.

APPENDIX 4.1. Inpatient Diary Card

Dialectical Behavior Therapy DIARY CARD	Name:		Date started:

Date	Alcohol		Over-the-Counter Medications				Street/Illicit Drugs		Suicidal Ideation (0–5)	Misery (0–5)	Self-Harm					Used skills (0–7)*
	#	Specify	#	Specify	#	Specify	#	Specify			Urges (0–5)	Action Yes/No				
Mon																
Tues																
Wed																
Thurs																
Fri																
Sat																
Sun																

*
0 = Not thought about or used	3 = Tried, but couldn't use them	6 = Didn't try, used them, they didn't help
1 = Thought about, not used, didn't want to	4 = Tried, could do them, but they didn't help	7 = Didn't try, used them, helped
2 = Thought about, not used, wanted to	5 = Tried, could use them, helped	

SKILLS DIARY CARD   INSTRUCTIONS: Circle the days you worked on each skill.

1. Wise mind	Mon	Tues	Wed	Thurs	Fri	Sat	Sun
2. Observe: just notice	Mon	Tues	Wed	Thurs	Fri	Sat	Sun
3. Describe: put words on	Mon	Tues	Wed	Thurs	Fri	Sat	Sun
4. Nonjudgmental stance	Mon	Tues	Wed	Thurs	Fri	Sat	Sun
5. One-mindfully: in-the-moment	Mon	Tues	Wed	Thurs	Fri	Sat	Sun
6. Effectiveness: focus on what works	Mon	Tues	Wed	Thurs	Fri	Sat	Sun
7. Objective effectiveness: DEAR MAN	Mon	Tues	Wed	Thurs	Fri	Sat	Sun
8. Relationship effectiveness: GIVE	Mon	Tues	Wed	Thurs	Fri	Sat	Sun
9. Self-respect effectiveness: FAST	Mon	Tues	Wed	Thurs	Fri	Sat	Sun
10. Reduce vulnerability: PLEASE	Mon	Tues	Wed	Thurs	Fri	Sat	Sun
11. Build MASTERy	Mon	Tues	Wed	Thurs	Fri	Sat	Sun
12. Build positive experiences	Mon	Tues	Wed	Thurs	Fri	Sat	Sun
13. Opposite-to-emotion action	Mon	Tues	Wed	Thurs	Fri	Sat	Sun
14. Distract	Mon	Tues	Wed	Thurs	Fri	Sat	Sun
15. Self-soothe	Mon	Tues	Wed	Thurs	Fri	Sat	Sun
16. Improve the moment	Mon	Tues	Wed	Thurs	Fri	Sat	Sun
17. Pros and cons	Mon	Tues	Wed	Thurs	Fri	Sat	Sun
18. Radical acceptance	Mon	Tues	Wed	Thurs	Fri	Sat	Sun

Note. Reprinted from Linehan (1993b). Copyright 1993 by The Guilford Press. Reprinted by permission.

Diary Card

Name: _____ Date Started: _____ Date of Admission: _____

STAGE OF TREATMENT: (circle)   Getting In   Getting in Control   Getting Out

GOALS FOR WEEK: (circle all relevant)   Orientation   Commitment   Behav. Control   Emotl. Regulation   D/C Planning   Discharge

Date	Level of Misery 0–5		Emotions (name them)		Suicidal/Self-Harm: Urges (0–5), Actions? Y/N		Alcohol or Drug Use: Urges (0–5), Actions? Y/N		Other Behaviors to Reduce __: Urges (0–5), Actions? Y/N		__: Urges (0–5), Actions? Y/N		Actions toward Goals		Skills Used
	AM	PM	AM	PM	AM	PM	AM	PM	AM	PM	AM	PM	Name Actions	Name Actions	
Mon	AM	PM	AM	PM	AM	PM	AM	PM	AM	PM	AM	PM			0 1 2 3
Tues	AM	PM	AM	PM	AM	PM	AM	PM	AM	PM	AM	PM			0 1 2 3
Wed	AM	PM	AM	PM	AM	PM	AM	PM	AM	PM	AM	PM			0 1 2 3
Thurs	AM	PM	AM	PM	AM	PM	AM	PM	AM	PM	AM	PM			0 1 2 3
Fri	AM	PM	AM	PM	AM	PM	AM	PM	AM	PM	AM	PM			0 1 2 3
Sat	AM	PM	AM	PM	AM	PM	AM	PM	AM	PM	AM	PM			0 1 2 3
Sun	AM	PM	AM	PM	AM	PM	AM	PM	AM	PM	AM	PM			0 1 2 3

0 = No attempt to use skills   1 = Tried skills without success   2 = Tried skills with success   3 = Used skills automatically

(continued)

From *Dialectical Behavior Therapy in Clinical Settings*, edited by Linda A. Dimeff and Kelly Koerner. Copyright 2007 by The Guilford Press. Permission to photocopy this appendix is granted to purchasers of this book for personal use only (see copyright page for details).

SKILLS DIARY CARD Instructions: Check the days you worked on each specific skill by filling in "Skills Used" scale.

	Mon	Tues	Wed	Thurs	Fri	Sat	Sun
Mindfulness Skills							
OBSERVE: JUST NOTICE							
DESCRIBE: PUT WORDS ON							
PARTICIPATE: IN PRESENT EXPERIENCE							
NONJUDGMENTAL							
MINDFULLY: IN THE MOMENT							
URGE SURFING							
ALTERNATE REBELLION							
WISE MIND							
Distress Tolerance Skills							
DISTRACT: WISE MIND "ACCEPTS"							
SELF-SOOTHE THE FIVE SENSES							
"IMPROVE" THE MOMENT							
RADICAL ACCEPTANCE							
PROS AND CONS							
BURNING YOUR BRIDGES							
ADAPTIVE DENIAL							
Interpersonal Effectiveness Skills							
OBJECTIVES EFFECTIVENESS: "DEAR MAN"							
RELATIONSHIP EFFECTIVENESS: "GIVE"							
SELF-RESPECT EFFECTIVENESS: "FAST"							
Emotion Regulation Skills							
REDUCE VULNERABILITY: "PLEASE"							
BUILD MASTERy:							
BUILD POSITIVE EXPERIENCES							
OPPOSITE TO EMOTION ACTION							

106

APPENDIX 4.3. Examples of Completed Diary Cards

Diary Card

| Name: C. H. | Date Started: April 15 | Date of Admission: March 30 |

STAGE OF TREATMENT: (circle) (Getting In) Getting in Control Getting Out

GOALS FOR WEEK: (circle all relevant) (Orientation) (Commitment) (Behav. Control) Emotl. Regulation D/C Planning Discharge

Date	Level of Misery 0–5	Emotions (name them)	Suicidal/Self-Harm: Urges (0–5), Actions? Y/N	Alcohol or Drug Use: Urges (0–5), Actions? Y/N	Other Behaviors to Reduce — Violence: Urges (0–5), Actions? Y/N	Other Behaviors to Reduce — Dissociate: Urges (0–5), Actions? Y/N	Actions toward Goals — Name Actions	Actions toward Goals — Name Actions	Skills Used
Mon 4/10	AM 3 / PM 4	AM numb / anxious PM	AM 4 / PM 3	AM 0 / PM 1	AM 1 N / 1 N PM	AM Y / Y PM	Agree to plan	Talk to staff	0 1 (2) 3
Tues 4/11	AM 2 / PM 3	AM OK / sad PM	AM 3 / PM 2	AM 0 / PM 1	AM 1 N / 1 N PM	AM N / Y PM	Reduce caffeine	Cry with staff	0 1 (2) 3
Wed 4/5	AM 4 / PM 5	AM fear / confused PM	AM 5 / PM 5	AM 2 / PM 3	AM 1 N / 4 N PM	AM Y / Y Y PM	Chain analysis	Therapy	(0) 1 2 3
Thurs 4/6	AM 4 / PM 3	AM sad / anxious PM	AM 5 / PM 5	AM 2 / PM 3	AM O N / 2 N PM	AM N / Y PM	Chain analysis	Family meeting	0 (1) 2 3
Fri 4/7	AM 3 / PM 5	AM sad / afraid PM	AM 3 / PM 5	AM 1 / PM 2	AM 1 N / 1 N PM	AM N / Y PM	Call friend	Good eating	0 1 (2) 3
Sat 4/8	AM 5 / PM 4	AM lonely / OK PM	AM 5 / PM 4	AM 1 / PM 3	AM 1 N / O N PM	AM Y / N PM	Organize room	Mindfulness	0 1 (2) 3
Sun 4/9	AM 5 / PM 4	AM lonely / angry PM	AM 4 / PM 5	AM 2 / PM 4	AM 1 / 5 PM	AM Y / Y PM	Call brother	Distract self	0 1 (2) 3

0 = No attempt to use skills   1 = Tried skills without success   2 = Tried skills with success   3 = Used skills automatically

(continued)

SKILLS DIARY CARD

Instructions: Check the days you worked on each specific skill by filling in "Skills Used" scale.

	Mon 4/10	Tues 4/11	Wed 4/5	Thurs 4/6	Fri 4/7	Sat 4/8	Sun 4/9
Mindfulness Skills							
OBSERVE: JUST NOTICE		✓				✓	
DESCRIBE: PUT WORDS ON							
PARTICIPATE: IN PRESENT EXPERIENCE		✓					
NONJUDGMENTAL							
MINDFULLY: IN THE MOMENT				✓	✓	✓	
URGE SURFING	✓	✓		✓	✓		✓
ALTERNATE REBELLION							
WISE MIND	✓				✓		
Distress Tolerance Skills							
DISTRACT: WISE MIND "ACCEPTS"	✓	✓	✓✓	✓	✓	✓	✓✓✓
SELF-SOOTHE THE FIVE SENSES		✓				✓	
"IMPROVE" THE MOMENT				✓	✓	✓	
RADICAL ACCEPTANCE	✓			✓	✓	✓	✓
PROS AND CONS				✓			
BURNING YOUR BRIDGES							
ADAPTIVE DENIAL							
Interpersonal Effectiveness Skills							
OBJECTIVES EFFECTIVENESS: "DEAR MAN"	✓	✓					
RELATIONSHIP EFFECTIVENESS: "GIVE"					✓		
SELF-RESPECT EFFECTIVENESS: "FAST"							
Emotion Regulation Skills							
REDUCE VULNERABILITY; "PLEASE"	✓	✓		✓		✓	
BUILD MASTERy:						✓	
BUILD POSITIVE EXPERIENCES		✓			✓		✓
OPPOSITE TO EMOTION ACTION							

(continued)

Diary Card

Name: C. H. | Date Started: April 19 | Date of Admission: March 30

STAGE OF TREATMENT: (circle) Getting In Getting in Control (Getting Out)

GOALS FOR WEEK: (circle all relevant) Orientation Commitment Behav. Control (Emotl. Regulation) (D/C Planning) Discharge

Date	Level of Misery 0–5	Emotions (name them)	Suicidal/Self-Harm: Urges (0–5), Actions? Y/N	Alcohol or Drug Use: Urges (0–5), Actions? Y/N	Other Behaviors to Reduce — Procrastinate: Urges (0–5), Actions? Y/N	Other Behaviors to Reduce — Dissociate: Urges (0–5), Actions? Y/N	Actions toward Goals — Name Actions	Actions toward Goals — Name Actions	Skills Used
Mon 4/24	AM 1 / PM 1	AM OK / PM happy	AM 0 / PM 0	AM 0 / 1 N PM	AM 2 Y	AM N / Y PM	Present d/c plan	See outside therapist	0 (1)(2) 3
Tues 4/25	AM 1 / PM 1	AM good / PM good	AM 0 / PM 0	AM 0 / 1 N PM	AM 1 N / 1 Y PM	AM N / Y PM	Visit parents	Stay on track	0 1 2 (3)
Wed 4/19	AM 1 / PM 2	AM fine / PM afraid	AM 0 / PM 0	AM 0 / 2 N PM	AM 4 Y / 4 Y PM	AM N / N PM	Made ther. appt.	Cleaned room	0 1 (2) 3
Thurs 4/20	AM 2 / PM 3	AM sad / PM afraid	AM 0 / 2 N PM	AM 1 N / 1 N PM	AM 4 Y / 3 Y PM	AM Y / Y PM	Call friends	None	0 1 (2) 3
Fri 4/21	AM 1 / PM 2	AM OK / PM sad	AM 0 / 1 N PM	AM 0 / 1 N PM	AM 2 Y / 2 N PM	AM N / N PM	Visit apartment	Talk to staff	0 1 (2) 3
Sat 4/22	AM 1 / PM 1	AM OK / PM OK	AM 0 / PM 0	AM 0 / 1 N PM	AM 0 N / 0 N PM	AM N / N PM	Write d/c plan	Long walk	0 1 (2) 3
Sun 4/23	AM 0 / PM 1	AM joy / PM angry	AM 0 / PM 0	AM 0 / 1 N PM	AM 0 N / 0 N PM	AM N / N PM	Mindfulness	Visit friends	0 1 (2) 3

0 = No attempt to use skills   1 = Tried skills without success   2 = Tried skills with success   3 = Used skills automatically

(continued)

SKILLS DIARY CARD Instructions: Check the days you worked on each specific skill by filling in "Skills Used" scale.

Mindfulness Skills	Mon 4/24	Tues 4/25	Wed 4/19	Thurs 4/20	Fri 4/21	Sat 4/22	Sun 4/23
OBSERVE: JUST NOTICE	✓	✓				✓	✓
DESCRIBE: PUT WORDS ON	✓						
PARTICIPATE: IN PRESENT EXPERIENCE		✓					✓
NONJUDGMENTAL							
MINDFULLY: IN THE MOMENT							✓
URGE SURFING							
ALTERNATE REBELLION							
WISE MIND	✓	✓				✓	✓
Distress Tolerance Skills							
DISTRACT: WISE MIND "ACCEPTS"				✓		✓	
SELF-SOOTHE THE FIVE SENSES		✓	✓			✓	✓
"IMPROVE" THE MOMENT	✓	✓	✓	✓	✓	✓	✓
RADICAL ACCEPTANCE							
PROS AND CONS							
BURNING YOUR BRIDGES							
ADAPTIVE DENIAL							
Interpersonal Effectiveness Skills							
OBJECTIVES EFFECTIVENESS: "DEAR MAN"			✓		✓	✓	
RELATIONSHIP EFFECTIVENESS: "GIVE"			✓		✓	✓	
SELF-RESPECT EFFECTIVENESS: "FAST"							
Emotion Regulation Skills							
REDUCE VULNERABILITY: "PLEASE"	✓	✓	✓		✓	✓	✓
BUILD MASTERy:	✓	✓	✓		✓	✓	✓
BUILD POSITIVE EXPERIENCES		✓				✓	✓
OPPOSITE TO EMOTION ACTION				✓			

110

APPENDIX 4.4. Milieu Correction/Overcorrection Protocol for Egregious Behavior

Use when: An episode of parasuicidal or egregious behavior occurs

Assign and orient to protocol
A. Clinical lead (or designated staff) assigns and orients patients to protocol.
B. Participation in protocol supersedes all other activities.
C. If patient incapable, at the moment, of doing protocol (in restraints, etc.), it is done ASAP.

Step 1: Chain analysis (C.A.)
A. Patient undertakes C.A., guided by worksheet.
B. Patient works on C.A. alone for 2 hours (minimum).
C. Patient presents C.A. to designated staff for feedback.

Step 2: Presentation of C.A. to peers
A. Patient describes incident and presents C.A. to peers in group meeting.
B. Peers give feedback.
C. Patient reviews peer meeting with designated staff and prepares for Step 3.

Step 3: Correction/overcorrection (C/O)
A. With designated staff, patient identifies what has been damaged or needs correction or repair.
B. Patient, together with designated staff, identifies C/O appropriate to damage caused or disarray caused.
C. Patient undertakes C/O (repairs damage, demonstrates change, discussions, community service, etc.).
D. *Patient reviews C/O with designated staff.*

Step 4: Patient returns to normal activities

Implementing Dialectical Behavior Therapy in Residential Forensic Settings with Adults and Juveniles

Robin A. McCann, André Ivanoff,
Henry Schmidt, *and* Bradley Beach

The percentage of severely disordered individuals who are incarcerated continues to grow in the United States. Although some are housed in forensic hospitals, where mental health treatment is a central focus, others are housed in correction facilities primarily for the purposes of retribution and specific deterrence. The notion of rehabilitation per se has become secondary, at least in adult correctional institutions in the United States. The mental health services that are offered are usually limited to those that are constitutionally required, and typically include only treatment of serious psychiatric disturbances such as psychoses or severe depression. The focus of treatment is on acute rather than on enduring symptoms or behaviors (Rotter, Way, Steinbacher, Sawyer, & Smith, 2002). Mental health treatment for the purpose of reducing recidivism, in the United States, has become rare, except within the juvenile justice system. Mental health programming in the U.S. juvenile justice system continues to include rehabilitation as part of its mandate, although in many cases resources have been reduced or diverted to capital projects. Evidence-based mental health programming targeting reductions in recidivism, as outlined in Andrews and Bonta (1998), is more typical of the Canadian justice system than of that in the United States.

In this chapter the terms *forensic* and *correctional* are used to broadly describe legally prescribed settings where mental health services are offered. Specifically, *hospitals* provide treatment for individuals who have committed crimes, but who are judged not guilty by reason of insanity. *Prisons* provide custody and confinement for individuals who have committed crimes and are judged wholly responsible for their behavior. While treatment and mental health services are the first priority in forensic hospitals, they also take place in correctional settings (i.e., prisons), but are considered secondary to safety and security. Where necessary, distinctions are made between forensic hospitals and correctional facilities.

Providing effective treatment in adult and juvenile justice settings is viewed by many as daunting. Research, however, does suggest what works and what does not work. Treatment aimed at reducing criminal recidivism does work to reduce reincarceration. Punishment, on the other hand, does not decrease recidivism (Andrews & Bonta, 1998). Recidivism rates, defined as rearrest within 3 years, are approximately 60% (U.S. Department of Justice, 2002) across types of adult offender groups.

Punishment-based programming such as intensive surveillance, shock incarceration (e.g., an intensive, highly structured boot-camp-like program that is generally shorter in length than a regular prison sentence), and "Scared Straight" programs (Andrews & Bonta, 1998) are positively correlated with recidivism (Andrews, 1997). These data suggest that punishment does not reduce recidivism and may even stimulate crime if one looks solely at recidivism. The most likely reason for recidivism, however, is not the fact that incarceration occurred, but that afterward these individuals return to the same criminogenical conditions, including high-poverty and high-crime neighborhoods, with the same risk factors as when they entered the system.

There is evidence that some correctional and forensic treatments can decrease recidivism among adolescent and adult offenders. Meta-analyses grouping all available published studies find that, on average, treated individuals recidivate 10% less than untreated individuals (Andrews, 1997). When treatment is consistent with known forensic treatment principals, studies suggest it is even more effective. Andrews, Bonta, Gendreau, and Cullen (1990) report that appropriate treatment decreases recidivism rates by 50%.

Given that appropriate treatment does reduce recidivism rates, we review the use of dialectical behavior therapy (DBT) as a promising option. We begin with reasons why DBT may be particularly useful and then describe two established models. The two implementation models we use are the Institute for Forensic Psychiatry at the Colorado Mental Health Institute (CMHIP) and the Washington State Juvenile Rehabilitation Administration (JRA). The realities of forensic and correctional management, client behavior, and staff reactions and concerns are uppermost in our minds as we write, and so are woven throughout this chapter.

Why Apply DBT in Forensic Settings?

There are at least four different reasons for applying DBT in forensic settings:

1. Current treatment of individuals with personality disorders in forensic and correctional settings is inadequate and fails to address both short-term management and adjustment issues and the longer term goals of behavior change, social readaptation, and recidivism reduction.
2. DBT is highly compatible with the best-practice principles for effective treatment in forensic settings treatment.
3. Biosocial theory, used in DBT to explain the etiology of borderline personality disorder (BPD), can also be used to explain the development of other personality disorders, especially antisocial personality disorder (ASPD) and psychopathy, as well as other disorders that are frequently found among correctional populations.
4. Staff burnout, common in highly restricted settings, may be ameliorated by DBT (McCann, Ball, & Ivanoff, 1996).

DBT May Remedy the Inadequate Treatment Currently Provided to Individuals with Personality Disorders in Forensic and Correctional Settings

Few studies target personality disorders, despite the high rates of these disorders in correctional populations. Rotter et al. (2002), who examined 4,700 inmates referred for psychiatric services, found that 21–36% met criteria for personality disorders. In regards to personality disorder subtype, 69% met criteria for ASPD, 10% met criteria for borderline personality disorder, 19% met criteria for not otherwise specified (NOS) personality disorders, and 5% met criteria for other personality disorders (paranoid and schizotypal).

There are no randomized studies targeting individuals with personality disorders in correctional or forensic facilities, despite high incidence rates (Warren et al., 2003). Randomized studies have targeted recidivism in offenders (Porporino & Fabiano, 2000). Nonrandomized studies have targeted symptoms such as anger, depression, coping (McCann et al., 1996), and self-injurious and suicidal behavior (Low, Jones, & Duggan, 2001) among individuals with personality disorders in correctional or forensic facilities.

In an exhaustive review of treatment for individuals with personality disorders in forensic settings, Warren et al. (2003) conclude the following:

1. There is some evidence for the effectiveness of cognitive-behavioral therapy, including DBT, at lower security levels.
2. There are no randomized studies of cognitive-behavioral therapy with individuals with personality disorders who meet criteria for psychopathy.
3. Despite the absence of controlled research, there is some evidence supporting the therapeutic community (TC) model for those with personality disorders. TC is a treatment milieu, not a specific treatment method. Staff and residents working in a TC have significant involvement in decision making and the practicalities of the day-to-day running of the community. The staff–resident hierarchy is flattened and the culture is democratic.
4. The evidence for pharmacological intervention is poor.
5. A range of treatments should be available at each level of security to facilitate consistency of treatment approach.

Given the plethora of individuals with personality disorders, particularly ASPD, in correctional and forensic settings, and the dearth of existing treatment, applying DBT may help remedy this gap.

DBT Is Compatible with Best-Practice Principles for Effective Forensic Treatment

Principle 1. Decreasing Risk of Recidivism

Forensic mental health treatment is most effective when treating the highest risk, or most severe, cases (Andrews & Bonta, 1998). DBT targets multidiagnostic, difficult-to-treat, high-risk individuals who engage in life-threatening behaviors, including those with BPD. Correctional populations are composed of difficult-to-treat, high-risk (to recidivate) individuals. Such individuals include multidiagnostic psychotic individuals with concomitant problems such as substance abuse or dependence, ASPD, or psychopathy.

Lifetime mental illness prevalence rates are reported to be between 50 and 100% in adult correctional populations (Andrews & Bonta, 1998). Teplin (1990), using the most severe diagnoses (schizophrenia, mania, or major depression), found a prevalence rate of 9.5%. A 1997 survey of inmates in state facilities identified 16% as mentally ill (Ditton, 1999). Recent evidence suggests that offenders diagnosed with the most severe mental disorders (e.g., psychotic or bipolar disorder), when symptomatic, are more likely to commit criminal offenses and to behave violently (Hodgins, 2002; Stueve & Lin, 1997). The generally cited figure is that 15% of correctional populations have significant need for mental health services. This, however, does not include personality disorders and it does not include relatively less severe disorders such as mild depression or posttraumatic stress disorder (PTSD). Most important, it does not include individuals whose only disorder is a substance use disorder. Rates of mental illness among juvenile correctional populations are similarly high. In Washington State juvenile settings, approximately 60% of juveniles in JRA custody are regarded as a target population who are broadly in need of mental health services.

As mentioned, some of the most-difficult-to-treat individuals are those with concomitant ASPD or substance use disorders (SUDs). ASPD and SUD are the most frequent diagnoses in adult correctional settings. In males, the prevalence of ASPD in correctional settings is between 27 and 65% (Andrews & Bonta, 1998), in contrast to community samples, where the prevalence is between 1 and 3% (American Psychiatric Association, 1994). In females, the prevalence of ASPD ranges from 12 to 65% in correctional facilities (Rotter et al., 2002). Contrary to common perception, not all incarcerated individuals meet criteria for ASPD. In one study, at least 50% of inmates were not identified as antisocial (Brinded & Mulder, 1999). In addition some "antisocial" behaviors such as lying, mistrust, and "doing your own time" may merely reflect adaptation to correctional culture (Rotter et al., 2002). Conversely, not all individuals with ASPD are incarcerated; clearly such individuals work in politics, academics, business, the church, and so on. Although antisocial characteristics and behaviors are likely found in most individuals in adult forensic settings, many also possess characteristics of the other two Cluster B personality disorders, BPD and narcissistic personality disorder. The overlap in characteristics and typical behavior patterns of individuals with these personality disorders is a primary reason why DBT was initially examined for use with adult forensic and correctional populations.

Substance-related disorders and depressive disorders commonly co-occur with ASPD (American Psychiatric Association, 1994). Most jail detainees with a severe mental disorder (schizophrenia or a major affective disorder) also meet criteria for ASPD (Abram & Teplin, 1991). ASPD and other Cluster B personality disorders also co-occur with psychotic and other major Axis I disorders. For example, in a sample of 107 inmates with either psychotic or major depression diagnoses, 71 carried a concomitant ASPD diagnosis. Individuals with ASPD and a severe Axis I disorder are also at higher risk of recidivism than those with only Axis I disorders (Hodgins & Cote, 1993).

Individuals diagnosed with ASPD, particularly those who meet criteria for psychopathy, are almost always difficult to treat, are frequently multidiagnostic (Blackburn, 2000), and are more likely to recidivate. Individuals who meet criteria for psychopathy compose 10 (Nolan, Volavka, Mohr, & Czobor, 1999) to 22% (Tengstrom, Grann, Langstrom, & Kullgren, 2000) of forensic patients and 11 (Simourd & Hoge, 2000) to 25% of incarcerated offenders (Hare, 1991). It is estimated that 20–30% of inmates with ASPD meet criteria for psychopathy (Hare, 1995).

Forensic patients with high psychopathy scores are more likely to violently recidivate. In other words, of those who have already committed violent offenses, individuals with high psychopathy scores are more likely to commit new violent offenses than individuals with low psychopathy scores. Tengstrom et al. (2000), in a 2-year follow-up of forensic patients, found that patients who met criteria for psychopathy recidivated violently 48% of the time. Patients who did not meet criteria for psychopathy recidivated 14% of the time. Harris, Rice, and Cornier (1991) followed postrelease behavior of mentally disordered offenders for 10 years. Offenders who met criteria for psychopathy recidivated violently 77%. Offenders who did not meet criteria recidivated violently 21%.

Until the advent of DBT, clinicians opined, based on woefully inadequate data, that clinical improvement was at best marginal for those diagnosed with BPD (Linehan, 1993a). Currently, clinicians opine, based on woefully inadequate data, that clinical improvement among individuals with high psychopathy scores is marginal, if not impossible (Hare, 2003). DBT may remedy such clinical pessimism.

Principle 2. Responsivity: Matching Treatment to Learning Styles of Offenders

DBT is a cognitive-behavioral treatment consistent with the second overarching best-practice forensic principle: responsivity. Most meta-analyses find behavioral or cognitive-behavioral treatments the most effective match for offenders with respect to their learning style (Andrews, 1997). In contrast, some nonbehavioral and insight-oriented treatments have been found to be "criminogenic," that is, they may actually stimulate crime (Andrews & Bonta, 1998; Quinsey, Harris, Rice, & Cormier, 1998). Research supporting cognitive-behavioral methods cite skills training, including behavior rehearsal, role plays (targeting self-control rather than external control), problem solving, and emotion regulation as recommended components (Bogue, 2002). Psychopathic individuals may also benefit from cognitive-behavioral treatments (Wong & Hare, 1998). Such individuals are difficult to treat and need intensive and more elaborate treatment, including both individual and group therapy (Salekin, 2002). In summary, DBT includes the cognitive-behavioral methods described and includes group, individual, and milieu modes of treatment.

Principle 3. Criminogenic Needs: Target Risk Factors Associated with Recidivism

Examples of criminogenic needs include substance abuse, poor problem solving, antisocial peers, anger, poor self-management, emotion dysregulation, and antisocial beliefs. Mental disorders represent a risk factor if they are associated with offending. Among other targets, DBT directly targets dysfunctional behaviors, including problems involving emotion regulation, problem solving, self-management, and substance abuse, while simultaneously increasing the behavioral skills and motivation needed to replace problem behaviors and increase functional behaviors. Additionally, DBT interpersonal effectiveness skills (see Linehan, 1993b) can be used to target antisocial beliefs and antisocial interactions through its emphasis on the acquisition of prosocial skills to replace antisocial behaviors, including lying, aggression, and stealing.

Extending Biosocial Theory to ASPD and Psychopathy

In addition to being consistent with forensic best-practice principles, a second reason to apply DBT in forensic settings is that its biosocial theory can be extended to ASPD and psychopathy. Behavioral dyscontrol, impulsivity, irresponsibility, angry outbursts, frequent lying, aggression, and violence toward self and others are common characteristics associated with ASPD and conduct disorder (Black, Baumgard, & Bell, 1995). Impulsivity, irresponsibility, aggression, poor anger management, and pathological lying are also characteristic of psychopathy (Hare, 2003). Some of these attributes, such as impulsivity, angry outbursts, and aggression, are diagnostic of BPD as well (American Psychiatric Association, 1994). Parallels may exist between violent behaviors directed toward others and suicidal behaviors (Fruzzetti, 2000). Empirical evidence suggests that interpersonal aggressiveness may be reinforced by both diminished negative emotional arousal and instrumental gains, similar to suicidal behaviors (Fruzzetti & Levensky, 2000; Rubio & Fruzzetti, 1999). Other possible parallels between the development and maintenance of BPD and ASPD syndromes are described below.

Emotional Vulnerability or Emotional Insensitivity

Biosocial theory views BPD as the result of the transaction of emotional vulnerability with invalidation over time (Linehan, 1993a). This also appears applicable to individuals with ASPD subtypes who exhibit affect dysregulation. Support for an affect dysregulation subgroup of ASPD individuals is found in several studies. Weiss, Davis, Hedlund, and Dong (1984) identified a subgroup of dysphoric antisocial individuals. Reich (1985) summarizes several studies reporting positive responses of antisocial individuals to treatments for affective disorders. Zlotnick (1999) found that affective dysregulation, particularly poor anger management, was significantly related to ASPD in women prisoners, after controlling for BPD.

Psychopathic antisocial individuals, however, appear emotionally insensitive and blunted, requiring more extreme levels of stimulation to regulate themselves than individuals with only characteristics of BPD. Their emotional insensitivity is characterized by sensation seeking (Quay, 1977), low arousal (Eysenck, 1977), low anxiety (Lykken, 1995), and low behavioral inhibition (Frick,1998), as well as with neurologically based difficulties in processing and understanding emotional material (Hare, 2003). They appear to have lower emotional arousal to distressing images and fail to demonstrate differential responses between neutral versus emotion-laden lexical tasks (Hare, 2003). Such temperaments provide significant challenges for parents, resulting in harsh and inconsistent parenting (Frick, 1998). Applying biosocial theory to psychopathic, emotionally insensitive individuals with ASPD, we suggest that ASPD results from the interaction between emotional insensitivity transacting with pervasive and severe invalidation over time.

Invalidating Environment

The invalidating environments of individuals with ASPD or psychopathy are characterized by (1) "disturbed caring," (2) reinforcement of antisocial behavior, and (3) models of antisocial coping and behavior in distressed and chaotic families. Disturbed caring is exemplified by the frequent experience and/or witnessing of physical abuse among inmates (Ditton, 1999) and psychopathic individuals (Weiler & Widom, 1996), as well as within ASPD populations (Waltz, Babcock, Jacobson, & Gottman, 2000). Disturbed caring typically involves harsh and inconsistent discipline, little positive parental involvement, and inadequate supervision; all these are notable family characteristics among children with conduct disorders (Patterson, DeBaryshe, & Ramsey, 1989). Similarly, parental rejection and lack of parental supervision is characteristic of the family background of psychopathic individuals (Hare, 2003). Sensation-seeking behavior on the part of the emotionally insensitive child may increase the frequency of harsh, inconsistent, neglectful, or rejecting parenting (Quay, 1977).

Invalidating environments are not only characterized by disturbed caring but by reinforcement of antisocial behaviors. Antisocial behaviors are often positively reinforced while prosocial skills are punished. Delinquent peers may provide each other with positive feedback for deviant behavior and negative feedback or even punishment for socially conforming behavior (Buehler, Patterson, & Furniss, 1966). Such sensation-seeking behavior may be self-reinforcing for emotionally insensitive children. Families may also negatively reinforce antisocial or coercive behaviors. Parents of children with conduct disorders have been observed to inadvertently negatively reinforce their children's more troubling behaviors (Patterson et al., 1989). In turn, children with conduct disorders negatively reinforce their parents' ineffective parenting (Patterson et al., 1989). Such negative reinforcement of disordered behavior and punishment of prosocial behavior over time serves to maintain conduct-disordered and antisocial behavior patterns. For example, when a parent says "No," the adolescent with conduct disorder may threaten the parent, resulting in the parent avoiding future assertion, which negatively and intermittently reinforces the adolescent's escalation of aversive emotional responses, that is, threats.

This same dynamic can be witnessed in forensic settings. Biosocial theory specifies that such invalidation plays a part not only in etiology, but also in the maintenance of disorder. For example, the same problematic reinforcement contingencies can be seen in forensic settings. When residents do something kind to help someone else, such as going out of their way to make sure someone else is treated fairly, it is common for staff to invalidate valid behavior by responding with suspicion, perhaps inaccurately accusing the antisocial resident of "manipulation" or "grooming," in this way punishing the helpful behavior.

However, prosocial behaviors in the free world may function as antisocial behavior in the correctional world and vice versa. For example, in the free world it is considered prosocial to "turn the other cheek" and even to do something nice for someone who has harmed you. In the correctional world, such behavior may be seen as weak and vulnerable. Similarly, in the free world it is considered prosocial and adaptive to ask for help from authority figures. In correctional settings, people who do this may be labeled "snitches" and threatened, injured, or even killed.

DBT May Reduce Staff Burnout

The final reason to consider DBT is its direct treatment of staff stress and burnout. Stress among staff in correctional facilities is widespread and severe (Schaufeli & Peeters, 2000). Burnout linked to stress is characterized by pessimism toward one's work, frequent apathy or anger directed toward patients, and withdrawal from patient contacts and job duties (Jones, 1981). Correlates of burnout include factors common in forensic settings, such as high patient-to-staff ratios, frequent direct care contact with difficult-to-treat patients (Maslach & Jackson, 1993), and less experienced staff (Morgan, Van Haveren, & Pearson, 2002). Intrarole conflict—for example, conflict between security and therapeutic roles—is also positively correlated with burnout (Allard, Wortley, & Stewart, 2003; Schaufeli & Peeters, 2000). Biosocial theory serves to help maintain a more compassionate, hopeful stance about working with individuals with antisocial or borderline behavioral disorders. Further, the use of a DBT case consultation group functions to address the challenge of remaining on therapeutic task, as well as maintaining motivation and hope.

For these reasons, it makes sense to consider DBT. We now turn to a description of two DBT program settings as examples, an adult forensic hospital, the CMHIP[1], and the youth correctional system in Washington State, the Juvenile Youth Administration JRA[2], to illustrate the adaptation of traditional DBT to highly restricted settings with adjudicated and mentally ill residents. Both of these programs are residential and long-term, with average lengths of stay of 1 year or longer. Although they manifest some differences, they share primary adaptations. The implementation of these programs took place over several years, and, as discussed in the final section of this chapter, administrative needs, supports, and resources figure prominently in their development.

The forensic model for adults developed at CMHIP has been previously described (McCann et al., 2000). The majority of the residents at the Institute for Forensic Psychiatry at CMHIP have been adjudicated not guilty by reason of insanity (NGRI) of generally violent crimes. Of these 180 individuals adjudicated NGRI, 160 patients are male. Most CMHIP patients carry Axis I diagnoses and approximately one-third carry a concomitant Axis II diagnosis (Colorado Department of Human Services, 1999). The majority of patients also have concomitant substance use disorders. The length of stay from maximum security to community placement is usually determined by the legal system and the patients' progress in treatment. The mean length of stay from maximum security to community placement is currently 6 years (C. Lewis, personal communication, October 13, 2004). The Institute for Forensic Psychiatry at CMHIP implemented comprehensive[3] DBT on one medium- and one minimum-security unit in 1995. McCann and colleagues collected uncontrolled data for 19 months. When outcomes for DBT residents were compared to a treatment-as-usual group, they demonstrated increased effective coping, decreased ineffective coping, and decreased hostility and depression (McCann, Ball, & Ivanoff, 1996). Currently, comprehensive DBT is implemented on one ward; DBT skills groups and correction/overcorrection protocols (see Swenson, Witterholt, & Bohus, Chapter 4, this volume, on inpatient DBT) are implemented on seven other wards.

Treatment of adolescents in long-term highly restrictive settings presents a formidable challenge due to a historical emphasis on retribution; accountability; lack of resources and training for staff, particularly relative to mental health inpatient facilities; and an environment that tends to exacerbate behaviors that are symptomatic of mental or emotional disorders. The Washington State JRA offers a continuum of care for adjudicated adolescents, ranging from large residential facilities (178–220 youth) to work camps, community group homes, and parole. A significant number of youth across these institutions have mental health problems (Cauffman, Scholler, Mulvey, & Kelleher, 2005).

In 1997 the JRA, in collaboration with the State Department of Social and Health Services, began a pilot project exploring the use of DBT to treat extreme mental health-related behaviors in its resident juvenile offender population. In an uncontrolled evaluation, promising results were found in reducing suicidal and assaultive behaviors when compared to other youth not enrolled in DBT. Further, important reductions in felony recidivism were found at 12 months postrelease for these difficult-to-treat youth (Washington State Institute for Public Policy, 2002). Based on the early success of this model, the expanding population of mentally ill and multiple-problem youth across the JRA population (i.e., chemically dependent, cognitively delayed, medically fragile, and/or sex offending), and JRA's commitment to the development of programming based on evidence-based cognitive-behavioral principles, DBT has since been incorporated into the integrated treatment model developed for all JRA youth. The pilot project adaptations of both JRA and CMHIP will be discussed here.

Forensic Application of DBT Stages and Targets of Treatment

Stage 1 Primary and Secondary Targets

DBT treatment stages were applied to the forensic treatment environment and the demands of the highly restricted residential treatment setting. Consistent with forensic risk and treatment principles and DBT, Stage 1 targets are conceptualized as two phases. Stage 1, Phase 1 targets include decreasing severe behavioral dyscontrol, that is, decreasing verbal threats and unit destructive behaviors, and increasing self-management (The Stage 1, Phase 1 primary treatment targets are summarized in Table 5.1.) Phase 2 targets include relapse prevention or "coping ahead."

Because forensic treatment must always target risk factors associated with violent recidivism (Hodgins, 2002), Phase 2 primarily targets relapse prevention. It is our experience that residents are unable to tolerate phase 2 until they have gained behavioral control (Phase 1). Relapse prevention is addressed through the DBT Crime Review Group outlined in Appendix 5.1.

The use of the Stage 1 primary behavioral target hierarchy helps staff accomplish several treatment objectives. First, given the variety of problem behaviors exhibited by residents in these settings, it provides an attention/selection algorithm for staff to utilize while working in the milieu. The hierarchy avoids potential conflict among staff about what priority behaviors are, thereby improving staff cohesion and teamwork. Intense focus of the entire staff team on egregious behaviors has facilitated rapid reductions in events high in medical risk and legal liability. Such reductions in egregious behaviors function to enhance staff motivation to engage in DBT.

Linehan (1993a) described secondary behavioral targets as rigid, ineffective behavior patterns functionally related to the Stage 1 primary treatment targets. Secondary targets common among patients with BPD during Stage 1 treatment include emotion vulnerability, self-invalidation, active passivity, apparent competence, unrelenting crises, and inhib-

TABLE 5.1. Stage 1, Phase 1 Primary Treatment Targets for Forensic DBT

Treatment target	Examples of targeted behavior
1. Decreasing imminently life-threatening behaviors	Suicidal, homicidal, and self-injurious behaviors, including thoughts, urges, and actions associated with these behaviors.
2. Decreasing unit-destroying behaviors	Using drugs and other substances; selling drugs; "setting up" other residents in "stings"; stealing; planting evidence; "paybacks"; sexual relationships with members of the same sex; destroying rooms or making them unsafe or uninhabitable; escapes, including executing or planning escape for self or others; and other behaviors requiring "clear the floor" security interventions, thereby shutting down the treatment program.
3. Decreasing treatment-interfering behaviors	Those that reduce the team's, the individual's, or other residents' ability to participate in treatment (e.g., using sensitive or embarrassing information to hurt another patient, "shining" [looking good at the expense of others]).
4. Decreasing quality-of-life-interfering behaviors	Offense-specific behaviors, specifically if seen on the unit (e.g., stealing, "grooming others for sex"); high-risk behaviors reported from the community (e.g., chemical dependency, criminal involvement, criminal peers, homelessness); behaviors related to Axis I disorders; other behaviors associated with risk for recidivism.

ited grieving (Linehan, 1993a; see Koerner & Dimeff, Chapter 1, this volume, for a description). Linehan (2000) suggests that different disorders will reflect different secondary treatment targets. Several of the original secondary targets Linehan identified apply well to forensic patients. *Apparent competence* versus *active passivity* has been particularly relevant for individuals with ASPD. Apparent competence occurs when other people (most often staff) erroneously assess a resident as more competent than he or she really is. A common cause of apparent competence among forensic residents in restricted settings is failure to generalize skills. A classic example is the resident with ASPD who demonstrates good interpersonal skills for years with many on the inpatient unit, a context where demands are relatively low compared to the demands of living in the community. Given the apparently competent appearance, staff do not assist in preparing the resident for obstacles he or she may encounter upon release as they might a client who appears less competent and more obviously "in need" of assistance with skills generalization.

While progressing toward release, the resident becomes quickly overwhelmed with problems such as job, food, finances, medications, transportation, housing, and loneliness. While behaviorally adept in the residential facility, behavioral skills and self-management strategies fail to generalize to this new context. For example, the resident applies for a job, but the job market is tight and few employers wish to hire someone with a criminal history. Functional behaviors in hospital (e.g., telling the truth to clinicians) are not reinforced in this context. For example, one inmate informed his potential employer, a church deacon, that, while psychotic, he had cannibalized his victim. Aghast, the deacon called the police.

Habitual dysfunctional behaviors, such as lying ("I have no criminal history") and grandstanding ("No, I don't need a referral to vocational services") are, in the short term, reinforced. An impervious job market, shame, and cognitions ("Staff don't care" and "I hope for a miracle") interfere with effective behavior such as using interpersonal skills to ask for help. The resident claims he is doing well, when he is not. Ultimately he concludes, "F_ _ _ it!" He engages in a variety of behaviors ensuring intervention by authorities: He obtains a job with false references, falsely claims he obtained a job, tells lies that will be quickly uncovered, mindfully steals in front of the Loaf and Jug convenience store security camera, purposely uses marijuana immediately prior to a tox screen, escapes for one night to voluntarily return the next day, and so on—in sum, he practices *active passivity*. Should this dilemma remain undetected, the individual may be at increased risk to resume higher target Stage 1 behaviors. Upon detection, clinicians, who believed the resident was more competent than he really was, may name call (e.g., liar, psychopath) and express anger, disappointment, and hopelessness. Invalidated, the resident once again becomes uncomfortable and oscillates to apparently competent behavior. Clinician failure to observe the forensic resident's secondary targets ultimately destroys the therapeutic alliance, results in premature progression to the community, and ultimately leads to life-threatening behaviors.

We added two secondary targets for individuals with ASPD or psychopathic characteristics: *decreasing criminal identification* and *increasing citizenship*. Criminal personality and criminal cognitions are highly correlated with both violent and nonviolent recidivism (Quinsey, Harris, Rice, & Cormier, 2006). Criminal personality is defined as a high score on the Psychopathy Checklist. Criminal cognitions include sentiments promoting illegal behavior, alienation, aggression, and a victim stance. In contrast, a "citizen" is a person who owes allegiance to society, and who is, in turn, entitled to its protection. How could those living in restricted settings not lose their allegiance to "citizens"? The real consequences of their egregious behaviors, which include reduced societal status, incarceration, involuntary treatment, involuntary medications, and often ambivalent treatment providers, lead forensic residents to view them as alienated victims. Custodial staff, administrators and treatment providers, perhaps as a function of declaring their own citizenship, will insist that residents are "nothing but criminals." Such a context fuels the residents' justification of criminal sentiments: "I won't get caught," "No one matters but me," "Only the strong survive," "An eye for an eye," and so on.

Without citizenship, belonging, attachment, and connection, a "life worth living" within society is not possible. Validation of the Herculean effort needed to become a "citizen" is essential. Given the challenge of becoming a "citizen" in a context that intermittently punishes such efforts, oscillation between criminal identification and citizenship is expected. Irreverence is helpful: "You murdered a child. Of course others dislike you!" On the one hand, everything is as it should be. On the other hand, "What skills can you use to tolerate your distress?"

In addition to the original secondary targets identified by Linehan and those developed specifically for forensic populations, others described in this book may also apply. The courts, mental health professionals, correctional officers, and others control the contingencies of highly restricted individuals. Adults control the contingencies of adolescents. Therefore, it holds true that the secondary targets of the nonincarcerated adolescent (see Miller, Rathus, DuBose, Dexter-Mazza, & Goldklang, Chapter 9, this volume; and Miller, Rathus, & Linehan, 2006) also apply to restricted adult and juvenile populations. The adolescent secondary targets of decreasing authoritarian control and increasing adolescent self-determination are of particular relevance.

Stage 2 Targets

Consistent with standard DBT, after forensic residents achieve behavioral control, treatment targets shift. We limit our treatment of the standard Stage 2 target, quiet desperation, for two reasons. First, there is no compelling evidence that emotional experiencing is related to reducing factors linked to criminal behavior. Second, despite common trauma histories, a majority of our patients appear to experience emotions fluidly after Stage 1 DBT. Nevertheless, when needed and feasible, we target emotional desperation via individual exposure therapy (see Foa & Rothbaum, 1998). To date, such exposure has not resulted in violence, consistent with the literature (Foa, Zoellner, Feeny, & Hembree, 2002).

Forensic Modification of Treatment Functions

Consideration of the functions (rather than the modes) of comprehensive DBT addresses the challenge of implementing DBT in forensic settings with poor staff-to-resident ratios. Chapter 1 overviews the standard functions of comprehensive DBT: enhancing capabilities, improving motivation, generalization of skills, improving the environment's motivation to provide effective treatment, and enhancing staff motivation and capabilities. In residential restricted settings, improving motivation, generalization of skills, and improving the environment's motivation to provide effective treatment are accomplished as part of milieu treatment.

Increasing Skills Capability

Consistent with standard DBT, skill acquisition and strengthening occur in skills training groups that are structured just as they are in a standard outpatient DBT program.

McCann et al. (2000) originally adapted the DBT skills for use in a forensic setting through extensive consultation with residents with antisocial characteristics. Adaptations target emotional insensitivity and concomitant apathy and criminal identification that is characteristic of antisocial patients. To ensure that residents actually *learned* the skills, skills acquisition was measured by both written and role-play quizzes. (See Figure 5.1 for examples.) Should a resident fail the written quiz, he has the opportunity to pass the role-play quiz and vice versa. When residents have completed two full cycles of DBT skills and have passed the final quiz, they are eligible to progress to advanced DBT groups (see below).

Staff who are most effective at teaching skills figure out how to incorporate fun and games into the practice. For example, when spiking a volleyball or dunking a basketball, yell out the name of a DBT skill! Create a rap song summarizing DBT skills. Identify mindfulness skills in the films *Crouching Tiger, Hidden Dragon* or *Finding Nemo*. Participate in a scavenger hunt accumulating items for a personalized distress tolerance kit (obviously we're not suggesting this in a maximum security facility). While it may appear naive to expect hardened criminals or disaffected oppositional adolescents to participate in such games, our experience is that they participate with creativity and gusto. One of the authors (R. M.) routinely integrates music and dancing with her forensic residents. Although many staff avoid dancing, most of the residents participate, at times adding hip-hop steps. A nonjudgmental stance and a willingness to risk feeling self-conscious and embarrassed (which is particularly difficult for staff) is essential.

Increasing Skills Generalization

Correctional research suggests that treatment is more effective in community than in residential environments (Andrews & Bonta, 1998). Further, risk assessment traditionally operates on the unsupported belief that residential behavior accurately predicts behavior postrelease. But we do not take that for granted in DBT. Instead we think of skill generalization as an important goal that cannot be assumed. Skills coaching, cue exposure, and advanced DBT groups in the milieu and the community help to increase skills generalization.

A common "teachable moment" in forensic settings is when a resident's goals are blocked by staff refusal to grant a request. Often, following this event, the resident quickly escalates and argues.

> Dee is a 16-year-old female diagnosed with BPD who places high demands on the unit staff. She becomes highly emotionally dysregulated when denied a request. Due to previous cutting, Dee has a deep open wound on her arm. When denied a request, she pulls out a vein out of her arm, eliciting shock and disgust from all who are near her. Active staff intervention is required or, at worst, security staff are required to physically move or restrain her.
>
> An effective intervention using skills coaching that occurred with Dee unfolded in the following way.

> DEE: Can I get an extra snack? I'm really hungry.
> STAFF: I don't know if I should answer that; if I say "no" are you going to pull the vein out of your arm? [irreverent communication]
> DEE: Well, no. [She probably would have if staff would have said no then.]
> STAFF: So, if I say no to your request what skill could you use?

Emotion Regulation Module

1. Robert drinks 20 cups of caffeine coffee per day, 20 Mountain Dew sodas per day and is up all night on his computer. He is irritable and anxious. What ABC PLEASE skill does Robert most need?
2. TRUE or FALSE? In order to use the DBT ACTING OPPOSITE TO THE CURRENT EMOTION skill you must ignore your true feelings.

Answers: 1. AVOID MOOD-ALTERING DRUGS, 2. FALSE

Mindfulness Module

3. Ed did not receive a Christmas present from his family. His roommate Jason received eight presents from his family. Ed flushes one of Jason's presents down the toilet. CIRCLE ONE: Ed's behavior is an example of:

    Wise Mind   Emotional Mind   Reasonable Mind

Answer: 3. EMOTIONAL MIND

Distress Tolerance Module

4. The parole board turned down Albert. Albert feels hopeless. He tries the DBT skill COMPARISONS. It doesn't work. He tries all the other DBT WISE MIND ACCEPTS skills. They don't work. What should Albert do?

Answer: 4. Albert should do WISE MIND ACCEPTS over and over again. Or Albert should try IMPROVE THE MOMENT over and over again.

Interpersonal Effectiveness Module

5. When Ed attends Community Therapy he becomes so angry he cannot think. Which of the following factors is most interfering with Ed's interpersonal effectiveness? CIRCLE ONE:

    a. Worry   b. Environment   c. Lack of Skill   d. Indecision   e. Emotion

6. Role-Play: DEAR MAN. Examinee Instructions: Sam always violates the phone rules. He doesn't log in his call. He doesn't keep to the 15-minute time limit. You are unable to use the phone to call your wife. Demonstrate how you might use the DBT DEAR MAN skill.

    Examiner instructions: Need two examiners. One examiner role-plays Sam. The second examiner checks and records how the examinee demonstrated each component of DEAR MAN.

Answer 5: EMOTION

Answer 6:   ✗ D: *Explains to Sam that wife is pregnant.*

               ✗ E: *Explains he is worried about wife.*

               ✗ A: *"Will you keep the time limit?"*

               ✗ R: "I'll give you a cigarette."

               ✗ M: Ignores Sam's rationalizations and verbal attacks.

               ✗ A: Good eye contact, audible speech, shoulders squared, and so on.

               ✗ N: When Sam says "No," examinee negotiates: "Just in the evenings."

FIGURE 5.1. Examples of DBT quiz items.

DEE: I don't know, radical acceptance?

STAFF: (*Gives her a high five.*) That's it, you got it. I know this is really hard, but do you think you could use radical acceptance in this situation?

DEE: I don't know, maybe, but I really need that snack.

STAFF: Of course [validation], but sometimes here we have rules or situations that we can't change at the time, and that's when you can use this skill.

DEE: But I really just want you to give me the snack.

STAFF: But if you have done your best to get me to give it to you and I say "No," what choice do you have? [commitment strategy]

DEE: I guess none but to accept it, but I don't think it's fair.

STAFF: You may be right! It may or may not be, but the point is you can get through this without making it worse if you use the skill. Are you willing to try?

DEE: I guess.

STAFF: I don't want to force you to use it, I can talk to you about it later if you want. Are you sure you want to try it? [commitment strategy]

DEE: Yeah, I want to do it.

STAFF: OK, now I want you to ask me for the snack and if I say "No," what skill are you going to use?

DEE: Radical acceptance.

STAFF: That's it! Now go ahead and ask! [cheerleading]

DEE: Can I have an extra snack?

STAFF: No, not now. We don't give out snacks until this evening.

DEE: (*getting visibly angry*) But . . .

STAFF: (*gently interrupting*) Use your skills, Dee, you can do it. [cheerleading]

DEE: I don't think that's fair and I don't like it, but I can accept it.

STAFF: That was it, nice job! I know that was hard. [reinforcement and validation]

DEE: Yeah, it was, but I can do it.

STAFF: You did! I knew you could! [reinforcement and cheerleading] Do you want to help me pass out the mail? [reinforcement and distraction to activities]

DEE: Sure.

The integration of dialectical, commitment, and behavioral strategies with skills is essential in facilitating progress. The following case illustrates such integration.

Steve is a 45-year-old African American man diagnosed with schizophrenia and alcohol abuse. He was convicted of sexual assault. While serving his sentence in the prison, he bit a correctional officer, resulting in his not guilty by reason of insanity (NGRI) adjudication. Steve describes a history of victimization: experiencing racism while growing up in the South, false conviction of sexual assault (records suggest that he is innocent), and victimization by Department of Correction guards. Steve does not believe he has schizophrenia and views this diagnosis and his court-ordered medications as additional evidence of white victimization. He has a 10-year history of medication noncompliance, paranoia, and assaults on staff and peers. He desperately wished to leave the hospital, as evidenced by unsuccessful yearly writs for release and escape.

When Steve perceives staff or peers as lying he becomes paranoid. On the one hand, given that he lives in a forensic hospital, his perception of lying is frequently correct. He views staff insistence that he accept his diagnosis and medication as lying. He believes that staff, following the orders of a corrupt military, have an ulterior motive, the desire to victimize black men. In response, Steve "cheeks" his medications, becomes increasingly paranoid, blames staff, blames peers, and eventually assaults someone. This results in emergency medication, restrictions, and court-ordered medications—and this is more evidence to Steve that he is a victim.

An intervention was implemented as follows. First, staff accepted that 10 years of pushing "change" had failed: Educating Steve regarding his mental illness, encouraging him to take medications, and so on was not working. Treatment strategies were balanced as follows. We clarified consequences (contingencies): When staff tell him he has schizophrenia, he feels victimized. When staff tell him he needs medication, he feels victimized. We clarified that we could not agree he did not need medication (observing limits). We agreed that when he feels victimized, Steve ultimately retaliates, victimizing others. This ultimately results in negative consequences for himself and others, which supports his belief that he is a victim.

We asked Steve what would be most effective in resolving this dilemma, that is, that our very attempts to help him caused him to feel victimized (i.e., we used entering the paradox). Steve thought about this for several weeks and then explained that if he were "a can of peas" and someone else labeled him "a can of asparagus," he still would be "a can of peas" (metaphor)." He decided that when others label him as "schizophrenic" (asparagus) he would still be "a can of peas, Steve," not a victim. Further, Steve applied the mindfulness skill of effectiveness. We determined that, given his assault history, it is unlikely a judge would release him from the hospital without medication compliance (highlighting absence of alternatives). Thus while Steve has not accepted the diagnosis of paranoid schizophrenia, he accepts that others call him such. Steve is voluntarily taking medications, without a victim stance; has safely resided in the community for more than 1 year; and is progressing toward unconditional release.

The following interventions, implemented in consecutive order, may help build the motivation and skills of staff to provide this type of milieu coaching:

1. Inclusion of milieu skills coaching in correctional staff job appraisal plans. Discipline territoriality and union regulations can interfere. Cordial and equitable relations with other disciplines and support from administration is crucial.

2. Teaching and modeling of skills coaching to staff by high-status nursing or correctional administrators. For example, the division chief or unit leader nurse could briefly review the DBT willingness skill in staff meetings, for example, at the "Monday Morning Meeting." As Monday progresses, supervisors and other staff continue to teach willingness to additional staff in 5-minute "teaching on the hoof" episodes. Throughout the week staff keep a tally of their willingness coaching frequency.

3. Skill of the week. Everyone coaches the same skill all week. Given the high rates of aggressive resident assault (26%; Scott, 2004) precipitated by staff request, staff are understandably reluctant to implement the protocol. The solution to this problem involves ensuring that residents are fully oriented to skills coaching prior to its use.

4. Contests. Staff record their frequency of DBT skills coaching on a staff DBT diary card. These staff diary cards are reviewed by the DBT case consult team. Whoever emits the highest frequency of coaching wins the dollar store grab bag. The grab bag includes

typical dollar store items: note pads, playing cards, food, inexpensive clothing items, cosmetics, and the like.

Ideally, staff coach residents to use skills to handle difficult situations (i.e., cues). Conversely, there are definitely times when staff must remove emotionally dysregulating cues. For example, if residents do not have the skill to handle a particular cue, staff may encourage them to take a time-out until their anger decreases. Alternatively, exposure to emotionally dysregulating cues, although perhaps counterintuitive, may be the most effective means of facilitating skills generalization.

Joe is a 40-year-old man with BPD, ASPD, bipolar disorder, and alcohol dependence who murdered five people and resides in a forensic hospital. He becomes emotionally dysregulated by schedule changes and interpersonal conflict. A counselor changed the time of group therapy. The next day when the counselor said "Good Morning," Joe screamed "F_ _ _ you! Stop playing games with my head!" Frightened, the counselor's first urge was to convince the team to send Joe to a higher security ward. The counselor's second urge was to avoid greeting Joe altogether. During DBT case consultation, the counselor's fear was validated in the context of Joe's violent history. In addition the consultation team noted that Joe had become a fear cue for the counselor and the counselor had become an anger cue for Joe. Because Joe's swearing was regarded as merely therapy-interfering, however, he was not transferred to a higher security ward. Given that Joe had not assaulted anyone in 10+ years, it seemed likely that he could learn to tolerate the counselor's greeting, without abusive tirades. The team's intervention plan included:

1. Orienting Joe. The counselor would continue to greet him, in order to expose him to a common cue in this and outside communities: greetings. Joe agreed that this intervention made sense as he wished to obtain a job in the community, ideally working in a supermarket.
2. Joe committed to blocking his aggressive or abusive responses. Initially, Joe appeared irritated and ignored greetings.
3. After repeated greetings with coaching, Joe reluctantly (with coaching) began to reciprocate the counselor's greeting (opposite action). He then moved to initiate greetings, and ultimately began to seek out the counselor for unscheduled chats.

At CMHIP, several additional "advanced" DBT Phase 2 groups have been added for residents who have already completed at least one cycle, but more typically two cycles, and "graduated" from all four DBT skills modules. The advanced groups include crime review group, behavior analysis group, skills integration group, and community placement group. Criteria for entry in advanced groups includes a passing score on the DBT written final exam (see Figure 5.1), no life-threatening or ward-destructive behavior for at least 6 months, and behavioral demonstration of skills use in the milieu.

The crime review group functions as a relapse prevention group. The resident first completes a thorough behavior analysis of his offense(s) including cross-reference with police and other official offense reports. He identifies links in the behavior analysis where he could have used skills. He articulates which skills he could have used. This becomes the basis of his relapse prevention plan. Appendix 5.1 provides a protocol for crime review group.

The behavioral analysis group can take place on a residential or community basis. Behavioral analyses are chosen according to their importance on the Stage 1 target hierarchy. Residents identify the prompting event, vulnerability factors, and effective and ineffective links, and the brainstorm solutions, corrections, and overcorrections. Residents troubleshoot solutions, choose a solution, and role play. (See Appendix 5.2 for a protocol for behavior analysis group.)

The skills integration group integrates skills from DBT and other relevant groups including the University of California Los Angeles Psychosocial Skills Training[4] (Clinical Research Center for Schizophrenia and Psychiatric Rehabilitation, 1988) and the Reasoning and Rehabilitation Cognitive Skills[5] training (Porporino & Fabiano, 2000). Clients structure the agenda, bringing in their current problems for assessment, solution analysis, and role play. Group members also propose (using the DBT interpersonal effectiveness skills of DEAR MAN) situations that they would like others to work on. Each group starts with an update from the group member who consulted with the group the prior week. The community placement group uses the same format as the skills integration group except the group occurs in community settings (e.g., a group member's apartment, boarding homes, clubhouses).

Increasing Resident Motivation Using Correction/Overcorrection Protocols

High-level Stage 1 target behaviors including suicidal, aggressive, and destructive behaviors usually result in application of correction/overcorrection protocols. Swenson, Sanderson, Dulit, and Linehan (2002) outline three steps of the correction/overcorrection protocol and they are explained further in Chapter 4 of this book.

Consistently implementing these protocols in forensic settings is a Herculean task. First, it is essential that the team have consensus on the list of behaviors that will result in a resident being placed "on protocol." The selection of behaviors should derive from and follow the Stage 1 target hierarchy. Second, given the high rates of aggressive resident assault (26%; Scott, 2004) precipitated by staff request, staff are understandably reluctant to implement the protocol. The solution to this problem involves ensuring that residents are fully oriented to the protocol prior to its use. Such "coping ahead" includes practicing skills such as radical acceptance prior to receiving an egregious protocol. Orientation decreases, but does not eliminate, resident opinion that the protocols are "punishment." Thankfully, over time, we have found that protocols become part of the culture. It is understood that gaining control over these problematic behaviors is linked to goals. Savvy residents learn to initiate protocols and ask for chain analysis forms, saving themselves and staff time and trouble. Similarly, it is mandatory that staff practice skillful assignment of the behavioral chain analysis in case consultation. Figure 5.2 outlines recommended steps staff should take in assigning protocols.

As is always the case in DBT, maintaining a dialectic of adherence versus flexibility is essential. Adherence means following the protocol. Flexibility means considering the context (e.g., staffing ratios, patient's current mental status, time of day) in which the protocol is administered. For example, Napa State Hospital found that the peak time for staff assaults is between 6:00 P.M. and 8:00 P.M. (Scott, 2004). This would suggest particular staff prudence and skillfulness when placing residents on egregious behavior protocol during this time period.

The primary tasks in responding to suicidal behavior are to keep residents safe and to respond in a way that decreases the probability of further suicidal behavior. Responding to suicidal behavior without inadvertently reinforcing it presents a difficult challenge. Unit staff are trained to respond in a manner that maximizes residents' safety. Policies require regular monitoring behavior, up to and including one-to-one observation.

_____ T orients P to Protocol

       _____ T nonjudgmentally OBSERVES and DESCRIBES PROBLEM BEHAVIOR.

       _____ T informs P that he is on protocol. T reminds P that the faster he completes the protocol, the faster he will resume his privileges and normal treatment programming.

       _____ T hands P "Chain Analysis Worksheet." If P throws worksheet on ground, T does not pick it up.

_____ T validates P's distress. T hypothesizes primary emotions other than anger; hopelessness or shame may be good bets. A Nonjudgmental Stance and Radical Genuineness is invaluable.

_____ If P is unwilling, T coaches commitment strategies.

       _____ T highlights P's freedom to comply (or not) with the protocol. It is not the job of any T to force P to complete the chain analysis.

       _____ T links protocol completion with P's goals.

       _____ T cheerleads.

       _____ T uses shaping, particularly important with irate, cognitively limited, or psychotic individuals.

       _____ T uses contingencies—for example, "I'd love to talk with you after you complete the chain analysis!"

_____ If P verbally abusive, or still unwilling, T politely walks away. Note, P is still on protocol even if he refuses or abuses T.

Anti-DBT Tactics

_____ Inflexibility. T gives chain even though staffing ratios are poor, the unit is "high," and such assignment will escalate P to assault. Conversely, T avoids giving chain in order to avoid name calling, verbal abuse, and interpersonal conflict.

_____ T is unwilling or unable to nonjudgmentally DESCRIBE problem behavior.

_____ T argues, tries to reason, threatens punishment, is unable or unwilling to ignore P's threats of grievances (and the like).

_____ T assigns chain as "revenge."

_____ T spends more than 5 minutes assigning chain.

FIGURE 5.2. Checklist for assigning behavioral chain analysis without getting assaulted.

Often the task of "logging" on residents or one-on-one observation falls to the most junior and therefore least-trained and least experienced staff. In these situations, boredom, inexperience, and the staff's own emotional response to suicidal and self-harm behavior may increase the likelihood that they will respond to reduce their own discomfort in a way that increases the likelihood of suicidal behaviors in the resident. Strict protocols are reviewed with staff defining interaction with residents during monitoring and one-on-one, and when possible, staff members are assigned who are known to be not reinforcing for that particular resident. Discussion is limited to use of skills or work on a correction/overcorrection worksheet, and the 24-hour rule[6] is enforced between residents and their primary staff.

> Serena is a 16-year-old who has many BPD criterion behaviors. She has an extensive history of severe self-mutilation that has been escalating over the past 6 months. She also has a history of destructive behaviors and assaults on others, including staff.

When not emotionally dysregulated, she is charming, bright, and engaging. Due to the consequences involved in confronting Serena, staff tend to avoid making behavioral demands on her (excessive leniency) until her escalation interferes with the overall functioning of the unit.

The staff then decide to "crack down" (authoritarian control) on her, which triggers an emotional response and severe self-harm and aggressive behaviors. Staff respond by relaxing behavioral demands and increasing social contact with Serena, spending a great deal of time talking with her and soothing her. This is effective at decreasing her emotional arousal and problematic behavior. In reality, staff are inadvertently cuing and reinforcing maladaptive behavior, that is, the self-harm and aggressive behaviors "work" while the resident inadvertently reinforces staff's maladaptive response to her.

The team's plan that finally helped Serena gain control of her behavior included:

1. *Behavioral analysis*: Serena was required to work on and complete an exhaustive behavioral chain analysis by herself prior to joining the rest of the unit for any activities (negative reinforcement).

2. *24-hour rule*: Serena was not allowed contact with her primary counselor in the unit for 24 hours after any major incident. Feedback on the behavioral chain analysis and all other needs and requests went through other unit staff.

3. *Behavioral rehearsal*: Serena practiced a replacement behavior or skill that would result in a more adaptive response and then practiced it with unit staff.

4. *Correction/overcorrection*: Serena corrected the harm that was done and made amends to the staff and possibly the whole unit if her behavior caused the loss of free time or the like, for other residents. In her next counseling session with her primary therapist, Serena then discussed her behavior analysis in detail, troubleshooting any problems with the solutions generated. Defining the behavior as *respondent* (under the control of the precipitant) or as *operant* (under the control of the consequence) plays a role in determining staffs' milieu response and subsequent intervention. In Serena's situation, this involved strict adherence to the egregious behavior protocol (extinction) and orienting the staff to expect a behavioral burst (increase in target behavior following an extinction intervention). The intervention also included teaching Serena distress-tolerance and emotion-regulation skills. Serena rehearsed these interventions with her therapist and then was reinforced in the milieu every time she made an attempt to use the skills in a real situation. Staff reinforced Serena's use of skills with principles of shaping, where successive approximations to the ultimate goal are coached and reinforced. She was given bonus points if she was able to use them when she was emotionally dysregulated, which eventually resulted in skill generalization. The combination of sound behavioral principles and teaching and reinforcing new, more skillful behavior, resulted in a gradual decline in her self-harm and assaultive behavior.

DBT Training and Implementation Recommendations

Administrative Support for Program Implementation

Forensic and correctional settings are faced with growing resource constraints. If optimal planning begins by asking "What do you need to do the job?", the more likely question heard today is, "How little can you get by with?" While some administrators are driven by a desire to provide treatment to vulnerable populations, administrative support for adopting new treatments is driven by necessity and cost. Patient suicide; negative high-profile publicity; litigation; staff burnout, turnover, and consequent training demands; and high incidences of self-harm or disruptive behaviors are common concerns motivating administrative action. Training forensic staff in new models of treatment often occurs, simply because the costs and risk of not changing are too high. Suicide, violence toward staff, lawsuits against the institution, and unit destructive behaviors clearly extract a high price from the system and from staff (Ivanoff & Schmidt, 2006).

Nonfatal self-harm, however, is also costly to institutional management in several ways. Immediate clinical and medical responses to self-harm incidents often involve expensive emergency medical or other crisis services. A disruption to unit security and management also occurs. Other residents may become distressed or use the disruption as an opportunity to engage in illegal or unit-destructive activities; both of these scenarios require increased vigilance. Nonfatal self-harm behavior may traumatize staff. As staff monitoring increases, other residents may be restricted or prevented from participating in treatment or other beneficial activities. Staff morale and sense of control then decrease, particularly when self-harm and other disruptive incidents occur frequently (Schmidt & Ivanoff, 2006a). These incidents can have a snowball effect, particularly when residents view them as opportunities to obtain desired changes such as housing. The unintentional reinforcing consequences of self-harm and other forms of disruption are particularly problematic in restricted settings, leaving administrators and clinicians alike flummoxed.

Implementing treatment in a restricted residential setting requires full support of the administrators and managers, and a good understanding of the principles underlying treatment (Ivanoff & Schmidt, 2006). Within these settings, one of the primary roles of administrators and managers is to facilitate the delivery of treatment. The higher in the organizational structure, the more that role is fulfilled in the securing of resources, direction of activity, and education of community and governmental stakeholders in the mission, advances, and ongoing struggles of the institution or agency. Understanding and support of the treatment model enables staff and administrators to "speak the same language" when discussing decisions, and to determine the consequences alternate decisions might have on ability to provide treatment to residents. Decisions can be evaluated based upon "effectiveness" in meeting the mission of the facility, concordance with the principles of skill development, likelihood of enhancing motivation of residents and staff, and other treatment-relevant parameters. Discussions of these principles naturally focus staff and administrators on a common goal, and diminish a sense that decisions are made arbitrarily or based upon personality.

Administrative Goals

Several administrative goals may be accomplished by introducing DBT. Prioritizing goals prior to training is important. The more clearly specified, the higher the likelihood of success. The most common administrative goals include:

1. Reduction of suicidal behavior, assaults, and severely disruptive behavior—that is, incidents falling into the egregious behavior protocol described earlier.
2. Improved presence of targeted treatment services, often related to improved Joint Commission on the Accreditation of Health Care Organization (JCAHO) compliance and to the standards set by the National Commission on Correctional Health Care (NCCHC).
3. Behavioral management, that is, the reduction in other problematic behaviors that may interrupt or delay treatment for an individual or for the group.

4. Desire for stimulating ideas to enhance existing treatment and program activities.

5. Increasing professional knowledge in general.

6. An interest in a new, possibly more effective, model for treating difficult patients.

Enhancing Therapists' Capabilities: Training the Willing *and* Willful

In forensic and correctional settings, safety and security sometimes exist in uneasy tandem with treatment goals. Luckily, DBT training can address both concerns simultaneously. The list that follows is not comprehensive but, in our experience, is a logical training order.

1. *Sell commitment by citing correctional treatment outcome research*. Many forensic staff, including professional staff, are unaware of the promising treatment outcome studies with correctional populations, as described earlier in this chapter. These data directly challenge the myth that "nothing works" with correctional patients, engendering hope in correctional and professional staff.

2. *Discuss the pros and the cons of implementing DBT*. One con is the fear, embarrassment, and other negative emotions staff experience by learning new skills. As one staff member ruefully stated, "I learned that I was doing everything wrong for 20 years!" Staff express fear of "letting their guard down," of becoming more vulnerable to dangerous patients. They are concerned that skills will help "psychopaths to become better psychopaths." They are concerned that administrators and other professional staff start new initiatives and "pet projects" with great enthusiasm, but ultimately leave them "holding the bag" with few resources yet full accountability. Such fears are valid. We advise that they should be discussed directly and dialectically. For example, "On the one hand you are right. There is a study, suggesting that [unstructured] treatment increased recidivism among psychopaths. On the other hand, one study is not conclusive, and only 10% of our patients meet criteria for psychopathy. Plus, DBT is a structured, not an unstructured, treatment." During these discussion, ask the questions, "What is the middle path here? What is the synthesis between these diametrically opposite or polarized positions?" In other words, apply the treatment and its principles to the process of deciding whether to systematically use the treatment.

3. *Implement skills training groups and milieu skills coaching*. Use shaping when implementing DBT skills. Both correctional and mental health staff view skills training as the treatment mode with the highest face validity. Because it is manualized, skills training is also the easiest mode to implement. Get a DBT "foot in the door" by training a few skills well on one unit. Crisis survival strategies are often the first skills taught because residents need them now. Reduce staff anxiety by first teaching the "Top Ten DBT Skills": in sum, either the most preferred or easiest skills for staff to coach. In our experience, the Top Ten DBT skills include DEAR MAN, GIVE, FAST, Mindfulness What and How Skills, ABC Please, Opposite Action, Radical Acceptance, and Willingness (Linehan, 1993b, 2005). First, encourage staff to role-play skills by using situations from their own professional or personal lives (also practicing genuineness). After staff acquire skills, practice coaching "patients" in role plays. Identify factors that interfere with staff coaching such as shame, fear, denigrating peers, catastrophizing, and the like, and then use the "Factors Reducing Interpersonal Effectiveness" handout from the interpersonal effectiveness module (Linehan, 1993b) to help trouble-shoot.

4. *Provide enough training to make a real difference*. Is a little staff training always better than none? Not necessarily. A study at Echo Glen found more punitive staff behav-

ior on the part of staff who received a small amount of DBT training, while the cottage staff who received at least 40 hours of training improved resident behavior and functioning (Trupin, Stewart, Beach, & Boesky, 2002). The temptation in many programs is to only teach residents and staff DBT skills and in doing so to conflate DBT skills with comprehensive DBT. While perhaps a fine approach to begin building a comprehensive DBT program (see Koerner, Dimeff, & Swenson, Chapter 2, this volume), it is important to note that our successes, as well as those evaluated in the randomized controlled trials of DBT, are based on comprehensive application of the model.

Finally, staffing needs must be reviewed and additional resources requested to enhance treatment effectiveness. The staffing ratios generally assigned to prisons (where safety and security are paramount) are insufficient for providing high-quality CBT. The ability to spot residents in the milieu trying to use skills or in situations in which skill usage is required is directly dependent upon staff being present on the floor in sufficient numbers to observe residents.

Partial Implementations and Modifications

Many programs choose to begin by implementing skills training. While this is realistically a good place to begin, skills groups alone do not cover the five essential functions of DBT described in Chapter 1. Failing to address these functions invalidates DBT as an evidence-based treatment and reduces the likelihood that it will produce change in the target behaviors. Based on no results, conclusions are then erroneously drawn about the failure of DBT rather than a failure to accurately implement it. Programs cite many reasons given for partial implementation and modifications in forensic settings. Among them are DBT's incompatibility with correctional treatment goals, its complexity, the unsupportiveness of the setting, unwilling staff, the cost of full implementation, or simply "Our clients don't need all of this!" (Ivanoff, Schmidt, & Finnegan, 2006).

Organizations in distress often identify urgent needs for programming and proceed quickly. Program pitfalls worth guarding against include (1) adapting materials with low fidelity or "cherry-picking" some skills and omitting others; (2) starting training prior to organized commitment, or training the wrong individuals first—for example, managers should be trained before line staff; (3) the use of nonintegrated treatment models for different problem areas (in one site eight different models are used on one unit!); and (4) the "flavor of the week"—moving to the next new thing in treatment models to address new problems rather than working within the existing model to improve fidelity.

Research on Forensic DBT

The first survey of DBT programs in correctional and forensic settings in the United States and the United Kingdom was conducted in 1998 (Ivanoff, 1998). At that time, while interest was growing, there was little shared information about DBT in these settings. Of the 14 programs who responded to that survey, 11 were forensic and four were strictly correctional; roughly half were inpatient. Most programs reported working to implement comprehensive DBT, including all major functions and modes. The most common obstacles reported involved staff who were not trained in mental health or behavior therapy, the difficulty of adapting the standard outpatient treatment to highly restricted settings, and adapting the treatment to address the needs of a more male population, often with distinct antisocial characteristics. All reported some activities directed at evaluation. Across the United Kingdom there is an organized, developed research effort and four of the 10 programs in the United States/Canada were already receiving funding for their efforts. Since then, programs using DBT components in correctional and forensic settings have dramatically increased in number.

Most recently, Berzins and Trestman (2004) reviewed program information from 10 correctional systems in the United States and Canada. Most of these programs turned to DBT to help manage their most dysfunctional residents, those with significant behavioral dyscontrol and personality disorders. Despite strong anecdotal support, they report widespread difficulty collecting data to document effectiveness. Again, overtaxed staff often isolated in institutional implementation structures make data collection beyond regular program monitoring—for example, incidents, segregation, and restraint—extremely difficult.

The two programs selected for inclusion in this chapter are prototypes and offer rich experience to others working in this area. Based on these examples of DBT, as well as numerous smaller efforts elsewhere, sufficient anecdotal evidence exists to support such adaptations. DBT is regarded as a useful part of treating these most difficult patients. To date, outcome data on residential cost-effectiveness have not been reported, but are expected soon. Whether identified by staff or administrators, the administrative and clinical problems cited above suggest DBT as a model of choice.

NOTES

1. The Colorado Mental Health Institute at Pueblo (CMHIP) operates as an agency of the Colorado Department of Human Services and provides services for approximately 3,000 citizens per year. The bed capacity is 500. The Institute for Forensic Psychiatry (IFP) is one of the CMHIP treatment programs, serving adults with mental illnesses referred by the criminal justice system. Evaluations and treatment services are provided to adults pretrial, postconviction, or following acquittal by reason of insanity.

2. The Juvenile Rehabilitation Administration (JRA) provides evidence-based services to youth committed by Washington State juvenile courts. Committed youth are typically adjudicated of serious or violent felony offenses or have histories of chronic offending. JRA treatment services for youth in residential programs include DBT, aggression replacement training, and an adaptation of multidimensional treatment foster care. Functional family parole services, functional family therapy, and family integrated transitions are provided to youth in the community setting.

3. Comprehensive DBT includes all five treatment functions: (1) increasing new skills in residents, (2) increasing resident generalization of skills, (3) enhancing resident motivation to persist with and practice new skills, (4) structuring the environment to support the use of new skills, and (5) enhancing staff motivation and skills to promote the above and to prevent burnout. In contrast, some partial DBT programs provide only skills training groups; such programs address only the first DBT function.

4. The University of California at Los Angeles (UCLA) Social and Independent Living Skills Program was developed for individuals with schizophrenia and other psychotic disorders. There are eight modules: basic conversation, recreation for leisure, medication management, symptom management, substance abuse, workplace fundamentals, friendship and intimacy, and community reentry. Each module consists of a trainer's manual, a participant workbook, and a demonstration video. Each module includes specific education objectives. For example, in the medication management module, there is a skill area on identifying benefits of antipsychotic medication that teaches participants how to politely negotiate medication with their physicians.

Meta-analysis of 27 studies suggests that patients who receive this therapy experience increased social function, decreased relapse, and increased hospital discharge.

5. Reasoning and Rehabilitation Cognitive Skills (Porporino & Fabiano, 2000) is a 36-session group therapy program focused on changing faulty thinking patterns associated with recidivism. Examples of such faulty thinking patterns include deficits in self-control, problem solving, social perspective taking, and critical thinking. There is evidence that this treatment decreases recidivism (Porporino & Robinson, 1995; Antonowicz, 2004).

6. 24-hour rule: The client is oriented to this rule prior to engaging in self-injurious behavior. Once self-injurious behavior occurs, the client is not allowed to contact his or her therapist for 24 hours afterward unless (1) injuries are life-threatening or (2) a contact was previously scheduled during this 24-hour period. Here the goal is to encourage the client to contact the therapist before self-injurious behavior occurs.

REFERENCES

Abram, K. M., & Teplin, L. A. (1991). Co-occurring disorders among mentally ill jail detainees: Implications for public policy. *American Psychologist, 46*, 1036–1045.

Allard, T. J., Wortley, R. K., & Stewart, A. L. (2003). Role conflict in community corrections. *Psychology, Crime, and Law, 9*, 279–289.

American Psychiatric Association. (1994). *Diagnostic and statistical manual of mental disorders* (4th ed.). Washington, DC: Author.

Andrews, D. (1997). Punishment, treatment, and treatment programs. In S. Wong & C. Di Placido (Eds.), *Risk assessment and management self study manual* (6-1-1-22). Saskatoon, SK: Correctional Service of Canada.

Andrews, D. A., & Bonta, J. (1998). *The psychology of criminal conduct.* Cincinnati, OH: Anderson.

Andrews, D. A., Bonta, J., Gendreau, P., & Cullen, F. T. (1990). Does correctional treatment work?: A clinically relevant and psychologically informed meta-analysis, *Criminology, 28*, 369–403.

Antonowicz, D. H. (2004). *The Reasoning and Rehabilitation Program: Outcome evaluations with offenders.* Unpublished manuscript.

Ball, E. M. (2004) *Crime Review Group protocol.* Unpublished manuscript.

Berzins, L. G., & Trestman, R. L. (2004). The development and implementation of dialectical behavior therapy in forensic settings. *International Journal of Forensic Mental Health, 3*, 93–103.

Black, D. W., Baumgard, C. H., & Bell, S. E. (1995). A 16- to 45-year follow-up of 71 men with antisocial personality disorder. *Comprehensive Psychiatry, 36*, 130–140.

Blackburn, R. (2000). Treatment or incapacitation?: Implications of research on personality disorders for the management of dangerous offenders. *Legal and Criminological Psychology, 5*, 1–21.

Bogue, B. (2002). *An evolutionary model for examining community corrections.* Boulder, CO: Justice System Assessment and Training.

Brinded, P. M., Mulder, R. T., Stevens, I., & Fairley, N. F. (1999). The Christchurch prisons psychiatric epidemiology study: Method prevalence rates for psychiatric disorders. *Criminal Behavior and Mental Health, 9*, 131–143.

Buehler, R. E., Patterson, G. R., & Furniss, J. M. (1966). The reinforcement of behavior in institutional settings. *Behavior Research and Therapy, 4*, 157–167.

Cauffman, E., Scholle, S. H., Mulvey, E., & Kelleher, K. J. (2005). Predicting first-time involvement in the juvenile justice system among emotionally disturbed youth receiving mental health services. *Psychological Services, 2*, 28–38.

Clinical Research Center for Schizophrenia and Psychiatric Rehabilitation. (1988). *Social and independent living skills.* Los Angeles: Author.

Colorado Department of Human Services. (2001). Colorado Mental Health Institute @ Pueblo: Institute for Forensic Psychiatry: Overview of division operations (9-4-01).

Ditton, P. M. (July, 1999). *Mental health and treatment of inmates and probationers* (Bureau of Justice Statistics Special Report, NCJ 174453). Washington, DC: U.S. Department of Justice.

Eysenck, H. J. (1977). *Crime and personality* (3rd ed.). London: Routledge.

Foa, E. B., & Rothbaum, B. O. (1998). *Treating the trauma of rape: Cognitive-behavioral therapy for PTSD*. New York: Guilford Press.

Foa, E. B., Zoellner, L. A., Feeny, N. C., Hembree, E. A., & Alvarez-Conrad. (2002). Does imaginal exposure exacerbate PTSD symptoms? *Journal of Consulting and Clinical Psychology, 70,* 1022–1028.

Frick, P. J. (1998). Callous unemotional traits and conduct problems: A two factor model of psychopathy in children. In D. J. Cooke, A. E. Forth, & R. D. Hare (Eds.), *Psychopathy: Theory, research, and implication for society* (pp. 161–188). Dordrecht, The Netherlands: Kluwer.

Fruzzetti, A. E., & Levensky, E. R. (2000). Dialectical behavior therapy for domestic violence: Rationale and procedures. *Cognitive and Behavioral Practice, 7,* 435–447.

Hare, R. D. (1991). *The Hare Psychopathy Checklist–Revised*. North Tonawanda, NY: MHS.

Hare, R. D. (1995). Psychopathy: A clinical construct whose time has come. *Criminal Justice and Behavior, 23,* 25–54.

Hare, R. D. (2003). *Hare PCL-R technical manual* (2nd ed.). North Tonawanda, NY: MHS.

Harris, G. T., Rice, M. E., & Cornier, C. A. (1991). Psychopathy and violent recidivism. *Law and Human Behavior, 15,* 625–637.

Hodgins, S. (2002). Research priorities in forensic mental health. *International Journal of Forensic Mental Health, 1,* 7–23.

Hodgins, S., & Cote, G. (1993). Major mental disorder and antisocial personality disorder: A criminal combination. *Bulletin of the American Academy of Psychiatry and Law, 21,* 155–160.

Ivanoff, A. (1998). *Survey of criminal justice and forensic dialectical behavior therapy programs in the U.S. and U. K.* Seattle: Linehan Training Group.

Ivanoff, A., & Schmidt, H., III. (2006). Administrative challenges. In G. Dear (Ed.), *Preventing suicide and other self-harm in prison*. London: Palgrave-Macmillan.

Ivanoff, A., Schmidt, H., III, & Finnegan, D. S. (2006, June). *Addressing DBT treatment functions and modes in criminal justice settings*. Paper presented at the International Association of Forensic Mental Health Service Meeting, Amsterdam, The Netherlands.

Jones, J. W. (1981). *The burnout syndrome. Current research, theory, and interventions*. Park Ridge, IL: London House Press.

Linehan, M. M. (1993a). *Cognitive-behavioral treatment of borderline personality disorder*. New York: Guilford Press.

Linehan, M. M. (1993b). *Skills training manual for treating borderline personality disorder*. New York: Guilford Press.

Linehan, M. M. (2000). Commentary on innovations in dialectical behavior therapy. *Cognitive and Behavioral Practice, 7,* 478–481.

Linehan, M. M. (2005). *Emotion regulation*. Seattle: Behavioral Tech, LLC.

Linehan, M. M. (2007). *DBT intensive training course*. Seattle: Behavioral Tech, LLC.

Low, G., Jones, D., & Duggan, C. (2001). The treatment of deliberate self-harm in BPD using DBT: A pilot study in a high security hospital. *Behavioral and Cognitive Psychotherapy, 29,* 85–92.

Lykken, D. T. (1995). *The antisocial personalities*. Hillsdale, NJ: Erlbaum.

Maslach, C., & Jackson, S. E. (1993). *Maslach Burnout Inventory*. Palo Alto, CA: Consulting Psychologists Press.

McCann, R. A., Ball, E. M., & Ivanoff, A. (2000). DBT with an inpatient forensic population: The CMHIP model. *Cognitive and Behavioral Practice, 7,* 447–456.

Miller, A. L., Rathus, J. H., & Linehan, M. M. (2006). *Dialectical behavior therapy with suicidal adolescents*. New York: Guilford Press.

Morgan, R. D., Van Haveren, R., & Pearson, C. A. (2002). Correctional officer burnout: Further analyses. *Criminal Justice and Behavior, 29,* 144–160.

Nolan, K. A., Volavka, J., Mohr, P., & Czobor, P. (1999). Psychopathy and violent behavior among patients with schizophrenia or schizoaffective disorder. *Psychiatric Services, 50,* 787–792.

Patterson, G. R., DeBaryshe, B. D., & Ramsey, E. (1989). A developmental perspective on antisocial behavior. *American Psychologist, 44,* 329–335.

Porporino, F. J., & Fabiano, E. (2000). *Programme overview of cognitive skills reasoning and rehabilitation revised: Theory and application.* Ontario, Canada: T3 Associates.

Porporino, F. J., & Robinson, D. (1995). An evaluation of the Reasoning and Rehabilitation Program with Canadian federal offenders. In R. R. Ross & R. D. Ross (Eds.), *Thinking straight: The Reasoning and Rehabilitation Program for delinquency prevention and offender rehabilitation.* Ottawa, Canada: AIR.

Quay, H. C. (1977). Psychopathic behavior: Reflections on its nature, origins, and treatment. In I. Uzgiris & F. Weizman (Eds.), *The structuring of experience.* New York: Plenum Press.

Quinsey, V. L., Harris, G. T., Rice, M. E., & Cormier, C. A. (2006). *Violent offenders: Appraising and managing risk.* Washington, DC: American Psychological Association.

Reich, J. (1985). The relationship between antisocial behavior and affective illness. *Comprehensive Psychiatry, 26,* 296–303.

Rotter, M., Way, B., Steinbacher, M., Sawyer, D., & Smith, H. (2002). Personality disorders in prison: Aren't they all antisocial? *Psychiatric Quarterly, 73,* 337–349.

Rubio, A., & Fruzetti, A. (2000). *Borderline and antisocial personality disorders: Gendered public vs. similar private and self behaviors.* Manuscript submitted for publication.

Salekin, R. T. (2002). Psychopathy and therapeutic pessimism: Clinical lore or clinical reality? *Clinical Psychology Review, 22,* 79–112.

Schaufeli, W. B., & Peeters, M. C. (2000). Job stress and burnout among correctional officers: A literature review. *International Journal of Stress Management, 7,* 19–48.

Schmidt, H., III, & Ivanoff, A. (2006a). Behavioral prescriptions for treating self-injurious and suicidal behaviors. In M. Piasecki & O. Thienhaus (Eds.), *Handbook of correctional psychiatry.* Washington, DC: Civic Research Press.

Schmidt, H., III, & Ivanoff, A. (2006b). Taking aim at a fuzzy target: *Challenges to reducing suicidal behaviors in correctional settings.* Unpublished manuscript.

Scott, C. L. (2004, November). *Studies of aggression at Napa State Hospital: From research to treatment.* Presentation at the Colorado Mental Health Institute at Pueblo.

Simourd, D. J., & Hoge, R. D. (2000). Criminal psychopathy: A risk and need perspective. *Criminal Justice and Behavior, 27,* 256–272.

Stueve, A., & Lin, B. G. (1997). Violence and psychiatric disorders: Results from an epidemiological study of young adults in Israel. *Psychiatric Quarterly, 68,* 327–342.

Tengstrom, A., Grann, M., Langstrom, N., & Kullgren, G. (2000). Psychopathy as a predictor of violent recidivism among criminal offenders with schizophrenia. *Law and Human Behavior, 24,* 45–58.

Teplin, L. A. (1990). The prevalence of severe mental disorder among male urban jail detainees: Comparison with the Epidemiologic Catchment Area Program. *American Journal of Public Health, 80,* 663–669.

Trupin, E. W., Stewart, D. G., Beach, B., & Boesky, L. (2002). Effectiveness of a dialectical behavior therapy program for incarcerated female juvenile offenders. *Child and Adolescent Mental Health, 7,* 121–127.

U.S. Department of Justice. (2002). *Reentry trends in the U.S. recidivism.* Washington, DC: Bureau of Justice Statistics.

Waltz, J., Babcock, J. C., Jacobson, N. S., & Gottman, J. M. (2000). Testing a typology of batterer. *Journal of Clinical and Consulting Psychology, 68,* 658–669.

Warren, F., McGauley, G., Norton, K., Dolan, B., Preedy-Fayers, K., Pickering, A., et al. (2003). *Review of treatments for severe personality disorder.* London, UK: Department of Health and Prison Service DSPD Programme, Home Office.

Washington State Institute for Public Policy. (2002). *Preliminary findings for the Juvenile Rehabili-*

tation Administration's Dialectical Behavior Therapy Program (Document No. 02-07-1203). Olympia: Washington State Institute for Public Policy.

Weiler, B. L., & Widom, C. S. (1996). Psychopathy and violent behavior in abused and neglected young adults. *Criminal Behavior and Mental Health*, 6, 253–271.

Weiss, J. M., Davis, D., Hedlund, J. L., & Dong, W. C. (1984). The dysphoric personality: A comparison of 524 cases of antisocial personality disorder with matched controls. *Comprehensive Psychiatry*, 24, 355–369.

Wong, S., & Hare, R. D. (1998). *Program guidelines for the institutional treatment of violent psychopathic offenders*. Unpublished manuscript.

Zlotnick, C. (1999). Antisocial personality disorder, affect dysregulation and childhood abuse among incarcerated women. *Journal of Personality Disorders*, 13, 90–95.

APPENDIX 5.1. DBT Graduate Group: Crime Review Group (Ball, 2004)

Duration: 90 minutes

Prerequisites: DBT skills graduate and demonstrating behavioral control

Membership: Two therapists and up to 10 patients (coed)

Room: Chairs set up U-shape facing large white board. Video camera.

Purpose: Consolidate DBT skills, increase insight into violence, and develop a relapse plan.

GROUP STRUCTURE

I. Before Group
   A. Set up video camera. All sessions are videotaped. Camera is aimed at presenter and white board.
   B. Review police reports and presenter's write-up.
   C. Presenter turns in presentation to group therapists at least 1 week prior to presentation.
   D. Presenter writes synopsis of presentation on white board.
II. Start Group (5–10 minutes)
   A. Determine future assignments, order of presentation.
   B. Determine roles for today's group
      1. Perpetrator
         a. Patient presenting offense
      2. Victim voice(s)
         a. Direct victim
         b. Indirect victims: family members, friends, etc.
      3. Victim empathy advocate(s)
         a. Direct presenter plays the role of a direct victim.
         b. Advocate role-plays district attorney, victim advocate, or close friend.
         c. Advocate plays Perpetrator. Presenter remains in role of Victim
      4. Disposition Committee Member(s) (Committee advising superintendent regarding patients' eligibility for release)
         a. Find discrepancies in presenter's report.
         b. Confrontational but professional style is acceptable.
      5. Emotion observer
         a. Observes, reads, and encourages emotional expression from presenter and other group members.
         b. Observes, describes, and labels group member emotions.
         c. Validates emotion.
         d. Cheerleads presenter.
      6. DBT skills coach
         a. Coaches presenter during difficult moments.
III. Presentations are completed in sections. Each presenter presents seven sections. Multiple offenses may require multiple presentations. Presenter completes each section 1 week prior to presentation. Presenter copies a synopsis of his presentation on the white board immediately prior to group.
   A. Section 1: Problem Behavior
      1. Prior to group presenter reads police reports and writes:
         a. The problem behavior specifically and behaviorally
         b. The prompting event
         c. Summary of most significant links culminating in offense.
      2. Patient attempts to resolve discrepancies between his report and police reports.
      3. All group members look for "what is left out," that is, discrepancies between the presenter's report and police reports. Purpose of this feedback is to increase presenter's insight into his offense.
      4. Warning: Access to collateral data such as police reports is mandatory in forensic treatment. "Clarity, precision and compassion are of the utmost importance" (Linehan, 2007, p. 30). Be sure to validate, or, if necessary, invalidate, patient self-report with collateral data.
   B. Section 2: Vulnerability Factors
      1. Autobiography summarizing family, legal, substance abuse, mental health, or other history leading up to offense.

2. Vulnerability factors prior to offense(s): answers question "Why then?"
3. Warning: Clinician access to collateral data such as police reports is mandatory in forensic treatment. Additional sources of data include interviews with family members, other agency mental health records, military records, school records, and department of correction records.

C. Section 3: Victim Point of View
1. Chain from victim's point of view
2. Presenter plays role of victim during group.
3. Block presenter's avoidance: running out of room, criticizing others, refusing eye contact, sitting slumped in chair, etc.
4. If > 1 victim, several presentations may be required
5. Warning: Do not allow patients to victimize each other during role play.

D. Section 4: Consequences
1. Consequences for self and victims.
2. Group members direct presenter to speak with victim voices.

E. Section 5: Repair
1. Presents repair plan.
2. Victim voices speak with presenter re: meaning, significance, and emotional response to perpetrator's repair plan.
3. Warning: remind presenter to obtain permission and clinical consultation prior to contacting real-life victims for repair.

F. Section 6: Target Behavior Hierarchy
1. Prior to group, presenter completes his own target hierarchy.
2. Group helps presenter describe target behaviors behaviorally.
3. No role-play.

G. Section 7: Summary Analysis of Causes of Problem Behavior Including
1. Skills deficits
2. Emotions interfering
3. Reinforcers and punishers of ineffective behavior
4. Reinforcers and punishers of effective behavior
5. Warning: be alert to victim–victimizer dialectical dilemma.

H. Section 8: Solutions*
1. Determining each link (in chain) where he could have done something effective.
2. Defining what skill he might have used.

I. Section 9: Relapse Plan*
1. Include target behavior hierarchy.
2. Include relapse signs of major Axis I mental illness (if relevant).
3. Include DBT skills that will decrease probability of relapse or recidivism.
4. Warning: patients must overlearn their relapse plans.

J. * Warning: If patients become fatigued, you may collapse sections 7, 8, and 9 into one session.

IV. Presentation (20–30 minutes)
A. Presenter uses white board to present materials.
B. Members do not interrupt, practicing Level 1 validation or staying awake: unbiased listening and observing.

V. Role-play (30 minutes): See IIB

VI. Ending Group (15 minutes)
A. Mindfulness practice (5 minutes).
B. Each group member provides presenter with oral feedback regarding
1. Presentation
a. Positive feedback
b. Corrective feedback
c. All asked to maintain ratio of 6 positive to 1 corrective feedback
2. Unit behavior
3. Treatment progress.
C. Immediate feedback decreases the probability that patients will abuse each other in role plays. Cotherapists provide written feedback to
1. Presenter
a. Insight into violence
b. Empathy for victim

  c. Remorse
 2. Group Member Roles
  a. Victim voice
   i. Use of feeling words
   ii. Perceived accuracy of empathy
  b. Emotion observer
   i. Accuracy of Observations
  c. Victim empathy advocate
   i. Perceived accuracy of empathy
   ii. Skill facilitating perpetrator's emotional connection to victim voices
  d. DBT skills coach
   i. Use of Nonjudgmental Observation
   ii. Use of skills
  e. Disposition committee members
   i. Use of nonjudgmental observations
   ii. Ability to empathize with authority figures
   iii. Awareness of risk factors
VII. Presenter reviews videotape with individual therapist or case manager.
VIII. Special Considerations
 A. Some offenses such as sexual offenses, filicide, cannibalism, and the like are emotionally dysregulating for most people. Therapists maintain a dialectic between acceptance and change, coaching skills and accepting an individual patient's (or therapist's) limits: an occasional need to abstain from a particular session.
 B. Ensure that group members reinforce prosocial (not antisocial) values.

APPENDIX 5.2. DBT Graduate Group: Behavior Chain Analysis Group

Duration: 75 minutes

Prerequisites: DBT skills graduate and demonstrating behavioral control

Membership: Two therapists and up to 10 patients (coed)

Room: chairs set up U-shape facing large white board

GROUP STRUCTURE

I. Before Group: Choose Behavior Analysis (BA)
   A. Written prior to group. Determine choice prior to group using Target hierarchy. Highest target behavior has highest priority.
   B. If resident is not a member of behavior analysis group, invite the day before group to visit as a "speaker."
   C. Ask resident for permission to photocopy the written BA for peers. If permission granted, copy outline of BA on white board and provide copies of BA to group members. If permission not granted, ask resident to write BA on the white board prior to group.
   D. Warning: Consider resident's mental status in context of group members. Is resident suspicious or paranoid? Given the group context, is suspicion justified or unjustified? Does resident have allies or enemies in the group? Will peers reinforce criminogenic attitudes? Is the speaker facing legal charges for problem behavior? Will reviewing BA in group increase speaker's vulnerability to prosecution? If negatives > positives, do not review this problem behavior in group.
   E. Problem: Will discussion of deviant sexual problems sexually arouse group members? Solution: If yes, do not review this problem behavior in group.
   F. Problem: Parasuicide. Solution: Do not review BA of parasuicide in group.
II. Start Group with Mindfulness (5–10 minutes).
   A. Led by therapist
   B. Concrete
      1. Stories: sports, news, 1–2 minute videoclips, tales of endurance or good sportsmanship
      2. Observe candy, each other's shoes, frequency of speech, etc.
III. Mindfulness Observer
   A. Resident volunteer
   B. Rings bell after:
      1. Judgmental language
      2. Mindlessness
      3. Elephant in the room
      4. Unresolved dialectic
   C. Problem:
      1. The bell cues criticism or anger for some residents. Some residents wish to throw the bell across the room, assault the mindfulness observer, and so on.
      2. Solution: Coach skills. Remind residents that the bell is a cue, not a command.
      3. Solution: If all else fails, ring bell noncontingently.
IV. Validation
   A. Offer group members an opportunity to praise or validate the speaker.
   B. One cotherapist begins modeling validation (vs. praise): "It makes sense that. . . ."
   C. Shape peer validation. In our experience peers tend to provide praise, not validation.
   D. Second cotherapist ends validation in order to supplement validation or to repair prior invalidation of valid behavior or validation of invalid behavior by peers.
V. Therapy-Interfering Behavior
   A. Problem: Speaker complains incessantly about staff or peer X's behavior. Solution: If X's behavior is part of BA, ask speaker to describe the behavior. If other group members saw the behavior, ask for feedback regarding accuracy. Never defend or criticize staff behavior. If staff behavior was problematic, be radically genuine: "Love to do a BA on X but he is not here! You are the only one here! Are you willing? Let's go!"
   B. Problem: Resident repeatedly complains that you are promoting the values of the majority culture, the white culture, the conservative culture, or the like. Solution: Acknowledge difficult dialectic

142

between functioning as a prosocial model, that is, doing one's job, and promoting one's own values.

C. Problem: Lying. Solution: Use Describe to note discrepancies between what resident says and does, between what resident says from one moment to the next moment, between what resident says and what peers say, between what resident says and records. Bring charts to group for cross-reference. For multiparty problem behavior, ensure that each resident completes BA separately, and then look for consistencies and discrepancies across BAs. Remain behavioral and nonjudgmental. Discuss lying as an escape behavior. Do not force residents to cry "uncle" or otherwise shame themselves.

D. Problem: Residents make judgmental statements regarding peer X who is always "talking the talk" by completing BAs but seems to never "walk the walk." Solution: Coach Describe and Nonjudgmental skills. Seriously consider whether peer X's problem is motivational.

E. Problem: You are confused. Solution: Ask patients to describe the dialectic in the room.

F. Problem: You are angry. Solution: Concoct and share a Level 5 validation.

G. Problem: Chronic therapy-interfering behavior. Solution: Refer problem group member to his individual therapist.

VI. Behavioral Chain Analysis (Linehan, 1993a)

A. Problem behavior: It is mandatory for the speaker and therapists to agree that the behavior in question is a problem. Collaboration is essential.

1. If, against all evidence (e.g., urinalysis positive for cocaine), resident denies engaging in the problem behavior (e.g., using cocaine), reframe the problem until you obtain agreement. For example, "Is it a problem that you have this positive urinalysis?"

2. Assess whether the problem behavior is consistent or inconsistent with resident's Wise Mind values. For example, a resident stated that "casual sex" was consistent with his values. Upon further exploration, he acknowledged that "unprotected sex" was inconsistent with his values. Thus we defined the problem as "unprotected sex."

3. Assess whether the problem behavior is a dynamic risk factor, or a link to higher-target life-threatening behaviors. Assess whether the problem behavior is a proxy variable for higher-target dangerous behaviors. Assess secondary targets. Articulate these links and targets.

4. Weave in Commitment strategies. Connect the current chain analysis with the resident's past commitment to decrease violence. Highlight resident's freedom to either work or not work on the problem behavior.

5. Warning: Never continue a BA until you have consensus on the problem behavior.

B. Vulnerability factors

1. Repeat that vulnerability factors answer the question "Why now?"

2. Elicit vulnerability factors from speaker and (importantly) peers. Peers tend to be more mindful of the speaker's vulnerability factors than the speaker himself!

3. Watch out for medication-, news media-, probation-, court-, or anniversary-related vulnerability factors.

C. Links!

1. Note both effective and ineffective links. Identify DBT (and other) skills in chain. Praise and validation maintain speaker willingness.

2. Use Describe skills: For example, just write, "Staff member told you DBT skills are crap." Never defend nor criticize another staff member. Remember, correctional environments by their very nature are invalidating environments.

3. Ask group members to distinguish difference between thoughts, feelings, body sensations, and events.

4. Use "broken record" when eliciting feelings from speaker. Quickly correct errors: for example, "Manipulated is not a feeling word but a thought word. Give us a feeling word."

5. Keep balance between structure (completing the BA) and group participation. Maintain balance between detailing links and group interest. Remind the shy to use their Participation skills. Remind the gregarious to use Observe skills and help elicit feedback from the shy.

6. Prompting event is usually easier to determine after obtaining all the links in the chain.

VII. Solution Analysis

A. Residents are the experts and brainstorm skills.

B. Include non-DBT skills.

C. Write options on white board.

D. Weave in relevant self-management skills—for example, Premack Principle, Reinforcement schedules, and the like.

E. Consider change versus acceptance skills. What is most effective given the situation? What does the guest speaker most need to practice?

F. Warning: If, despite prior problem consensus, speaker wishes to remain miserable (see Options for Responding to Problems), and is not committed to changing problem behavior, do not proceed to VII. Dialectical strategies such as Entering the Paradox, Extending, or Devil's Advocate may be useful. If the mindfulness observer does not ring the bell, remind him. Use guidelines for treating willfulness—for example, "Are you willing to not act willful even though you feel willful?"

VIII. Role Play Practice

A. Collaboratively determine what skill to practice.

B. Set up role-play scene. Be clear regarding when each "take" begins and ends.

C. Provide feedback.

D. Warning: Keep your sense of humor when residents mimic staff behavior, including your own. Have fun, laugh, and joke! Never defend or criticize staff.

IX. Observations (5–10 minutes)

A. Each member shares one nonjudgmental observation about himself or the group.

B. Elicit observation from all members, including staff and speaker.

C. Therapists share observations last in order to supplement or repair.

CHAPTER 6

Dialectical Behavior Therapy for Individuals with Borderline Personality Disorder and Substance Dependence

Shelley McMain, Jennifer H. R. Sayrs,
Linda A. Dimeff, *and* Marsha M. Linehan

Overview of the Problem

Substance use disorders (SUDs) commonly co-occur with borderline personality disorder (BPD; Trull, Sher, Minks-Brown, Durbin, & Burr, 2000) and result in serious and complex behavioral problems. The co-occurrence of SUDs and BPD is second only to the co-occurrence of mood disorders and antisocial personality disorder in comorbidity prevalence (Trull & Widiger, 1991). In their extensive review of BPD and SUDs comorbidity data gathered from studies published between 1987 and 1997, Trull and colleagues (2000) found that among those seeking substance abuse treatment, rates of BPD ranged from 5.2% (Brooner, King, Kidorf, & Schmidt, 1997) to 65.1% (Dejong, Van den Brink, Harteveld, & Van der Wielan, 1993). Estimates of prevalence of current SUDs among patients receiving treatment for BPD range from a low of approximately 21% (Miller, Belkins, & Gibbons, 1994) to a high of 67% (Dulit, Fyer, Haas, Sullivan, & Frances, 1990). Subsequent studies confirm a significant overlap (Darke, Williamson, Ross, Teesson, & Lynskey, 2003; Swadi & Bobier, 2003; Skinstad & Swain, 2001; Zanarini, Frankenburg, Hennen, Reich, & Silk, 2004; Becker, Grilo, Anez, Paris, & McGlashan, 2005). This overlap is not unexpected—after all, impulsiveness in areas that are potentially self-damaging (such as substance abuse) is one of the diagnostic criteria for BPD. However, the high comorbidity between BPD and SUDs is not entirely explained by this overlap in criteria. For example, Dulit et al. (1990) found that 67% of current patients with BPD met criteria for SUDs. When substance abuse was not used as a criterion of BPD, the incidence dropped to 57%, which is still a very significant portion of the population.

Individuals with BPD and SUDs are difficult patients to treat and have a wider range of problems compared to those with either SUDs or BPD alone (Links, Helsegrave, Mitton, & Van Reekum, 1995). For example, rates of suicide and suicide attempts, already high among individuals with BPD (Frances, Fyer, & Clarkin, 1986; Stone, Hurt, & Stone, 1987) and substance abusers (Beautrais, Joyce, & Mulder, 1999; Links et al., 1995; Rossow & Lauritzen, 1999) are even higher for individuals with both disorders (Rossow & Lauritzen, 1999). Furthermore, substance abusers with BPD are uniformly more disturbed than substance abusers without a personality disorder. Studies comparing substance-abusing patients with and without personality disorders have reported that those with personality disorders have significantly more behavioral, legal, and medical problems, including alcoholism and depression, and are more extensively involved in substance abuse than patients without personality disorders (Cacciola, Alterman, Rutherford, & Snider, 1995; Cacciola, Alterman, McKay, & Rutherford, 2001; McKay, Alterman, Cacciola, Mulvaney, & O'Brien, 2000; Nace, Davis, & Gaspari, 1991; Rutherford, Cacciola, & Alterman, 1994). In one study, remission of BPD was found to be impeded by the presence of a SUD (Zanarini et al., 2004). A few studies of substance abusers that have compared those with BPD with those with other personality disorders found that patients with BPD had more severe psychiatric problems than patients with other personality disorders (Kosten, Kosten, & Rounsaville, 1989; Skinstad & Swain, 2001).

How do we account for the high rates of overlap between SUDs and BPD? A multitude of interacting factors, including biological, psychological, and sociocultural components, contribute to the development and maintenance of substance abuse in conjunction with BPD. Evidence for a genetic predisposition to abuse psychoactive substances in individuals with BPD is suggested by the high rates of addiction problems in family studies of individuals with BPD (Anokhina, Veretinskaya, Vasil'eva, & Ovchinnikov, 2000). There is also evidence of a relationship between trait impulsivity and substance abuse (Levenson, Oyama, & Meek, 1987). Substance-abusing individuals with BPD have been shown to exhibit higher levels of impulsivity relative to their non-substance-abusing BPD counterparts (e.g., Kruedelbach, McCormick, Schulz, & Greuneich, 1993; Morgenstern, Langenbucher, Labouvie, & Miller, 1997), which may largely account for the high rates of concurrent SUDs (Trull et al., 2000). People with BPD are at an increased risk for addiction problems due to the pervasive emotion dysregulation that underlies their disorder (Linehan, 1993c; Marziali, Munroe-Blum, & McCleary, 1999). The reliance on psychoactive substances, like other problematic behaviors (e.g., cutting, hand banging, excessive spending, binge eating), functions (albeit dysfunctionally) to regulate out-of-control negative emotions. Indeed, many people with BPD report that their use of drugs is an attempt to manage their overwhelming affective states, including sadness, shame, emptiness, boredom, rage, and emotional misery. At a biological level, the escape from negative emotions through the use of drugs is reinforced by a dopamine spike in an individual with otherwise low levels of dopamine in the mesolimbic area of the midbrain following extensive drug use over time (Leshner, 1997; Leshner & Koob, 1999). Whereas initial substance abuse produces pleasure because of increases in the dopamine system, prolonged use makes it harder to experience sensations of pleasure because the dopamine system is altered (Leshner & Koob, 1999), resulting in what Leshner and Koob (1999) refer to as a "changed brain." Finally, environmental factors also play an important role in the development and maintenance of addictive behaviors for individuals with BPD. Adverse family experiences such as poor communication, conflict, and abuse are often observed to characterize the histories of individuals with BPD (Herman, Perry, & van der Kolk, 1989; Zanarini & Frankenburg, 1997). Effective treatment must attend to the multitude of factors that interact to maintain addictive behavior.

Rationale for Applying Dialectical Behavior Therapy for Individuals with BPD and SUDs

The decision to use and evaluate dialectical behavior therapy (DBT) for individuals with BPD and SUDs was influenced by a number of developments. Within the broader mental health and addiction treatment systems, there has been a growing recognition over the past two decades of the limitations of traditional approaches in the treatment of people with concurrent disorders. Historically, many clinicians held that addiction problems must be overcome before mental health problems could be successfully treated. This perspective contributed to a long-standing differential approach to the treatment of people with concurrent mental health problems and SUDs compared to those with mental health problems without SUDs. Many individuals were barred from accessing specialized mental health services until their substance abuse problems were stabilized.

In recent years, a heightened awareness of the limitations of sequential approaches to treatment has promoted a growing movement toward the use of integrated approaches for concurrent disorders—that is, treatments in which both addiction problems and mental health problems are addressed by the same clinicians. To support the development of integrated treatment models, increased funding opportunities have been made available through major organizations, including the National Institute on Drug Abuse (NIDA) and the National Institute on Alcohol Abuse and Alcoholism (NIAAA). The adaptation of DBT for substance-dependent individuals with BPD was developed in the context of a study funded by the NIDA to evaluate DBT for substance-dependent individuals with BPD (Linehan et al., 1999; Linehan & Dimeff, 1997).

A number of other compelling reasons existed to justify the extension of DBT to the treatment of comorbid BPD and substance abuse. First, studies emerged that indicated that DBT was effective in reducing the impulsive behaviors associated with BPD, most notably suicidal behaviors (Linehan, Armstrong, Suarez, Allman, & Heard, 1991; Koons et al., 2001). The finding that DBT could be successfully used to treat multidisordered individuals who did not respond well to standard treatment protocols raised hope that it could help to reduce other impulsive behaviors, such as substance abuse. Furthermore, the theoretical underpinnings and core treatment strategies of DBT shared many commonalities with prominent addiction treatments. According to one popular theory of addictive behavior, known as the "self-medication hypothesis," individuals use drugs and alcohol to modulate their emotional states (Khantzian & Schneider, 1986). This premise is consistent with DBT's biosocial theory, which maintains that emotion dysregulation is at the core of BPD-criterion behaviors. The view that substance abusers have difficulties regulating affect, and that negative emotional states precipitate substance use, is supported by a large body of empirical evidence (Kushner, Sher, & Beitman, 1990; Bradley, Gossop, Brewin, & Phillips, 1992; Cummings, Gordon, & Marlatt, 1980). Finally, at the level of clinical practice, the core strategies of DBT, which draw upon cognitive-behavioral models and acceptance-based traditions, figure centrally in prominent addiction treatment models. Cognitive-behavioral strategies are the basis of relapse prevention, a widely established, effective treatment for addictive behavior. Core techniques in DBT, including cue exposure, skills training, and contingency management, are also the cornerstone of addiction treatment. The extensive use of validation in DBT is similar to Miller and Rollnick's (1991) motivational interviewing approach. The dialectical balance in DBT between problem solving and a fundamental acceptance of current reality, including things that may not be possible to change, has similarities to a core philosophy of 12-step approaches.

DBT is the first integrated treatment model developed for people with concurrent substance abuse and BPD. Since the development of the original treatment manual, DBT has evolved through research and clinical practice. To date, it has been implemented and evaluated by research groups in a number of countries, and with diverse groups of people with BPD and SUDs.

Empirical Findings

In recent years, findings from a growing number of studies provide empirical support for the effectiveness of DBT in the treatment of concurrent SUDs and BPD. To date, four randomized controlled trials have been conducted. They are described below.

In the first study of DBT for BPD and SUDs, Linehan et al. (1999) randomized 28 substance-dependent women with BPD to 1 year of DBT ($n = 12$) or a community treatment-as-usual (TAU) control group ($n = 16$). The majority of the sample (74%) were polysubstance users who met substance-dependence criteria for a range of psychoactive substances, including opiates, methamphetamine, and marijuana; the primary substances of choice were alcohol (52%) and cocaine (58%). DBT was more effective than TAU in reducing drug abuse throughout the treatment year and at 16-month follow-up, and was more effective in retaining participants over the 1-year treatment period (64% vs. 27%). As well, DBT participants showed greater social functioning and global adjustment at 16-month follow-up compared to those receiving TAU.

In a second study that targeted a more specific group of substance abusers and used a more rigorous control condition than the first trial, Linehan et al. (2002) evaluated the efficacy of DBT in the treatment of 23 opiate-dependent women with BPD. Polysubstance abuse was prevalent in this sample, with many participants also meeting the criteria for dependence on cocaine (52%), sedatives (13%), cannabis (8.7%), and alcohol (26%). Subjects were randomly assigned to either 1 year of DBT or comprehensive validation therapy (CVT) with 12-step intervention. Developed by Linehan and her colleagues (Linehan, Tutek, Dimeff, & Koerner, 1999), the CVT condition included individual therapy and encouragement to attend 12-step meetings. CVT treatment emphasized the application of DBT acceptance strategies within a disease model/12-step frame much like 12-step facilitation treatment used in Project MATCH (Nowinski & Baker, 1992). Study results indicated that both treatments were significantly effective in reducing opiate use during the first 8 months of active treatment. However, there was a divergence between the groups by the 8-month assessment point. Between the 8-month point and the end of the 12-month active treatment, subjects receiving the CVT + 12-step intervention significantly increased their opiate use compared to subjects in the DBT group, who maintained their reductions. There were significant differences between groups on treatment retention. All 12 subjects assigned to the CVT + 12-step intervention remained in treatment whereas four out of 11 DBT subjects dropped out of treatment.

The first published independent replication study of DBT with drug-addicted individuals with BPD was conducted by researchers in the Netherlands. Verheul and colleagues (2003) conducted a randomized trial to evaluate the effectiveness of standard DBT versus TAU control. Participants consisted of 58 women diagnosed with BPD, including those with and without SUDs. Results showed that DBT was more effective than TAU in reducing treatment dropouts, frequency of self-mutilating behaviors, and self-damaging impulsive behaviors, including alcohol abuse. Interestingly, there were no differences between conditions on other drugs of abuse. In contrast to Linehan's research with substance-dependent individuals with BPD, this study did *not* make use of the modifications to DBT for substance-dependent individuals, but instead made use of standard DBT. Moreover, addiction problems were not targeted.

In another independent randomized controlled trial of DBT (i.e., DBT with modifications for SUD; McMain et al., 2004), 27 women with concurrent SUDs and BPD were randomized to DBT or to a TAU control treatment that involved a nonmanualized treatment for patients with concurrent addiction and mental health problems. In terms of alcohol use outcomes, the results favored DBT: Use of alcohol did not change significantly among TAU subjects, while alcohol severity scores were substantially decreased in DBT subjects—roughly one-third lower than at pretreatment. Both groups showed improvements in drug use outcomes: DBT subjects had greater initial reductions in drug use, though by final outcome TAU subjects revealed an overall greater improvement. The results of this study showed that DBT had the most impact on reducing self-damaging behaviors and alcohol use. Similar to the findings in the Verheul et al. (2003) study, DBT was not more beneficial than standard treatments for addiction problems in reducing drug use. Although more research is needed, these findings suggest that whereas DBT may be equivalent to standard treatments in reducing drug use, it may have an added advantage of improving other behavioral problems related to BPD such as impulsivity and self-harm behavior.

Whom is DBT Designed to Treat?

DBT was originally developed for the treatment of chronically suicidal individuals with multiple and severe behavioral problems. The specific adaptation for substance dependence was designed and evaluated as a treatment for similarly severe substance-dependent individuals with BPD. The population of individuals with BPD and SUDs for whom this adaptation was based is largely heterogeneous in terms of drugs of abuse and demographic variables (e.g., race/ethnicity, gender, education, marital status). The majority of individuals who participated in the above-noted randomized control trials (RCTs) on which the adaptations are based were polysubstance-dependent with extensive histories of substance abuse and multiple unsuccessful attempts at getting off drugs prior to beginning DBT.

Might DBT be useful for other substance-dependent individuals without BPD? No studies have been conducted to date evaluating DBT's efficacy for substance-dependent individuals without a concurrent diagnosis of BPD. As clinical decisions are often required before findings are available from controlled clinical trials, a few principles may assist in determining whether DBT may be an appropriate intervention. First, clinical decisions and treatment planning should be guided by what is known from the empirical literature. Is there an already proven treatment for the particular problem(s) your patient has? Second, be parsimonious. All things being equal, consider beginning with a more simple and efficient treatment than one as complex and comprehensive as DBT. While DBT no doubt contains elements that will be therapeutic for most patients, it is also likely that it is considerably more extensive than most patients with SUDs require. Third, consider the extent to which emotion dysregulation plays a role in the individual's continued use of drugs. Because DBT was developed specifically for individuals with pervasive emotion dysregulation, it may be a good fit for people whose use of drugs is associated with affective dyscontrol. But DBT may be ineffective for individuals whose emotions contribute little, if any, to sustained use of drugs. Finally, given that it was developed for a population of usually difficult-to-treat patients with multiple Axis I and Axis II problems, DBT may be well suited to address the problems of the patient who though non-BPD is a multidiagnostic SUD patient who has failed on multiple occasions in other evidence-based SUD therapies.

What is DBT for Concurrent Substance Abuse and BPD?

The standard DBT protocol was developed by Linehan (1993a, 1993b) for the treatment of BPD. In DBT for the treatment of BPD and SUDs, an integrative approach to treatment is adopted to concurrently address addiction problems and other behavioral problems that are unique to individuals with BPD. DBT for concurrent BPD and SUDs differs from standard DBT in only one respect: It provides more focus on addictive behaviors and associated problems. Otherwise the treatments are identical. It is designed for the treatment of multidisordered individuals with concurrent BPD and substance abuse problems. Consistent with the standard DBT treatment, the overarching goals of treatment are (1) to reduce serious behavioral dyscontrol (e.g., substance abuse, suicidal behavior, nonsuicidal self-injurious behaviors, excessive and extreme behaviors that interfere with therapy, and other behaviors that significantly interfere with the patients' quality of life), and (2) to promote more adaptive, skillful behaviors for functioning in life. As with other impulsive behaviors associated with BPD, addictive behaviors are conceptualized as learned behaviors that function as a means to regulate emotions and that may occur in the midst of the chaos of dysregulation. All modes of the treatment protocol (i.e., individual therapy, skills group, telephone coaching, therapist consultation team) are delivered just as they are in standard DBT.

Several additional features were incorporated into DBT for patients with both BPD and SUDs in order to facilitate the treatment of substance abuse. The treatment modifications are drawn from interventions discussed in the substance abuse treatment literature, as well as from clinical experience gained from applying DBT to substance-using individuals with BPD in a number of settings. DBT for patients with BPD and SUDs is distinguished from standard DBT only by the addition of (1) a conceptual framework for understanding the overlap between BPD and substance abuse, (2) a dialectical philosophy to define treatment goals related to addictive behaviors and to address relapse, and (3) a modified treatment target hierarchy that includes a focus on substance abuse. In addition, a number of special treatment strategies were added to address the unique needs of patients with concurrent BPD and SUDs including a set of attachment strategies developed to enhance treatment engagement and retention in this notoriously difficult-to-engage population and specific examples of the DBT skills tailored to the SUDs population.

Dialectical Abstinence

DBT stresses the message that to get the most satisfaction in life, abstinence from drug use is the most appropriate ultimate goal in a Stage 1 treatment. Why? Because drug use significantly interferes with building a life worth living in severely disordered individuals, including those with BPD and SUDs. However, focusing solely on abstinence often leaves a real gap when patients fall short—a phenomenon described initially by Marlatt and Gordon (1985) as the "abstinence violation effect" (AVE): The intense negative emotions that patients typically feel in response to a slip or relapse can themselves create the very conditions for continued drug use. Particularly among severely disordered individuals with problems of pervasive emotion dysregulation, addressing the AVE often requires support and coaching from the therapist to help them safely return to abstinence. A dialectical stance on drug use was developed in recognition of the findings that, on the one hand, cognitive-behavioral relapse prevention (RP) approaches based largely on harm reduction principles (Marlatt & Donovan, 2005) are effective in reducing the frequency and intensity of drug use following a period of abstinence from drug use, and that, on the other hand, "absolute abstinence" approaches are effective in lengthening the interval between periods of use (Hall, Havassy, & Wasserman, 1990; Supnick & Colletti, 1984). "Dialectical abstinence," which seeks to balance these positions, is a synthesis of unrelenting insistence on total abstinence before any illicit drug abuse and radical acceptance, nonjudgmental problem solving, and effective relapse prevention after any drug use.

While the ultimate goal in DBT is to get and keep patients completely free of their problem drugs of abuse, for many individuals the goal of abstinence seems out of reach. The essence of the absolute abstinence end of the dialectic involves teaching clients specific cognitive self-control strategies that allow them to turn their minds fully and completely to abstinence. Specifically, patients are taught how to anticipate and treat willfulness, hopelessness, and the waffling on one's commitment to get off drugs that commonly arises and complicates treatment once an individual makes a commitment to give up a dysfunctional habit. Patients learn that the key to absolute abstinence lies in making a strong commitment to rule out drug use entirely. This can be best accomplished by making a commitment to stay abstinent for a specified period that is no longer than he or she can commit to with 100% certainty that abstinence will be maintained. Like the popular 12-step slogan "Just for Today," the commitment to 100% abstinence may be for only 1 day, or for a whole month, or just for 5 minutes, depending on what the individual can commit to with 100% certainty of success. The commitment, then, is an act of mental "slamming the door shut" for that specified period of time. Upon expiration of the original commitment period, the individual recommits again to abstinence. In this sense, absolute abstinence is achieved by a series of recommitted "slamming the door shut." Hence, abstinence is sought only in the moment and only for a given set of moments. Like pearls that comprise a pearl necklace, a lifetime of abstinence is achieved a moment or a day at a time—just this one moment, then the next, and so on. The ultimate goal of this strategy is to block the ability to make half-hearted commitments (or to deny the reality that one has been made), while simultaneously limiting the commitment duration to a period that is perceived by the person's brain, so to speak, as achievable.

Other absolute abstinence cognitive self-control strategies used to trick the individual's brain during this phase include immediate "adaptive" denial of desires and options to use during the specified period of commitment, practicing radical acceptance of the absence of drug use and the difficulties involved, making an inner deal with oneself that the option to use drugs is left open for the future, as well as the promise to oneself of using drugs when close to death or upon learning of a terminal illness. Individuals with SUDs are also taught how to look ahead, plan for danger, and be proactive in order not to use again. For example, they are coached to "burn bridges" so they no longer have access to drugs; they learn what cues are dangerous for them and how to avoid those cues; and they learn skills for tolerating urges and cravings, as well as skills for changing their social environment to be more conducive to staying drug-free. Determining which strategy to utilize depends on which is most effective in promoting abstinence and the willingness to maintain it.

While remaining fully committed to abstinence, DBT, like RP, recognizes that all new behaviors, including those associated with abstinence, take time and practice to solidify, and that as a consequence of this reality slips are likely to occur along the way. While maintaining that a commitment to abstinence is essential, the therapist simultaneously prepares the patient for doing the least amount of damage if and when a slip does happen and provides assistance for returning to abstinence as quickly as possible. As in RP, a lapse is viewed as a problem to solve, not as a treatment failure. Instead, the emphasis is on acquiring and strengthening the skill of "failing well," which involves admitting that drug use has occurred and learning from one's mistakes by conducting a thorough chain analysis and identifying solutions for future use should the event that prompted use of drugs occur again. In teaching how to fail well, emphasis is placed on "what if" and "just in case" skills should a crisis occur. Consistent with RP (Marlatt & Donovan, 2005), the therapist and the patient discuss realistic skills and game plans the client can use should he or she be faced with a similar situation in the future. Rather than be caught off guard by an inevitable high-risk situation that could threaten an individual's hard-earned abstinence, DBT, like RP, focuses on precaution, planning, and preparedness as means of enhancing the individual's behavioral control, resulting ultimately in better treatment outcomes. Much like how a flight crew prepares their passengers for *the unlikely event of* a loss of cabin pressure or a water landing, DBT and RP prepare people to effectively manage the inevitable high-risk situation, including a potential slip, so that the response is swift and effective (e.g., a slip is indeed only a slip and does not progress to a full-blown relapse). Such "drop and roll" emergency strategies include calling the DBT therapist, having reminders about why they want to get clean, and getting rid of drugs so they cannot use them again. Failing well includes analysis of and reparation for the harm done from using drugs. The emphasis on correcting the harm caused to others and to oneself is similar to making amends in 12-step programs.

Other harm reduction strategies (Marlatt, 1998) incorporated into DBT include educating patients about HIV/AIDS and hepatitis C transmission, infections related to IV drug use, and other ways to minimize harm should they use drugs. In this respect, DBT is helping patients to use drugs more safely when they do use, but this approach is taken only on an as-needed basis, always working toward returning to abstinence.

The concept of dialectical abstinence is similar to the actions of a running back in football. In each play, the running back is never fully content to obtain a few extra yards for a first down: He is always striving to score a touchdown. Once the play is initiated, all his efforts are oriented toward moving the ball the full distance to the goal (abstinence) unless he is tackled. The DBT therapist adopts a similar approach, "running" with the patient like mad in the direction of abstinence, stopping only if the patient falls and even then only long enough to get the patient back on his or her feet, and then running again with the full intent to score a touchdown on the next play.

Hierarchy of Targets in the Treatment of Concurrent BPD and Substance Abuse

The hierarchy for DBT with patients with SUDs remains the same as in traditional DBT. While there are special considerations to be made regarding prioritizing substance use and related behaviors, the hierarchy remains a guide to treating patients with multiple, high-risk, difficult behaviors.

Pretreatment

In DBT, the therapist communicates the expectation of abstinence by asking the patient to commit to stop using in the very first session. This commitment is strengthened via the DBT commitment strategies, and is discussed frequently during treatment. Obtaining initial commitment in the first few sessions can be accomplished with the standard DBT commitment strategies. In brief, the patient and the therapist explore the patient's goals and values, and the therapist points out that the patient cannot accomplish those goals or live within those values while the patient is abusing substances. At this point, the therapist asks for a commitment to complete abstinence. Using the "door in the face" (asking for a very large commitment, such as "Do you agree never to use again?," which can increase the likelihood of agreement to smaller goals) and "foot in the door" (obtaining a relatively small agreement, which then opens the door for the therapist to ask for more) techniques strategically, the therapist can eventually elicit the longest period to which the patient can commit to abstinence. This initial commitment may be for the course of treatment (a year) or just for 24 hours. What is important is that a commitment to abstinence—the goal of Stage 1 DBT—is made, and that the therapist conveys the message that this commitment will be taken very seriously.

In the initial commitment to treatment, the therapist seeks a commitment to abstinence: Is the patient willing to get off drugs, is abstinence the goal of DBT? Or is the client expecting and preferring a pure harm-reduction approach, where the goal is *not* necessarily to get off drugs but to experience fewer negative consequences while using drugs? As with trip planning, you want to be sure you know your destination before you purchase your airplane tickets. Better that you and your patient are clear what DBT will and won't offer than discover a fundamental difference in preferred approach during the midst of treatment. Only after a patient has committed to abstinence would the therapist make use of the "absolute abstinence" commitment strategy (e.g., committing to a period of abstinence that the person knows he or she can achieve with absolute certainty). This specific strategy is designed to help the individual achieve his or her goal of abstinence by breaking down the task into smaller and more manageable steps.

In DBT a patient is in pretreatment until he or she makes a commitment to work on eliminating all life-threatening behaviors and to engage in treatment. The same expectation is true in DBT with patients with SUDs. But should a patient be expected to make a commitment to abstain from all illicit problematic substances prior to starting DBT? With patients with BPD, abstinence is the most appropriate choice of goals since teaching controlled use is not likely to lead to positive results. However, the problem with requiring abstinence before treatment begins is that some people will initially refuse such a goal. For example, a patient beginning DBT for opiate dependence may be unwilling to stop using marijuana, though eager to begin treatment for opiates. In such situations, requiring abstinence from all substances is not necessarily effective. Instead, the therapist may focus on obtaining a commitment to abstain from the substance that presents the greatest threat to the patient's quality of life (and any others that the patient can be convinced to give up), while obtaining an agreement that other, lower priority substances will be negotiated later in therapy. It is often the case that once patients have had success with one problematic substance, they become much more engaged in addressing another. Because the others are lower on the treatment hierarchy, they can be focused on at a later point. In other cases, complete abstinence may not be essential. For example, individuals who do not meet the criteria for alcohol dependence but express concern over their drinking may be able to learn to control their use of alcohol. Similarly, individuals maintained on methadone may not seek abstinence from methadone but may be able to dramatically improve their quality of life.

Upon obtaining a commitment from a patient to abstain, the therapist then moves to the role of devil's advocate. The therapist points out all of the reasons why one might want to stay on drugs, and asks, "Why on earth would you want to make this commitment?" This helps the patient pinpoint reasons why he or she uses, and generate reasons why it would be worthwhile to give up those "benefits" (e.g., short-term emotion regulation). Getting the patient to generate these arguments is important so he or she can re-create these reasons when alone and faced with temptation. More on commitment strategies can be found in Linehan (1993a).

In the first several sessions, the therapist and the patient may return to this discussion many times. Until the patient actually stops drug use for any length of time, the patient is considered to be in the "pretreatment commitment" phase and the commitment strategies are the main focus of the sessions. During this period, the therapist focuses heavily on the patient's values and priorities—their "Wise Mind" reasons to get off drugs. Many times these patients have never looked toward the future or considered what their values are. But with sufficient discussion patients generally can determine at least some of their own values. The consistent message from the therapist is that a person cannot live in line with his or her values, or meet his or her life goals, while he or she is living the life of someone who is addicted to substances. This lays the groundwork for increasing investment in abstinence when the patient may falter later in treatment, as well. Linehan (in press) has developed a series of skills handouts and homework sheets aimed at elucidating patients' values and helping them determine priorities to work toward those values, which are used in the initial phases and throughout treatment.

For example, one adolescent patient had not been drug-free for any period of time in his late childhood or adolescent years. He had never given any thought to what he valued or what he wished to work toward. With coaching from his therapist, he realized that he strongly valued his family relationships (which he had neglected for several years). He became very motivated to become drug-free in order to nurture these ties. This discussion strengthened his investment in the treatment and changed his focus from drugs to his family. After this discussion, the therapist reminded him of his values and related goals when he was not in Wise Mind, which helped him return to effective behaviors in many cases.

As soon as the patient has stopped drug use (even if only for a very brief period of time, such as a week), the therapist then switches strategies from commitment to problem solving following a lapse. Should a slip occur, chain analysis and solution analysis are the primary tools. In the spirit of failing well, effort is made to determine the factors that led to the slip as a means of generating alternative, effective solutions to avert another slip. A common treatment error in DBT and other substance abuse treatments is to use maintenance strategies (i.e., chain analysis) *before* cessation of the behavior has occurred. We have found that moving to chain analysis prematurely, before commitment has been secured, is much less effective because the patient is less likely to implement the solution. Given this reality, it is only *after* patients are abstinent and "throwing themselves into treatment" that therapists move to problem-solving, change-focused strategies. This is not to say that the therapist does not analyze patterns and assess the functions of the behaviors in the commitment phase, but the therapist does so in the service of helping the patient see the pros and cons of using drugs, as well as the consequences of doing so. Only once the patient and the therapist are functioning as a team in the service of the same goals, as evidenced by commitment and at least a brief cessation of drug use, does the dyad move into traditional DBT treatment strategies.

Stage 1

Treating a Stage 1 patient with concurrent BPD and SUDs typically involves targeting multiple, extreme problems. This can overwhelm the therapist and contribute to an unfocused treatment in which the emphasis is on the "crisis of the week," with little progress on any goals. To address this problem, DBT follows the target hierarchy delineated in the standard protocol (refer to Linehan, 1993a, for a more detailed description). The therapist is not expected to focus on only one behavioral target in each session; rather, the hierarchy is used to set session agendas and prioritize behavioral foci. This targeting system allows the therapist to attend to the problems that are of utmost importance without getting drawn off track by the unremitting crises that arise between sessions.

In DBT substance abuse is considered a quality-of-life behavior, and is therefore ranked below life-threatening and therapy-interfering behaviors. This means that in a given therapy session, a patient's substance abuse behavior may not be the top priority. For example, if a methamphetamine user becomes suicidal, the therapist may choose to target the drug use only briefly, or even to postpone discussion of it, in order to assess and minimize the risk of suicide. As long as the patient is refraining from engaging in life-threatening and therapy-interfering behaviors, the substance abuse behavior can take top priority. If there is a concern that the patient may not survive until the next session, or is behaving in a manner inconsistent with the progress of treatment, substance abuse must take a back seat to these other targets. This does not mean the therapist should ignore substance use in any session with higher-order targets. Rather, the DBT therapist needs to stay mindful of keeping the patient alive and participating in treatment rather than placing the main focus of the session on substances. While this may be an implicit rule of thumb of most other evidence-based therapies for addictive behaviors, it is made explicit in DBT because of the severity of patients treated in DBT.

If careful analysis reveals that lower-order targets are closely related to higher-order primary behavioral targets, the lower-order targets may take on more importance early in treatment as well. For example, a therapist may discover that drinking is a precipitant to suicide attempts. In this case, alcohol intake would be targeted immediately in an attempt to change the chain of events toward suicide. Similarly, cigarette smoking would generally be placed lower on the treatment hierarchy; however, if it were closely linked to illicit substance abuse, it would take higher priority. One of the authors (L. D.) had a heroin-dependent patient who often arrived late (more than 1 hour late in most cases) to nearly all his sessions. Targeting the tardiness by conducting chain analyses and problem solving was not yielding any changes. The consultation team discussed the problem and decided that because the patient's heroin use was nearly always related to his tardiness, the heroin use needed to be considered as therapy-interfering behavior. Targeting heroin use instead of one outcome of heroin use (tardiness) was more effective in this case.

In another case, one of the authors (S. M.) had a patient who drank one or two beers a day, a problem behavior that in ordinary circumstances might be very low on the treatment hierarchy. However, this patient had pancreatitis and had been informed by her doctor that a single beer could actually kill her. In this case, we chose to move the "drinking beer" target up to "life-threatening behavior" (any time a dangerous behavior becomes *imminently* life threatening it moves up the hierarchy; for this particular patient the behavior was also intentional self-harm in that the pain from drinking functioned to regulate her emotions), meaning that it took precedence over all else except her other self-harm behaviors. By using the data we had regarding pancreatitis and alcohol intake as our guides, we could tailor the hierarchy to her needs much more successfully.

Prioritizing various substances of abuse can be a challenge as well. Decisions regarding which problem substances are higher priority and which are lower priority should be made on a case-by-case basis. A focus on effectiveness and on the treatment hierarchy helps the therapist and the patient make decisions regarding priorities. Illicit substances are targeted first in most cases because they present a more significant threat to an individual's quality of life (not only the sequelae of the abuse specifically, but also the threat of legal problems). Replacement medications, particularly for opiates, are recommended if the severity of the drug use warrants their use. Although they may compromise quality of life somewhat, treatment outcome studies suggest that this is less of a risk than having no replacement (Dole, 1988). Decisions on how to prioritize substance targets with polysubstance users are made based on a patient's individual situation, taking into account the severity of abuse and the extent to which the substance increases the chances of a compromised quality of life (with substance abuse and in other areas of the patient's life as well).

The Path to Clear Mind

Using drugs is but one behavior targeted under the general category of decreasing substance abuse; other behaviors related to substance abuse must be prioritized as well. Within the behavioral target of substance abuse, DBT has additional targets specifically aimed at behaviors needed for getting off drugs. These targets related to decreasing substance use are collectively known as the *DBT Path to Clear Mind*. The path begins with the overarching substance abuse target of decreasing substance abuse, then places equal focus on other important steps necessary in becoming and staying clean. In contrast to the standard DBT hierarchy, the targets that form the Path to Clear Mind are *not* hierarchically arranged with the exception of the first, logical target: to decrease substance abuse. The Path to Clear Mind targets include:

• *Decrease substance abuse*. This is the first step in the Path to Clear Mind. This target includes stopping all use of illegal drugs and all abuse of prescribed drugs.
• *Decrease physical discomfort*. This target is particularly focused on decreasing discomfort due to withdrawal symptoms, but also includes other causes of physical discomfort. Because most people are not fully aware of the physical and psychological withdrawal symptoms that correspond to their specific drugs of abuse, it is critical to educate them about the effects of each substance used. For example, one woman who was dependent on crack believed that her use was under control because she managed to abstain for 3 days between each period of use. She didn't realize that her crack use corresponded to intense feelings of withdrawal including insomnia, irritability, and emptiness. Despite

being committed to the goal of abstinence, whenever she experienced the first hint of withdrawal she would run out to use crack in order to alleviate her discomfort. DBT readily incorporates replacement medications such as methadone, buprinorphine, or ativan when appropriate, in an effort to reduce the physical discomfort due to withdrawal while maximizing the chances of abstinence. Nonopiate forms of pain management may be effective as well.

• *Decrease urges, cravings, and temptations to use drugs.* Research has demonstrated that urges—in particular, urge intensity from the previous day, duration of urge, and urge intensity upon awakening—are predictive of lapse (Shiffman, Engberg, Paty, & Perz, l997). Patients are taught a variety of skills (Linehan, in press) to help them tolerate urges, cravings, and temptations and to be more proactive in preventing lapses. Strategies include observing and labeling an urge as "only an urge," reviewing the long-term pros and cons of using, and using distress tolerance skills. Examples of distress tolerance skills for SUDs include imagining oneself being effective and not using; distracting oneself from urges and cravings; soothing oneself; focusing on one moment at a time; immersing one's face in ice water to elicit the "dive response" (Hiebert & Burch, 2003), which may help to regulate emotion (Porges, Doussard-Roosevelt, & Maita, 1994); and reminding oneself that urges and cravings are temporary and do not need to result in action (Porges et al., 1994).

• *Decrease the option to use drugs.* This target involves decreasing the likelihood that the patient will be able to turn to psychoactive substances even when the temptation is great. To achieve this, the patient is coached to systematically eliminate opportunities to use drugs—to "burn (his or her) bridges" to his or her previous life of using drugs. Actions taken may include moving away from dealers, destroying phone numbers for drug contacts, changing one's phone number to prevent those people from making contact, stopping all lying and stealing, making public commitments to be clean, telling others (particularly one's therapist) how to detect signs of use, and identifying oneself as someone who has quit using. Coaching patients in how to assert themselves effectively by using interpersonal effectiveness skills is important at this stage. Coaching distress tolerance skills too is important to help patients purposefully end destructive, drug-focused relationships. For example, one patient purposefully angered a former boyfriend so that he would stop dropping by unannounced with free drugs. Breaking completely with this former boyfriend was extremely difficult but necessary for her to obtain abstinence. This approach can help patients prevent drug use even when they temporarily lose their commitment and decide to use again. It is similar to removing lethal means for suicidal patients. The objective is to help prevent the individual from acting when in a state of "Emotion Mind." This is a state during which the patient's thoughts, desires, and behaviors are ruled only by emotion (Linehan, 1993a), and he or she is less inclined to follow through with commitments. Cutting off options forces the patient to find other ways to tolerate urges and distress, rather than falling off the wagon.

• *Decrease contact with cues for drug use.* These cues serve to remind the patient of previous drug use (often out of the individual's awareness). Additionally, drug use cues may actually elicit withdrawal symptoms, in turn increasing the likelihood of relapse (Siegel & Ramos, 2002). Cues that have been paired repeatedly with drug use can actually operate to make the individual "expect" the drug. The brain then reacts as if the drug has been administered, and counteracts the drug's effects in order to maintain homeostasis. When such counteraction occurs in the absence of the drug, withdrawal sensations are experienced, increasing the likelihood of use to alleviate physical discomfort (Siegel & Ramos, 2002). It is important to carefully assess what the patient's cues for drug use are, as they vary according to each person's drug use pattern. Examples for such cues may include particular individuals, locations, thoughts, music, or even sitting in the back row of a Narcotics Anonymous meeting. By helping patients avoid contact with cues for drug use, their urges, cravings, and actual use can be reduced. Patients are coached to get rid of drug paraphernalia and other reminders of drug use, not to enter situations related to previous use, and to avoid individuals who may be associated with drugs. For example, one patient realized that she had an overwhelming urge to use cocaine whenever she was in her bathroom. It was important to help her understand that her bathroom was a cue because it was the place she escaped to for privacy to use crack. Changing the cues in the bathroom by painting the room, putting in soaps with a new fragrance and changing the color of the towels was instrumental in decreasing her urges to use.

• *Increase reinforcement of "Clear Mind" behaviors.* Patients who succeed in getting clean will not stay clean if their new, skillful behaviors are not reinforced. It is important for them to arrange their environments such that they receive reinforcement, not punishment, for engaging in these changes. A patient who manages to get clean, but still spends time with friends who use, will likely experience punishers (such as "I can't believe you're seeing a therapist" or "This won't last") that can threaten treatment success. This target focuses on helping the patient find new friends, social activities, vocational settings, and other environments that will provide support for clean behaviors, and withdraw support or even punish behaviors related to drug use. The interpersonal effectiveness skills (Linehan, 1993a, in press) are particularly important to help in building these new relationships.

• *Clear Mind.* "Clear Mind" is the ultimate goal of the substance abuse targets in DBT. It is a prerequisite to getting into "Wise Mind" (Linehan, 1993a, 1993b), in which the patient can synthesize the poles of "Reasonable Mind" (where one is influenced only by logic without the benefit of emotion) and "Emotion Mind" (where one is influenced only by emotions without the benefit of logic) to incorporate all ways of knowing. Wise Mind is by definition a state where one is able to make the wisest decisions possible, knowing just what is needed in any given moment. Clear Mind is itself a dialectic: it is the synthesis of "Addict Mind" and "Clean Mind." Substance-abusing patients start treatment in Addict Mind, in which their thoughts, beliefs, actions, and emotions are controlled by craving drugs, finding drugs, and using drugs. This is the state where one is "chasing the bag," impulsive, and willing to sacrifice what is important just to obtain and use the desired substance. After some clean time, patients often move to Clean Mind. In Clean Mind, the patient is not using, but forgets that he or she may be in danger of using again. This state can be thought of as being "blinded by the light," or having one's judgment clouded by the fact that one has finally managed to get off drugs. Patients in this state may become reckless, thinking they are immune from future problems because they have succeeded in getting clean. As a result they may fail to manage pain appropriately, ignore temptations or cues that increase vulnerability to use, and keep options open to use drugs.

In Clear Mind, the patient has achieved a state of Clean Mind *and* remains very aware that Addict Mind could return at any time. Cues may still lead to intense cravings and, without intervention, to actual drug use. The patient not only stops to enjoy success, but also prepares for future problems and has plans for what to do if staying clean becomes difficult. A metaphor that may help patients understand this point is as follows: Being in Clear Mind is like going for a hike up a mountain. As you near the peak, you may get excited and feel the hard work is done. When you get to the top, you stop working, rest, and enjoy the view. Without taking away from the thrill and relief of reaching the top, to be effective, you need to remember that there is still a return trip: you will need to leave the peak while there is still enough daylight to get back to the car; you will need to make sure you have enough food and water for the return trip; and you will need to be sure you have enough energy to get back. The point is, while you are enjoying your success, you must remember and prepare for the remaining challenges of hiking down the mountain. Thus, in Clear Mind, you work hard at *getting clean* and really appreciate the success of *being clean*, but you do not forget that getting clean isn't the end point. There is still a journey after getting clean that involves *staying* clean. Additionally, the planning for the return trip can't be put off until you reach the top of the mountain. If you make it to the peak and *then* realize you don't have enough food for the return trip, you will be in trouble. Planning for *staying* clean needs to begin *now*, just as planning for the entire hike begins before you leave home.

Balancing the many targets on the Path to Clear Mind can be challenging. Therapists may find many of the targets in this hierarchy are intertwined. As with the standard DBT treatment hierarchy, the Path to Clear Mind, coupled with detailed assessment, can provide much-needed structure. For example, one patient had committed to stop using, and in fact had successfully switched from heroin to suboxone and maintained several weeks of clean urine samples (i.e., she had successfully decreased her use and her physical discomfort associated with withdrawal). However, she was in a very tumultuous relationship, and was raising two small children with very little money. She continued to have strong urges that were most commonly associated with strong emotions related to her boyfriend and the stresses of parenting and poverty. Even when she was experiencing no urges, she had friends who would "check in" on her, and often bring her free heroin and cocaine. To the therapist, this was an overwhelming set of problems to tackle (i.e., strong urges related to her conflict with her boyfriend, poverty, stress of parenting, visits by drug-using friends). Using the Path to Clear Mind lent some order to their sessions, as they would choose one or two targets to focus on at any given time. At times their assessment would lead them to put high priority on items lower in importance—for example, they discovered that her strongest urges arose whenever she was presented with the cue of her boyfriend's crack pipe. As there was a relatively simple solution to the problem (having him hide his pipe better), this target was given precedence over others. The Path to Clear Mind is meant to provide structure, not to add to the confusion of complex problems or create unnecessary rigidity.

Special Treatment Strategies

The specific intervention strategies that were added to DBT for concurrent BPD and SUDs can be grouped into three main categories: (1) a set of attachment strategies designed to address the increased difficulties with becoming attached to treatment (the "butterfly" problem); (2) specific examples for the DBT skills for dealing with urges, cravings with attendant slips, or relapses (the "addiction" problem); and (3) self-management strategies to deal with the consequences of having a lifestyle built on a foundation of substance abuse (the "getting a normal life" problem).

Attachment Strategies

Engaging patients in the treatment process is vital to successful therapy. While the retention of any patients with BPD in treatment is notoriously difficult (Linehan, 1993a), it is even more difficult with those who have concurrent substance abuse problems. Though some patients will attach to treatment readily, Linehan et al. (1999) characterize others as "butterflies" who attend sessions intermittently, fail to return phone calls, and "flit" in and out of treatment unexpectedly. A number of factors can contribute to problems with treatment engagement. Many substance-abusing individuals with BPD lead chaotic lifestyles as a consequence of their pervasive drug use: They may be unemployed, unable to support themselves financially, and have resorted to criminal activities. Some individuals lack adequate housing and may live on the street or in crack houses. Some may stay in dysfunctional and even abusive relationships because they lack the financial means to move to a new environment. Drug abuse can interrupt the organization of routines in day-to-day living, making it difficult to attend scheduled appointments. Further, it usually involves denial and lying about one's behavior. Patients often minimize their problems and are reluctant to acknowledge problematic behaviors to themselves or others because of their ambivalence about change. For example, one woman, only after being treated for months, revealed that she was working as a prostitute. A general reluctance to discuss problematic behaviors can stem from fear about disclosing illegal activities or shame about drug use.

Anecdotally, many DBT therapists who begin treating substance abusers have found this to be a difficult adjustment. Therapists often comment that they feel they have much less leverage with their patients with SUDs. Whereas in standard DBT, they are often the sole source of reinforcement for their patients, including warmth, encouragement, praise, and validation, with patients with SUDs they feel as if they need to "compete" with the drugs. Traditional DBT patients often become very attached to the therapeutic relationship, but patients with SUDs may not, at least at the start of treatment. Drugs simply offer more powerful, immediate changes in emotion than the therapist can. Attachment strategies can counteract this problem when applied diligently, early in treatment.

A primary treatment task in DBT is to enhance the patient's motivation and engagement in treatment. Lack of motivation or disengagement is viewed as a problem to be solved rather than as an obstacle that needs to be resolved before treatment can be initiated. The therapist is challenged to engage the patient, and must be prepared to assume an active role in doing so. Similar to a skilled fisherman, who must use different bait, rods, and lines, and eventually may need to grab a net to reel in the catch, the therapist must be steadfast and patient in these efforts. Ideally, the process of catching the fish will be as gratifying as the victory of the catch. However, if it is a long wait without a catch, the process may be experienced as arduous and frustrating. Like the fisherman, the DBT therapist may require support from others in order to continue the pursuit.

DBT incorporates a number of specific attachment strategies (see Table 6.1) to facilitate treatment engagement with substance-abusing patients with BPD, in order to influence the probability of their entering, engaging in, and successfully completing treatment. The therapist must begin by orienting the patient to the problem. During this orientation phase, it is crucial to openly discuss potential barriers to treatment engagement, including anticipating the obstacles early, discussing the early warning signals, and developing a plan for handling these when they arise. Meeting jointly with other treatment providers (e.g., a pharmacotherapist) should occur during the orientation phase, to ensure that everyone is working together to support the patient. Supportive family or friends should also be engaged early into treatment to ensure that they are reinforcing effective behaviors. For example, one of our patients was under strong pressure from her father to enter a 60-day residential substance abuse facility, which would have meant that she would miss four consecutive sessions of DBT and therefore would have been dropped from the program. It was important to have a joint family meeting to discuss the rationale for her

TABLE 6.1. Strategies to Enhance Attachment to Treatment

- Orient the patient to the problem.
- Increase contact.
- Provide therapy *in vivo*.
- Build connections to the social network.
- Provide shorter or longer sessions as necessary.
- Actively pursue patients when they get lost.
- Mobilize the team when the therapist gets demoralized.
- Build the patient's connection to the treatment network.

remaining in an outpatient DBT program. It is also necessary during the orientation phase to develop a crisis plan with the patient, including details of where the patient may go if he or she "gets lost" (is in danger of missing four consecutive sessions), and who may be called upon to pull the patient back into treatment. In the first few sessions, the therapist can find out where the patient typically goes when he or she is using, where he or she will sleep, eat, take showers, and the like, and who will know how to find him or her. The therapist can also get written permission to talk to key people in the patient's life, in the event the patient stops attending sessions.

In the first several months of therapy, it is helpful to have as frequent contact with the patient as possible, in order to increase the patient's positive feelings about therapy and the therapeutic relationship. Furthermore, early on in treatment, extra contact can help patients reduce the chaos in their lives more quickly. Increasing contact by scheduling extra sessions, lengthening sessions, or adding phone and/or text messages can help patients manage multiple crises when they may not be able to wait a week for help, and can help them feel that there is a supportive community available to help. Some patients may benefit from shorter, more frequent sessions.

If the patient "gets lost," the primary therapist and the team must actively work to reengage him or her. This may involve pursuing the patient by sending cards or a token gift (e.g., a packet of forget-me-not seeds), or even searching for the patient in his or her own environment such as a neighborhood or a favorite coffee shop. For example, with one patient who failed to show to sessions, the therapist took some glue to the patient's workplace, a strip club, with an attached note stating "Stick with us." It is critical to try and prevent deleterious consequences from building while the patient remains out of contact. For example, one patient, who missed 3 weeks of sessions because he went on a crack binge, ended up in a physical altercation with police that led to eviction from his apartment, criminal charges, and jail time. In our experience, actively pursuing patients in their own environment if they become lost often has a powerful impact, with patients typically surprised that anyone cares enough to pursue them.

With patients who are hard to engage, it is not uncommon for therapists to feel burned out and to lack the energy to actively find the patient. The treatment team needs to remain alert to the fact that hard-to-engage patients are likely to demoralize even the most skilled therapist, and to work actively to support the therapist. The entire team goes into alert and mobilizes when a patient misses three consecutive sessions. For example, when these authors were about to lose a patient due to the four miss rule, many members of the team tried to visit the patient at home and bring her a dose of suboxone so she would not use again. The therapist coordinated the effort, but several team members attempted to make contact with the patient, which energized the therapist and strengthened team relationships.

Using Skills to Cope with Urges and Cravings and to Reduce Risk of Relapse

The standard DBT treatment protocol for BPD includes four core skills modules (Linehan, 1993b), which are as relevant to the treatment of addictive problems as they are for other problems associated with BPD. With patients with SUDs, these core skills are taught as prescribed in the standard format. Our original expectation was that the development of new skills would be necessary, but we have found that the standard DBT skills (Linehan, 1993b, in press) are sufficient, with only one exception. The mindfulness skill of Clear Mind is a new skill aimed at addiction in particular.

Clean Mind

The concept of Clear Mind was described above, in the Path to Clear Mind section. Essentially, the therapeutic task is to help the patient facilitate the synthesis of two poles: (1) being clean (Clean Mind) and (2) staying wary of the dangers of addictive thoughts, emotions, and behaviors (Addict Mind). To do so, the skills trainers and individual therapist highlight moments when the patient may be in "Addict Mind, when he or she is" seeking drugs and not working toward abstinence, or in "Clean Mind," when he or she is clean and believing the struggle is over. Our patients helped to generate examples of these poles. Examples of Addict Mind behavior included any behavior involving looking for, buying, or otherwise seeking drugs; lying; stealing; not making eye contact; "acting like a corpse"; "not having any life in my eyes"; avoiding doctors; glamorizing drugs; and thinking "I don't have a drug problem." Examples of Clean Mind behaviors included thinking it is not dangerous to dress like a drug addict, returning to drug environments and relationships, believing one can handle the problem alone, stopping medication, thinking "I can use just a little," carrying around extra cash, and thinking "I can't stand this." Individual therapists and skills leaders who are vigilant to these signals can help move the patient back into Clear Mind, in which the patient is abstinent and acutely aware that without skills and vigilance temptation and intense urges can return at any moment.

Tailoring the Skills to Your Patient

When teaching DBT skills to patients with SUDs, the therapist must be able to aim the skills specifically at drug use behaviors, and have many relevant examples and stories to clearly and concretely illustrate each point. It is essential to clearly demonstrate how the skills can be useful to the specific problems and difficulties the patient with SUDs is struggling with. If one has never treated this population before, one can obtain examples from other therapists or other sources in order to effectively deliver this treatment to the population with SUDs.

Mindfulness Skills

Mindfulness skills are essential for treating addiction. An example of tailoring mindfulness skills is the use of the observe and describe skills to help patients acknowledge and deal with their cravings and urges to use substances. Urges and cravings to use substances are among the primary precipitants to substance use. Not uncommonly, there is tremendous anxiety associated with urges and cravings because they are perceived as a sign of failure or an indication of inevitable relapse. In an effort to cope with overwhelming anxiety and discomfort, and to reduce the risk of relapse, the addicted individual may try to ignore or avoid thoughts and feelings related to substance use. Unfortunately, while this strategy can reduce anxiety in the short term, it generally intensifies urges to use and increases the risk of relapse in the long run.

In the mindfulness module, patients are taught that urges are natural occurrences of chronic substance abuse that typically last no longer than an hour and diminish in intensity over time if they are simply noticed, and not resolved via substance use. "Urge surfing," a technique described by Marlatt (1985), is a metaphor for the observe and describe skills used to reduce the anxiety associated with urges and thereby decrease vulnerability to relapse. The skill involves helping patients detach from their urges by using observe and describe skills in a nonjudgmental, effective way, which makes the urges more tolerable and reminds the patient that the urge will simply pass with time. The surfing metaphor captures the strategies necessary to successfully cope with urges. Surfing requires keen alertness to every feature of the constantly changing wave. The surfer must make constant subtle adjustments to stay on the crest of the wave without being "wiped out" by it. If one can stay on top of the wave, the wave will eventually die out as it nears the shore. Denial is the opposite of mindfulness, and is analogous to surfing with one's eyes and ears closed while ignoring physical, emotional, and cognitive changes. Ignoring the waves will not make them go away. By accepting the inevitability of urges and cravings, the patient can develop a capacity to observe urges in a detached manner and can learn to wait for the wave to crest and pass.

"Alternate rebellion" is another example of a SUDs-oriented use of a mindfulness skill, specifically the "effectiveness" skill. Many, though not all, substance abusers report that an important aspect of their substance use is that it allows them to express their rebellion against authority, conventionality, and the boredom of abiding by laws. Unfortunately, many borderline individuals, as a result of experiences of invalidation by others, engage in self-destructive, rebellious behaviors in an effort to validate these beliefs. Alternate rebellion involves helping patients to effectively satisfy their urge to rebel without succumbing to the defeat of "cutting off one's nose to spite one's face." Alternate rebellion involves remaining focused on doing what works and staying focused on long-term goals. Patients are instructed that rebellion against conventionality is not inherently bad, but that expressing it through drug abuse is ineffective because it destroys their ability to get a life worth living. For these patients, using drugs can be replaced with safer ways to rebel, such as changing one's style of clothing, getting a tattoo or a body piercing, dyeing one's hair a shocking color, or finding new "hip" but safe places to hang out. Alternative ways of expressing rebellion can be effective particularly if they are secret. For example, a young woman who went to Disney World with her friends was refused admission for wearing a Mickey-the-Rat T-shirt. She returned to the car and put a blouse over her T-shirt so that she could still feel that she was expressing contemptuous rebellion but was now able to enjoy the day with her friends.

Distress Tolerance Skills

Many distress tolerance skills are needed in the course of substance use treatment. Again, the emphasis is on using the skills to foster abstinence and maintain a substance-free lifestyle. Using concrete examples to illustrate how to apply the skills will be of most use to patients. One example of such a focus is using radical acceptance and willing behavior to "burn bridges" that facilitate returning to substance use. This skill is especially useful in the initial stage of addiction treatment, in which the goal is to help the patient refrain from substance abuse and become stabilized. After the patient achieves abstinence, and the focus shifts to maintaining stability, it is appropriate to encourage some exposure to normal cues that may be associated with substance use (e.g., attending parties at which liquor is served), but first abstinence needs to be achieved and maintained for a period of time.

"Burning bridges" involves teaching patients to cut off all options to use drugs as the patient moves from Clean Mind to Clear Mind. It is important to assess the availability of psychoactive substances in the individual's environment. For example, is the patient selling drugs, or working or living with others who use them? The therapist must ask directly about what bridges need to be burned because many patients are reluctant to volunteer this information. Examples of strategies to reduce access include telling one's dealer never to make contact again, or intentionally damaging relationships with dealers so that they do not want to provide drugs anymore. In a more extreme example, Linehan suggested to one patient that she tell her drug dealer that her therapist would report him to the authorities if he provided her with any more drugs—a fairly sure way of cutting off one's supply.

"Adaptive denial" is an example of "pushing away" that turns the hallmark weakness of substance use—self-deception, or the ability to fool oneself—into an asset. One of the biggest challenges faced by substance abusers is that they are being asked to refrain from something they intensely desire. Abstaining requires the patient to replace maladaptive behaviors with behaviors that are less immediately rewarding. Adaptive denial involves blocking out or pushing away potentially accurate but distressing information through self-deception. For example, the thought "I can never use drugs again" is often so overwhelming that it makes the patient want to give up treatment. By avoiding this thought—denying its existence, so to speak—the patient may be more likely to succeed in treatment. It is important to note that patients may be confused by this approach because it contradicts other skills in DBT that focus on decreasing avoidance and thought suppression. This presents yet another dialectic in the treatment: therapists and patients can determine when denial might in fact be effective. One example of adaptive denial is an alcoholic who persuades himself that he cannot wait to have a refreshing glass of cranberry juice and soda water. He is tricking himself away from focusing on the distress of not seeking relief from alcohol. Similarly, the marijuana smoker who persuades herself that she wants to relax in a steaming bubble bath and the cocaine abuser who goes to horror movies because he loves the excitement are examples of engaging in skillful self-deception.

Reviewing "pros and cons" is another skill that can help patients manage intense cravings. When overcome by powerful urges, substance abusers typically have difficulty recalling the negative consequences of their drug use and tend to experience strong euphoria associated with the physiological and psychological aspects of addiction. Patients can be encouraged to make a written list of the negative consequences of substance abuse and the positive consequences of abstinence. This list can be a useful concrete reminder not to act on the urge. Skills group leaders can even drill patients on these lists so their arguments are memorized.

Emotion Regulation Skills

Just as in standard DBT, where many target behaviors function to regulate emotions, substance abuse behaviors with patients with BPD can be quite similar. As a result, the emotion regulation skills remain central to DBT treatment with substance-abusing patients. Many of our patients use drugs at the first sign of difficult emotions, so a strong focus on mindfulness to current emotions is essential. "Opposition action" to emotion helps these patients keep from "falling into the abyss" when they begin experiencing these difficult emotions. And the PLEASE skills are important to address problems with physical pain, malnutrition, sleep, and the many other vulnerabilities these patients often acquire.

For example, one patient had such strong tooth pain, she used opiates (heroin as well as pain medication) to tolerate it. Focusing on PLEASE skills became a high priority because the pain was consistently a cue for using. Getting her to visit the dentist, visit the physician, and attend to regular dental care and nutrition reduced her pain, which in turn reduced her drug use.

Interpersonal Effectiveness Skills

With patients with SUDs, the main focus of the interpersonal skills tends to be on changing one's environment so effective changes are supported. A great deal of time is spent role playing how to say "No" to drugs in a variety of situations, from strangers on the street, known dealers, significant others, and any other source of substances one may find. Helping patients burn bridges, as mentioned above, is also helpful, ensuring that they do not lose their self-respect in the process.

Interpersonal effectiveness skills also help one to create opportunities and increase the frequency of reinforcement for effective behavior. Rehearsing how to build new drug-free relationships and how to impress interviewers for a new job are excellent examples of how these skills can help move a patient toward abstinence. DEAR MAN can also help one to "train up" loved ones to reinforce effective behavior. Environmental support for substance-free behaviors is an extremely powerful intervention in and of itself (e.g., Myers & Smith, 1995), and interpersonal effectiveness skills are essential to making the environment more conducive to clean behavior.

For example, the patient mentioned above with consistent, intense tooth pain also spent a great deal of time practicing DEAR MAN so she could tell her dentist she did not want opioid pain relievers. She and the individual therapist rehearsed how to tell the dentist without providing too much information and while keeping the dentist invested in treating her. She also practiced telling her heroin dealer "No" at various levels of intensity. The therapist provided guidelines for knowing how intense to be in the face of different responses.

Self-Management Strategies

Too often, substance abuse leads to an array of problems that impact all aspects of a person's life, including interpersonal relationships, time management, leisure activities, health, finances, and family. However, individuals vary dramatically in terms of the extent to which their lifestyle is dominated by substance problems: some may lead chaotic lifestyles that may center on turning tricks and scoring drugs on the street, while others may be more stable and function in a job while actively pursuing their drug habit privately. Most programs for substance abuse recognize that the rehabilitation of addicted individuals goes beyond helping them give up drug use. It is also essential to help them take steps toward building a healthy lifestyle. This necessitates assessing the extent to which an individual's current lifestyle supports or impedes the recovery process. Helping a patient get a "normal" life often requires providing assistance in developing self-management skills and building structure to support the recovery process. The process of transitioning from a crisis-oriented lifestyle associated with drug use to a more mundane lifestyle can be very difficult.

Increasing self-management includes teaching the patient how to apply the principles of behavior change to oneself, as is essential in standard DBT. DBT patients are essentially taught to be their own behavior therapists, implementing change strategies out of session just as their DBT therapist does in session. For this reason, DBT patients are encouraged to record each time they reinforce their own effective behavior, in an effort to strengthen that behavior. For example, one patient would place a large check mark on her diary card (a reinforcer itself) and allow herself time to read a novel (a luxury she had rarely indulged in prior to this intervention) every time she used a skill in response to an urge.

Consequences are not the only area of intervention when implementing change principles; managing the antecedents/cues to urges and cravings to use drugs is also an important self-management strategy on the path toward building a drug-free lifestyle. For example, one woman had cravings to smoke marijuana every evening. Over the past several years, she had smoked pot every day after returning home from work. Although she removed the drugs and drug paraphernalia from her apartment, she continued to experience strong urges to use every day after work. It was important to help her schedule activities every evening as a way of distracting herself from her urges. She signed up for kickboxing classes and started going to the gym after work. As long as her cravings were not followed by substance use, the association between the cues and substances would diminish over time. In this regard, it was important for the therapist to discuss the concept of extinction. These strategies are all methods of helping the patient understand ways of applying self-management tools.

Lifestyle interventions may also consist of helping patients build structure, as in securing accommodation, developing healthy relationships, gaining education/employment, and attending to physical health issues. It may not be possible for the primary therapist to assist with all patient problems. The patient may be best served by enlisting the help of an ancillary case manager who is a resource to the therapist or who consults directly to the patient. For example, one opiate-addicted individual who was employed as a health care aide had resorted to stealing pain medications from her patients. She was advised to leave her job and pursue work in a less risky setting. Unable to think of alternative career choices, she was referred to an employment counselor who assisted her in identifying a more appropriate job. In DBT, the primary goal is to coach the patient on handling crises and accessing essential supports. Developing self-management skills and structuring the environment are inextricably related since they involve being mindful of and reducing the factors that lead to substance use.

Comparing DBT to Other Standard Addiction Treatments

DBT shares much in common with therapeutic approaches that have stood the test of time and rigorous scientific scrutiny, including three prominent approaches to treating drug dependence: cognitive-behavioral relapse prevention (Marlatt & Gordon, 1985), motivational interviewing (Miller & Rollnick, 1991), and the 12-step-based approaches (Alcoholics Anonymous, 1981). The key similarities and differences between DBT and these three approaches are highlighted in Table 6.2.

TABLE 6.2. DBT Contrasted with Major Addiction Treatment Models

Model	Similarities with DBT	Differences from DBT
Relapse prevention	• Development and maintenance of drug dependence is based on biopsychosocial model. • Based on cognitive-behavioral, problem-solving approach. • Idiographic, principle-driven treatment that arises out of thorough behavioral (functional) analyses of problem behaviors. • Attends to proximal factors (attending to "high-risk situations" is similar to use of chain analysis following drug use or other problem behavior in DBT); proximal factors (global lifestyle imbalance in RP is like vulnerability factors in DBT).	• RP was developed initially as an "aftercare" maintenance treatment for substance abusers who had achieved abstinence; DBT is a comprehensive, integrated psychosocial treatment for cessation of maladaptive behaviors and maintenance of those behaviors. • RP principles can be applied to both the goal of abstinence and the goal of harm reduction (e.g., moderation); DBT emphasizes abstinence for Stage 1 multidisordered patients.
Motivational interviewing	• In MI, treatment focuses on enhancing motivation to change; in DBT, attention to patient motivation and the factors inhibiting motivation permeate treatment. Both treatments include similar strategies for managing ambivalence or reluctance to make behavioral changes. For example, "psychological judo" in MI is similar to extending in DBT; use of self-motivational statements in MI is similar to use of "devil's advocate" in DBT; both treatments use evaluation of pros and cons. • MI is rooted in Rogerian, patient-centered therapy; DBT's validation strategies similarly involve adherence to Rogers's core concepts of empathy and acceptance of the individual.	• MI was developed as a brief intervention for unidisordered substance-using patients; DBT was developed for multidisordered people with BPD. • MI is typically conducted within a few sessions; standard DBT lasts a minimum of 1 year. • In MI, motivation is understood as an internal state; in DBT, motivation refers to the constellation of variables controlling whether behavior is emitted in a particular context. • MI offers a nonconfrontational approach and is opposed to confrontation; DBT is a synthesis in which the therapist is benevolently confrontational.
12-step approach	• Both treatments emphasize abstinence as the goal of treatment. • In both treatments, there is a focus on enlisting the support of the therapeutic community to facilitate the recovery process. • Both approaches draw from spiritual traditions, with AA being an outgrowth of the Christian Oxford Group movement, and DBT emphasizing aspects of Zen Buddhism. The spiritual dimensions of 12-step programs that emphasize "change what you can and accept the rest" intersect with the Eastern philosophical influence in DBT and the concept of radical acceptance when a "person, place, thing, or situation" cannot be changed. • Both models include an emphasis on initial behavior change, development of activities incompatible with drinking and drug use, and identification and change of dysfunctional behaviors and cognitions (McCrady, 1994). Both make use of contingency management and operant learning strategies, including the use of reinforcers to increase abstinence (e.g., keychains to recognize different lengths of sobriety).	• In DBT, substance abuse is a learned behavior that is precipitated by multiple and sometimes unrelated factors; 12-step approaches conceptualize substance abuse as a disease characterized by denial and loss of control. • In contrast to 12-step approaches, DBT does not require that patients contract to stop all drug use as a condition of starting treatment, nor are patients required to label themselves as an addict or an alcoholic. • Twelve-step approaches strongly advocate abstinence as the only reasonable treatment goal, since any return to use will result in relapse because it triggers the latent disease; DBT is not opposed to harm reduction approaches, including moderation. DBT emphasizes the dichotomy of abstinence versus harm reduction. • Twelve-step approaches focus on removing patients from the environment associated with drug use to a residential treatment facility to get clean; DBT favors eliciting change in the natural environment. • In 12-step approaches, the fellowship is considered an important, if not the primary, agent of change; in DBT, the individual is considered the agent of change.

With its strong basis in cognitive-behavioral and problem-solving principles, DBT shares much in common with Marlatt's *RP approach* (Marlatt & Gordon, 1985). Both are principle-driven approaches that focus on targeting and treating the controlling variables, including the proximal (i.e., immediate high-risk) and distal vulnerability factors that prompt and maintain alcohol and/or drug use problems. In both models, addiction is viewed as a complex process involving multiple interacting determinants (e.g., genetic, biological, learning history, sociocultural norms) that vary in their influence over time. Both models view behavioral change as a continuous process. There is an emphasis on developing new behavioral skills to replace maladaptive behaviors, while also attending to other important variables, such as cognitive expectancies and environmental factors that may trigger substance use. Treatment is focused on identifying the problematic links in the chain that led to substance abuse or other problematic behaviors. Treatment strategies include the teaching and modeling of coping skills, development of self-monitoring, behavioral assessment, didactics, cognitive restructuring, relapse rehearsal, the identification of early warning signals for relapse risk, and the development of prevention plans. Specific coping strategies include helping patients make changes in their lifestyle to support their recovery such as balanced daily living, replacing unhealthy habits with healthy ones (e.g., jogging, playing piano, meditation), developing a social network that supports recovery, substituting "adaptive wants" (e.g., recreational activities) for dysfunctional indulgences, labeling apparently irrelevant decisions as warning signals, and using avoidance strategies (Dimeff & Marlatt, 1995). In both models, difficult situations such as slips or relapses are reframed as opportunities for learning from one's mistakes. A main distinction between the models is that RP, which was developed as an aftercare program to promote maintenance of abstinence from addictive behaviors, does not include a specific program for the initiation of abstinence. In contrast, DBT was developed as a comprehensive treatment, and incorporates a range of interventions to treat individuals with multiple problematic behaviors.

Similar to *motivational interviewing* (MI; Miller & Rollnick, 1991), DBT also addresses patients' motivation to make changes. The fundamental difference between MI and DBT concerns the definition of "motivation." In MI motivation is conceptualized as an internal state, whereas in DBT it is defined behaviorally as the constellation of variables controlling an individual's behavioral repertoire in a particular context that relate to the probability of a behavior's emission. Despite this conceptual difference, at the level of clinical practice attention to motivational factors permeates the delivery of treatment in both models. Both treatments offer creative strategies for effectively managing a patient's ambivalence about or reluctance to make behavioral changes. In DBT there is an extensive focus on getting a commitment from the patient to participate in treatment and abstain from problematic substance use. Many of the strategies used in MI, such as evaluating pros and cons and "rolling with the resistance," are similar to DBT commitment strategies. Both approaches have deep roots in Rogers's client-centered approach (Rogers & Wood, 1974), which forms the bedrock of MI and of validation strategies in DBT. Unconditional positive regard (e.g., in DBT, radical acceptance of the patient), genuineness, and accurate empathic understanding are necessary and essential aspects of both treatments. How these treatment strategies are applied, however, varies considerably. A significant difference is that MI involves a nonconfrontational approach with the patient in which the therapist decidedly avoids confrontation, whereas in contrast, DBT opts for a synthesis. The DBT therapist communicates warmth to and acceptance of the individual but is simultaneously benevolently confrontational, often "going belly to belly" with the patient to elicit a commitment to stop using drugs and to participate in treatment.

Twelve-step approaches include the program initially developed by Alcoholics Anonymous (1981) and later adapted by fellowships such as Narcotics Anonymous, Cocaine Anonymous, Gamblers Anonymous, and many others. Also included here are 12-step facilitation therapy and 12-step counseling. Similar to these programs, DBT emphasizes abstinence from problematic substance use. The basic premise of 12-step approaches is that addiction is a chronic and progressive disease, and denial and loss of control over the use of drugs are the hallmarks of the disease process. In contrast DBT, like RP, holds that the initiation and maintenance of the problem are caused by many complex and transacting factors, with biology being simply one of many factors.

Many 12-step-based treatment approaches recommend the removal of the patient from the environment associated with substances, and a retreat to a residential environment in order to "get clean." In contrast, DBT generally favors helping patients make changes within the context of their natural environment. This approach is based on considerable data that show that drug-dependent individuals often quickly resume drug use once they return to their own environments (Marlatt & Gordon, 1985), as well as on the knowledge that the most powerful method of learning occurs when individuals develop new behaviors in the context in which they are expected to apply those behaviors.

Similar to 12-step approaches, DBT is an abstinence-based treatment. DBT adherents recognize the value of harm-reduction approaches, including moderation, but are aware of strong empirical evidence suggesting that the people most likely to fail at moderation efforts are those with the vulnerabilities typical of BPD (i.e., a high degree of psychopathology and high impulsivity; Klein, Orleans, & Soule, 1991). While DBT discourages substance use, DBT practitioners also carefully examine instances of use in order to discover the relevant contextual factors that are involved in maintaining drug use behaviors. Because behaviors learned in a particular state are recalled and used with greater success in similar states, DBT encourages patients to practice behavioral skills even during states of intoxication. Thus, the patient who arrives at a skills group under the influence of drugs is encouraged to remain in the group and to use skills to stay alert and engaged throughout the session. In DBT patients are not required to contract to stop all drug use as a condition of starting treatment, nor are they expected to label themselves as addicts or alcoholics, as is the practice in 12-step approaches. The DBT therapist works on gaining a verbal commitment to total abstinence during the first session. However, like other commitments obtained in DBT, this commitment is viewed as a public act that increases the probability of the behavior in the future, not as a contract that if violated threatens the continuation of treatment.

Both approaches draw from spiritual traditions. Alcoholics Anonymous is an outgrowth of the Christian Oxford Group movement, while DBT emphasizes aspects of Eastern and Western contemplative practices. Similarities include a common philosophical base that emphasizes radical acceptance when a "person, place, thing, or situation" cannot in fact be changed, and a perception that the current moment is indeed the perfect moment (Alcoholics Anonymous, 1976). Here, the spiritual dimensions of 12-step programs intersect with the Eastern philosophical influence in DBT. The Serenity Prayer, with its change what you can and accept the rest premise, speaks to this common basis.

Another area of overlap between the two models is that both emphasize the importance of the therapeutic community (for both therapists and patients) to derive support from others in the recovery process. Additionally, in both approaches there is an emphasis on initial behavior change, development of activities incompatible with drinking and drug use, and identification and change of dysfunctional behaviors and cognitions (McCrady, 1994). Both make use of contingency management and operant learning strategies, including the use of reinforcers to increase abstinence (e.g., chips and medallions to recognize different lengths of sobriety).

Summary

In recent years an effort was made to modify DBT to address the unique needs and capacities of substance-using individuals with BPD. DBT for individuals with BPD and SUDs incorporates the essential elements of the standard DBT protocol in addition to specific techniques designed to address problems associated with problematic substance use. DBT for substance abusers assumes that, similar to other dysfunctional behaviors associated with BPD, an individual's substance use functions as a means to regulate negative mood states. Consequently, the focus of treatment is to help the individual eliminate problematic substance use through the development of more effective strategies to regulate emotions. The goals of DBT for substance abuse include eliminating problematic substance use, reducing other maladaptive behaviors (e.g., self-harm behaviors), building structure, eliminating environmental stressors, and improving overall life functioning. DBT for substance abuse makes use of a number of new strategies such as a modified hierarchy of targets, a set of attachment strategies, examples of the DBT skills tailored to address urges and cravings to use drugs, and the concept of dialectical abstinence. DBT has been used in the treatment of individuals with BPD and diverse types of substance use problems. Research on DBT has shown it to be generally effective in reducing substance use and enhancing adaptive functioning in many troubled substance-using individuals diagnosed with BPD.

REFERENCES

Alcoholics Anonymous. (1976). *Alcoholics Anonymous*. New York: Alcoholics Anonymous World Services.

Alcoholics Anonymous. (1981). *Twelve steps and twelve traditions*. New York: Alcoholics Anonymous World Services.

Anokhina, I. P., Veretinskaya, A. G., Vasil'eva, G. N., & Ovchinnikov, I. V. (2000). Homogeneity of the biological mechanisms of individual predispositions to the abuse of various psychoactive substances. *Human Physiology, 26,* 715–721.

Beautrais, A. L., Joyce, P. R., & Mulder, R. T. (1999). Cannabis abuse and serious suicide attempts. *Addiction, 94*(8), 1155–1164.

Becker, D. F., Grilo, C. M., Anez, L. M., Paris, M., & McGlashan, T. H. (2005). Discriminant efficiency of antisocial and borderline personality disorder criteria in Hispanic men with substance use disorders. *Comprehensive Psychiatry, 46,* 140–146.

Bradley, B. P., Gossop, M., Brewin, C. P., & Phillips, G. (1992). Attributions and relapse in opiate addicts. *Journal of Consulting and Clinical Psychology, 60,* 470–472.

Brooner, R. K., King, V. L., Kidorf, M., & Schmidt, C. W. J. (1997). Psychiatric and substance use comorbidity among treatment-seeking opioid abusers. *Archives of General Psychiatry, 54*(1), 71–80.

Cacciola, J. S., Alterman, A. I., McKay, J. R., & Rutherford, M. J. (2001). Psychiatric comorbidity in patients with substance use disorders: Do not forget axis II disorders. *Psychiatric Annals, 31*(5), 321–331.

Cacciola, J. S., Alterman, A. I., Rutherford, M. J., & Snider, E. C. (1995). Treatment response of antisocial substance abusers. *Journal of Nervous and Mental Disease, 183*(3), 166–171.

Cummings, C., Gordon, J. R., & Marlatt, G. A. (1980). Relapse: Strategies of prevention and prediction. In W. R. Miller (Ed.), *The addictive behaviors: Treatment of alcoholism, drug abuse, smoking, and obesity* (pp. 291–321). London: Pergamon Press.

Darke, S., Williamson, A., Ross, J., Teesson, M., & Lynskey, M. (2004). Borderline personality disorder, antisocial personality disorder, and risk-taking among heroin users: Findings from the Australian treatment outcome study (ATOS). *Drug and Alcohol Dependence, 74*(1), 77–83.

DeJong, C. A., Van den Brink, W., Harteveld, F. M., & Van der Wielen, E. G. (1993). Personality disorders in alcoholics and drug addicts. *Comprehensive Psychiatry, 34*(2), 87–94.

Dimeff, L. A., & Marlatt, G. A. (1995). Relapse prevention. In R. K. Hester & W. R. Miller (Eds.), *Handbook of alcoholism treatment approaches: Effective alternatives* (2nd ed., pp. 176–194). Boston: Allyn & Bacon.

Dole, V. P. (1988). Implications of methadone maintenance for theories of narcotic addiction. *Journal of the American Medical Association, 260,* 3025–3029.

Dulit, R. A., Fyer, M. R., Haas, G. L., Sullivan, T., & Frances, A. J. (1990). Substance use in borderline personality disorder. *American Journal of Psychiatry, 147,* 1002–1007.

Frances, A., Fyer, M., & Clarkin, J. (1986). Personality and suicide. *Annals of the New York Academy of Sciences, 487,* 281–293.

Hall, S. M., Havassy, B. E., & Wasserman, D. A. (1990). Commitment to abstinence and acute stress in relapse to alcohol, opiates, and nicotine. *Journal of Consulting and Clinical Psychology, 58*(2), 175–181.

Herman, J. L., Perry, J. C., & van der Kolk, B. A. (1989). Childhood trauma in borderline personality disorder. *American Journal of Psychiatry, 146,* 490–495.

Hiebert, S. M., & Burch, E. (2003). Simulated human diving and heart rate: Making the most of the diving response as a laboratory exercise. *Advances in Physiology Education, 27,* 130–145.

Khantzian, E. J., & Schneider, R. J. (1986). Treatment implications of a psychodynamic understanding of opioid addicts. In R. Meyer (Ed.), *Psychopathology and addictive disorders* (pp. 323–333). New York: Guilford Press.

Klein, R. H., Orleans, J. F., & Soule, C. R. (1991). The Axis II group: Treating severely characterologically disturbed patients. *International Journal of Group Psychotherapy, 41,* 97–115.

Koons, C. R., Robins, C. J., Tweed, J. L., Lynch, T. R., Gonzalez, A. M., Morse, J. Q., et al. (2001). Efficacy of dialectical behavior therapy in women veterans with borderline personality disorder. *Behavior Therapy, 32,* 371–390.

Kosten, T. A., Kosten, T. R., & Rounsaville, B. J. (1989). Personality disorders in opiate addicts show prognostic specificity. *Journal of Substance Abuse Treatment, 6*(3), 163–168.

Kruedelbach, N., McCormick, R. A., Schulz, S. C., & Grueneich, R. (1993). Impulsivity, coping styles, and triggers for craving in substance abusers with borderline personality disorder. *Journal of Personality Disorders, 7*(3), 214–222.

Kushner, M. G., Sher, K. J., & Beitman, B. D. (1990). The relation between alcohol problems and the anxiety disorders. *American Journal of Psychiatry, 6,* 685–695.

Leshner, A. I. (1997). Addiction is a brain disease, and it matters. *Science, 278,* 45–47.

Leshner, A. I., & Koob, G. F. (1999). Drugs of abuse and the brain. *Proceedings of the Association of American Physicians, 111,* 99–108.

Levenson, R. W., Oyama, O. N., & Meek, P. S. (1987). Greater reinforcement from alcohol for those at risk: Parental risk, personality risk, and sex. *Journal of Abnormal Psychology, 96*(3), 242–253.

Linehan, M. M. (1993a). *Cognitive-behavioral treatment of borderline personality disorder.* New York: Guilford Press.

Linehan, M. M. (1993b). *Skills training manual for treating borderline personality disorder.* New York: Guilford Press.

Linehan, M. M. (1993c). DBT for treatment of BPD: Implications for the treatment of substance abuse (pp. 201–215). In L. Onken, J. Blaine, & J. Boren (Eds.), *Research monograph series: Behaviour treatments for drug abuse and dependence.* NIDA Research Monograph No. 137 (pp. 201–216). Rockville, MD: U.S. Department of Health and Human Services.

Linehan, M. M. (in press). *Skills Training Manual for Treating Borderline Personality Disorder* (2nd ed.). New York: Guilford Press.

Linehan, M. M., Armstrong, H. E., Suarez, A., Allman, D., & Heard, H. L. (1991). Cognitive behavioral treatment of chronically parasuicidal borderline patients. *Archives of General Psychiatry*, *48*, 1060–1064.

Linehan, M. M., & Dimeff, L. A.(1997). *Dialectical behavior therapy manual of treatment interventions for drug abusers with borderline personality disorder*. Seattle: University of Washington.

Linehan, M. M., Dimeff, L. A., Reynolds, S. K., Comtois, K. A., Welch, S. S., Heagerty, P., et al. (2002). Dialectal behavior therapy versus comprehensive validation therapy plus 12-step for the treatment of opioid dependent women meeting criteria for borderline personality disorder. *Drug and Alcohol Dependence*, *67*(1), 13–26.

Linehan, M. M., Schmidt, H., Dimeff, L. A., Craft, J. C., Kanter, J., & Comtois, K. A. (1999). Dialectical behavior therapy for patients with borderline personality disorder and drug-dependence. *American Journal on Addictions*, *8*, 279–292.

Linehan, M. M., Tutek, D. A., Dimeff, L. A., & Koerner, K. (1999). *Comprehensive validation therapy for substance abuse (CVT-S) for clients meeting criteria for borderline personality disorder: Treatment manual*. Unpublished manuscript.

Links, P. S., Heslegrave, R. J., Mitton, J. E., & Van Reekum, R. (1995). Borderline personality disorder and substance abuse: Consequences of comorbidity. *Canadian Journal of Psychiatry*, *40*(1), 9–14.

Marlatt, G. A. (1985). Cognitive assessment and intervention procedures for relapse prevention. In G. A. Marlatt & J. R. Gordon (Eds.), *Relapse prevention: Maintenance strategies in treatment of addictive behaviors* (pp. 201–279). New York: Guilford Press.

Marlatt, G. A. (Ed.). (1998). *Harm reduction: Pragmatic strategies for managing high-risk behaviors*. New York: Guilford Press.

Marlatt, G. A., & Donovan, D. M. (Eds.). (2005). *Relapse prevention: Maintenance strategies in the treatment of addictive behaviors* (2nd ed.). New York: Guilford Press.

Marlatt, G. A., & Gordon, J. R. (Eds.). (1985). *Relapse prevention: Maintenance strategies in the treatment of addictive behaviors*. New York: Guilford Press.

Marziali, E., Munroe-Blum, H., & McCleary, L. (1999). The effects of the therapeutic alliance on the outcomes of individual and group psychotherapy with borderline personality disorder. *Psychotherapy Research*, *9*, 424–436.

McCrady, B. S. (1994). Alcoholics Anonymous and behavior therapy: Can habits be treated as diseases? Can diseases be treated as habits? *Journal of Consulting and Clinical Psychology*, *62*, 1159–1166.

McKay, J. R., Alterman, A. I., Cacciola, J. S., Mulvaney, F. D., & O'Brien, C. P. (2000). Prognostic significance of antisocial personality disorders in cocaine-dependent patients entering continuing care. *Journal of Nervous and Mental Disease*, *188*(5), 287–296.

McMain, S., Korman, L., Blak, T., Dimeff, L., Collis, R., & Beadnell, B. (2004, November). *Dialectical behavior therapy for substance users with borderline personality disorder: A randomized controlled trial in Canada*. Paper presented at the annual meeting of the Association for the Advancement of Behavior Therapy, New Orleans.

Miller, N. S., Belkin, B. M., & Gibbons, R. (1994). Clinical diagnosis of substance use disorders in private psychiatric populations. *Journal of Substance Abuse Treatment*, *11*, 387–392.

Miller, W. R., & Rollnick, S. (1991). *Motivational interviewing: Preparing people to change addictive behavior*. New York: Guilford Press.

Morgenstern, J., Langenbucher, J., Labouvie, E., & Miller, K. J. (1997). The comorbidity of alcoholism and personality disorders in a clinical population: Prevalence and relation to alcohol typology variables. *Journal of Abnormal Psychology*, *106*(1), 74–84.

Myers, J. E., & Smith, A. W. (1995). A national survey of on-campus clinical training in counselor education. *Counselor Education and Supervision*, *35*(1), 70–81.

Nace, E. P., Davis, C. W., & Gaspari, J. P. (1991). Axis II comorbidity in substance abusers. *American Journal of Psychiatry*, *148*(1), 118–120.

Nowinski, J., & Baker, S. (1992). *The twelve-step facilitation handbook: A systematic approach to early recovery from alcoholism and addiction*. San Francisco: Jossey-Bass.

Porges, S. W., Doussard-Roosevelt, J. A., & Maita, A. K. (1994). Vagal tone and the physiological regulation of emotion. *Monographs of the Society for Research in Child Development, 59,* 167–186.

Rogers, C. R., & Wood, J. K. (1974). Client-centered theory: Carl R. Rogers. In A. Burton (Ed.), *Operational theories of personality* (pp. 211–258). Oxford, UK: Brunner/Mazel.

Rossow, I., & Lauritzen, G. (1999). Balancing on the edge of death: Suicide attempts and life-threatening overdoses among drug addicts. *Addiction, 94*(2), 209–219.

Rutherford, M. J., Cacciola, J. S., & Alterman, A. I. (1994). Relationships of personality disorders with problem severity in methadone patients. *Drug and Alcohol Dependence, 35*(1), 69–76.

Shiffman, S., Engberg, J. B., Paty, J. A., & Perz, W. G. (1997). A day at a time: Predicting smoking lapse from daily urge. *Journal of Abnormal Psychology, 106*(1), 104–116.

Siegel, S., & Ramos, B. M. C. (2002). Applying laboratory research: Drug anticipation and the treatment of drug addiction. *Experimental and Clinical Psychopharmacology, 10,* 162–183.

Skinstad, A., & Swain, A. (2001). Comorbidity in a clinical sample of substance abusers. *American Journal of Drug and Alcohol Abuse, 27,* 45–64.

Stone, M. H., Hurt, S. W., & Stone, D. K. (1987). The PI 500: Long-term follow-up of borderline inpatients meeting DSM-III criteria: I. global outcome. *Journal of Personality Disorders, 1*(4), 291–298.

Supnick, J. A., & Colletti, G. (1984). Relapse coping and problem solving training following treatment for smoking. *Addictive Behaviors, 9*(4), 401–404.

Swadi, H., & Bobier, C. (2003). Substance use disorder comorbidity among inpatient youths with psychiatric disorder. *Australian and New Zealand Journal of Psychiatry, 37*(3), 294–298.

Trull, T. J., Sher, K. J., Minks-Brown, C., Durbin, J., & Burr, R. (2000). Borderline personality disorder and substance use disorders: A review and integration. *Clinical Psychology Review, 20*(2), 235–253.

Trull, T. J., & Widiger, T. A. (1991). The relationship between borderline personality disorder criteria and dysthymia symptoms. *Journal of Psychopathology and Behavioral Assessment, 13*(2), 91–105.

Verheul, R., van den Bosch, L. M. C., Koeter, M. W. J., de Ridder, M. A. J., Stijnen, T., & van den Brink, W. (2003). Dialectical behaviour therapy for women with borderline personality disorder: 12-month, randomised clinical trial in the Netherlands. *British Journal of Psychiatry, 182*(2), 135–140.

Zanarini, M. C., & Frankenburg, F. R. (1997). Pathways to the development of borderline personality disorder. *Journal of Personality Disorders. Special Issue: Trauma and Personality Disorders, 11*(1), 93–104.

Zanarini, M. C., Frankenburg, F. R., Hennen, J., Reich, D. B., & Silk, K. R. (2004). Axis I comorbidity in patients with borderline personality disorder: 6-year follow-up and prediction of time to remission. *American Journal of Psychiatry, 161,* 2108–2114.

CHAPTER 7

Dialectical Behavior Therapy and Eating Disorders

Lucene Wisniewski, Debra Safer, *and* Eunice Chen

Since its inception, dialectical behavior therapy (DBT) has been adapted to address a variety of problematic behaviors associated with emotion dysregulation. This chapter focuses on how DBT has been adapted to treat clients with primary eating disorder (ED) diagnoses as well as clients with comorbid borderline personality disorder (BPD) and EDs.

An ED, according to the fourth edition of the *Diagnostic and Statistical Manual of Mental Disorders* (DSM-IV; American Psychiatric Association, 1994) and the tenth revision of the *International Classification of Diseases* (ICD-10; World Health Organization, 1998), involves extreme forms of eating behavior accompanied by an excessive dependence upon weight and shape as a means of self-evaluation. These lead to significant impairments in health and psychosocial functioning. ED diagnoses are classified into anorexia nervosa (AN), bulimia nervosa (BN), and, for those who meet neither criteria but who still have significant distress or impairment related to eating, a diagnosis of eating disorder not otherwise specified (EDNOS) (DSM-IV) or "atypical EDs" (ICD-10) is given. The EDNOS criteria also include clients meeting the binge-eating disorder (BED) research criteria (DSM-IV).

The aim of this chapter is to describe to the reader how three independent treatment sites adapted standard DBT for use with clients with EDs. The three models are comprehensive DBT for individuals with BPD and ED; DBT for serious, complex, and treatment-resistant EDs; and DBT for binge eating disorder and bulimia nervosa. Each model meets the functions of a comprehensive DBT treatment in terms of enhancing the capabilities of clients, improving motivational factors, assuring generalization to the natural environment, and enhancing therapist capabilities and motivation to treat effectively and to structure the environment. Through focusing on how each program's adaptations were tailored to specific treatment settings and client populations, this chapter intends not only to present the models but to illustrate the principles behind their design. Readers can then choose which model is most suitable for their own treatment settings.

We first review the rationale for applying DBT to clients with EDs, then compare and contrast the three different adaptations of DBT, and finally provide an overview of the biosocial model as well as the stages and target hierarchy for clients with EDs. Each individual section describes how the model was adapted for particular treatment settings and client populations followed by specific descriptions of (1) stages and target hierarchy, (2) the DBT program structure, (3) therapist strategies, and (4) core strategies.

This chapter does not cover basic information about EDs nor does it present details regarding other efficacious treatments for EDs such as cognitive-behavioral therapy (CBT) and interpersonal psychotherapy (IPT). We recommend texts such as Brownell and Fairburn (2002) and Garner and Garfinkel (1997) to readers who are seeking further information.

Why Apply DBT to the Treatment of Clients with EDs?

While helpful for significant numbers of clients with primary EDs, empirically derived treatments such as CBT and IPT are ineffective for about 50% of patients with BN and BED (e.g., Fairburn, Marcus, & Wilson, 1993). Treatment effects for AN are thought to be even more modest (Fairburn & Harrison, 2003). Some predictors of poor outcome in CBT for eating disorders include severity of symptoms (e.g., high rates of binge eating or purging, low body weight) and comorbid personality disorders or other Axis I disorders (for a detailed review, see Wilfley & Cohen, 1997). DBT, an approach designed for the "difficult-to-treat" client, represents a viable option for clients who have failed more traditional forms of therapy.

DBT, unlike CBT or IPT, is based on an emotion regulation model of ED symptoms. There is evidence that affect is a frequent precursor to binge eating (e.g., Greeno, Wing, & Shiffman, 2000) and that binge eating and other types of eating pathology (e.g., vomiting, restrictive eating) may provide a means, albeit maladaptive, of regulating emotions (see, e.g., Waller, 2003; Telch, Agras, & Linehan, 2000). Clients who turn to ED behaviors to modulate affective states may be triggered by thoughts of food, body image, perfectionism, or interpersonal situations (Chen & Linehan, in press; Waller, 2003). Furthermore, the factors that maintain the behaviors may change over time. For example, binge eating, in the absence of other adaptive emotion regulation skills, may become negatively reinforced as an escape behavior (Heatherton & Baumeister, 1991). Likewise, the behavior of binge eating may result in secondary emotions such as shame or guilt, and these emotions can prompt further ED behaviors (e.g., Sanftner & Crowther, 1998). In addition, for some clients restriction of intake may be viewed as a form of escape from the distress of experiencing aversive primary *or* secondary emotions in the absence of more adaptive emotional regulation skills. The fact that DBT is specifically designed to teach adaptive affect regulation skills and to target behaviors resulting from emotional dysregulation provides a theoretical rationale for applying DBT to treating EDs (McCabe, La Via, & Marcus, 2004; Telch et al., 2000; Telch, Agras, & Linehan, 2001; Wisniewski & Kelly, 2003).

In addition to its use of the affect regulation model, DBT—with its grounding in behavioral principles, dialectics, and Eastern philosophy—contains other elements that make it a particularly suitable treatment for clients with EDs. For example, EDs, especially AN, differ from other behavioral disorders such as depression and anxiety, in the significant degree of ambivalence clients with EDs maintain about changing behaviors required to treat their ED. Treatment of ED problem behaviors therefore requires a sophisticated use of commitment strategies and must focus not only on helping clients change their specific behaviors but also on the relationship of these behaviors to their long-term treatment goals. This dialectical tension is an inherent component of DBT and is its focus on both change- and acceptance-based therapeutic strategies. For clients with EDs, who must accept their current progress in treatment, their weight and shape, and other difficult-to-change aspects of their current situation, DBT's acceptance strategies are especially valuable. The focus on acceptance is equally important for the therapist and family members in that it provides a useful framework for relinquishing control over the time course for change.

Other key elements of DBT, such as the case management strategies of consultation to the client and consultation to the therapist, are similarly suited for work with clients with EDs. For example, the DBT strategy of consultation to the client promotes respect for the client's capacity to learn new behaviors in all relevant contexts. While enabling the teaching of new, effective skills, the consultation-to-the-patient strategy further serves the function of enhancing the client's self-efficacy to manage his or her environment and enhances the therapeutic relationship between therapist and client. This is particularly important for clients with EDs, as it is with clients with BPD, as the DBT therapist has greater capacity to leverage the therapeutic relationship to resolve ambivalence about necessary behavioral change in the service of the client's long-term goals. Through coaching clients to manage an often extensive health provider network, DBT therapists develop the client's sense of control and self-efficacy and reinforce the collegial nature of the therapist–client relationship.

The inclusion of a consultation team in DBT to enhance the therapist's capability and motivation to effectively treat patients is another unique component of DBT that has particular utility when working with individuals with chronic EDs. Given the tendency for clients with EDs and their problem behaviors to evoke intense emotions in their treatment providers, the therapist consultation team provides a context for therapists to receive support, assistance, and expertise from a multidisciplinary group of professionals (e.g., medical doctors, nutritionists). The consultation team also helps to ensure that the primary therapist remains committed to treating the client and remains maximally effective in his or her treatment.

Similarities between how the environment responds to BPD- and ED-criterion behaviors make DBT especially relevant for the treatment of EDs. For example, ED symptoms are often minimized despite the fact that some ED problem behaviors may be life-threatening behaviors and/or significantly impair functioning (Hayaki, Friedman, Whisman, Delinsky, & Brownell, 2003). Some ED behaviors (e.g., not accurately reporting bingeing and purging behaviors, hiding food, or drinking large amounts of water before being weighed) can be perceived as scheming, deceitful, and superficial by therapists, family, and friends. If held by professional consultants, such negative attributions can lead to both clients and therapists feeling invalidated while simultaneously interfering with thorough behavioral assessment of the client's actual problems. This can in turn lead to decreased motivation and burnout in clients and therapists alike. DBT, however, places an emphasis on clients as well as therapists working within a nonjudgmental framework, where behaviors are understood nonpejoratively and simply as problems to be solved.

The final basis for using DBT with clients with EDs is the existence of overlap between BPD and ED populations, with suicidal and nonsuicidal self-injurious behaviors common to both. For example, studies of patients with BN suggest that 15–40% attempt suicide (Dulit, Fyer, Leon, Brodsky, & Frances, 1994). Clients with both BPD and BN compared to those without BPD are up to four times more likely to self-injure (Dulit et al., 1994) and are twice as likely to attempt suicide (Herzog, Keller, Sacks, Yeh, & Lavori, 1992). Additionally, the presence of BPD is a predictor of poor treatment outcomes in CBT for clients with BED and BN (Grilo, Masheb, & Berman, 2001; Stice & Agras, 1999; Stice et al., 2001; Wilfley et al., 2000). Furthermore, there appears to be a significant association between suicide and AN, with reports that 20–58% of deaths in AN may be related to suicide (Herzog et al., 2000; Keel et al., 2003; Steinhausen, 2002). Given that DBT is the treatment of choice for clients with BPD (Lieb, Zanarini, Schmahl, Linehan, & Bohus, 2004; Linehan, Comtois, Brown, et al., 2002), standard DBT is currently a reasonable treatment choice for clients with BPD who also have an ED. Unlike other cognitive-behavioral treatment for EDs, DBT has clear guidelines for treating multiple problem behaviors, including suicidal and nonsuicidal self-harm behaviors as well as ED behaviors.

In summary, DBT represents a viable, research-based option for clients with primary EDs who have failed other efficacious treatments such as CBT or IPT (Fairburn, 1997; Wilson, Fairburn, & Agras, 1997). Given the treatment outcome literature on the efficacy of DBT for BPD, standard DBT may be considered for people with BPD who also have an ED.

Comparison of Three Adaptations

The first model described is comprehensive DBT for clients with both an ED (specifically BN or BED) and BPD. As a standard, comprehensive form of DBT, it includes weekly individual psychotherapy, skills training groups, consultation team meetings for therapists, and after-hours phone consultation. Modifications to standard, comprehensive DBT were made to make the content relevant to the needs of multidisordered individuals with BPD and EDs. The second model, DBT for individuals with severe and complex EDs, describes a model for using DBT to enhance existing CBT treatments for the EDs in order to treat clients diagnosed with AN, BN, and EDNOS in intensive outpatient and partial hospital group settings. This combination of DBT and CBT adds elements of the standard DBT approach to compliment the empirically validated CBT for the EDs. Finally, the model established for DBT for binge eating and bulimia was developed for higher functioning individuals with EDs. This manual-based, 20-session, outpatient program uses DBT skills training with nonsuicidal clients meeting a diagnosis of BED or BN.

A comparison of the three models with regards to the diagnostic criteria of the clients enrolled, the modes of therapy offered, and the treatment setting is described in Table 7.1.

Each of the programs described below has modified the standard DBT diary card in order to accommodate ED symptoms. Each program description includes a discussion about their program's diary card. Table 7.2 compares the diary cards for the three models with regards to which specific behaviors are monitored.

TABLE 7.1. Comparison of Variables among the Treatment Models

Model	Program setting	Treatment stage	Inclusion/exclusion criteria	Program modes or functions	Length of treatment	Other
Comprehensive DBT for BPD and ED	Outpatient treatment	Stage 1	*Inclusion*: BPD and either BED or BN (DSM-IV); 18–60 years; female only; willingness to consent to research procedure. *Exclusion*: Body mass index 19 and below (i.e., AN), schizophrenia or other psychotic disorder or bipolar mood disorder, court-mandated, or pregnant.	Group skills training, individual DBT, consultation team, telephone consultation	6 months	Based on standard DBT
DBT for severe and complex EDs	Intensive outpatient; partial hospital program	Multiple stages	*Inclusion*: AN, BN, BED, EDNOS; meeting criteria for intensive outpatient or partial hospitalization program as per APA criteria.[a] *Exclusion*: ED symptoms meeting for inpatient treatment as per APA criteria.[a]	Group skills training multiple times/week, consultation team, telephone coaching	Determined by symptoms and APA criteria.[a]	Group treatment only. Motivation/commitment and CBT groups in addition to DBT skills group.
DBT for BED and BN	Outpatient treatment	Stage 3	*Inclusion*: BED or BN; females between 18 and 65 years. *Exclusion*: suicidality within past month, psychosis or bipolar, psychotropic meds, unstable within past 3 months, meds affecting weight/appetite (e.g., amphetamines, topiramate, sibutramine), concurrent psychotherapy, pregnancy.	Group format (BED), individual format (BN), consultation team, no formal telephone consultation	20 weekly sessions 2 hours/week for BED, 1 hour/week for BN	Combines elements of individual and skills training into one session

[a] *The Practice Guidelines for the Treatment of Patients with Eating Disorders* (American Psychiatric Association, 2000) can be found at *www.psych.org/psych_pract/treatg/pg/prac_guide.cfm.*

TABLE 7.2. Targets Tracked on Diary Cards, According to Treatment Model

Model	Binge eating	Purging	Secondary eating targets (e.g., mindless eating, capitulating, AIBs)	Parasuicide	Drugs and alcohol	Food intake	Emotions	Skills practice (side 2)
Comprehensive DBT for BPD and ED	Yes	Yes	No	Yes	Yes	No	Yes	Yes
DBT for severe and complex EDs	Yes	Yes	No	Yes	Yes	Yes	Yes	Yes
DBT for BED and BN	Yes	Yes (for BN)	Yes	No	No	No	Yes	Yes

Adaptation of DBT's Biosocial Theory to EDs

Linehan's biosocial theory of BPD has been well described (Linehan, 1993a). While there are no data examining the goodness of fit of the biosocial model to individuals with EDs who do not have comorbid BPD, it is the authors' experience that conceptualizing EDs as a problem of pervasive emotion dysregulation based on the biosocial model of DBT is both applicable and relevant to clients with EDs.

To better accommodate clients with EDs, the standard biosocial theory for BPD has been adapted in a number of ways. First, in addition to its grounding in a belief in the individual's biological vulnerability to pervasive emotion dysregulation, the DBT biosocial model for understanding the development of EDs includes an awareness of a special nutritional vulnerability (Wisniewski & Kelly, 2003). Nutrition-related vulnerabilities that increase the risk for developing an ED include a disruption in the body's ability to appropriately signal hunger and satiety. This disruption, which may occur prior to or be a result of disordered eating behavior (e.g., Wisniewski, Epstein, Marcus, & Kaye, 1997), may make it especially difficult to eat effectively.

The emotionally invalidating environment for a client with an ED may be expanded from standard DBT to include body shape and weight-related teasing by peers and family (Fairburn et al., 1998; Streigel-Moore, Dohm, Pike, Wilfley, & Fairburn, 2002), as well as overconcern with weight and a familial history of dieting (e.g., Pike & Rodin, 1991). It can also include Western cultural expectations for beauty that may be experienced as invalidating by the majority of women. Such expectations may be promoted by images of women in movies, in magazines, in certain sports and arts such as ballet and gymnastics, and by the consistent message from the diet industry that one must lose weight. In clients with comorbid BPD and ED, dysregulation of the self—an important criterion behavior for BPD—may make these clients particularly vulnerable to turning to body image-focused environments as sources of information about what the self "should" be. Clients with EDs may also experience invalidation with respect to their specific ED symptoms when asked "Why can't you just stop eating?" or, conversely, "Why can't you just eat?" This conceptualization of the invalidating environment, although untested, may explain the greater degree of self-dysregulation often seen clinically in clients with both BPD and ED. Possessing both BPD and an ED may set the stage for clients to engage in more extreme behaviors (e.g., purging at very low weights) as a way of eliciting attention and positive reinforcement.

Adaptations of Standard DBT Treatment Targets

While standard DBT includes four stages of treatment for four levels of disorder (see Koerner & Dimeff, Chapter 1, this volume), the adaptations to date have focused primarily on clients in Stage 1 and Stage 3 of treatment. Specifically, the DBT program model for individuals with BPD and an ED describes an adaptation of standard DBT for people in Stage 1, the DBT program model for serious, complex, and treatment-resistant EDs describes an adaptation for people in Stages 1 to 3, and the DBT program model for binge eating and bulimia describes an adaptation for clients in Stage 3.

Target 1: Life-Threatening Behaviors

As in standard DBT, suicidal and other imminent life-threatening behaviors (nonsuicidal self-injurious behaviors, assaultive behavior, and homicidal behavior) are the first targets to be addressed in treatment. ED behaviors are Target 1 behaviors when they pose an *imminent* threat to the client's or another person's life. Examples might include fluid restriction in a low-weight bradycardic client, vomiting despite significant electrolyte imbalance, and bingeing and purging in an insulin-dependent diabetic client, as all of these conditions can lead to imminent, whether intentional or not, death.

Several difficulties arise when trying to determine whether a particular behavior meets the criteria for a Target 1 behavior or is instead a quality-of-life-interfering behavior (described below). In contrast to treating suicidal clients with BPD where Target 1 behaviors are easily identifiable (e.g., a suicide attempt regardless of actual behavior or its lethality; intentional, self-injurious behavior), there are no definitive guidelines to designate which ED behaviors pose *imminent* danger to life. Even clients with similar clinical presentations may vary in terms of underlying severity. For example, electrolyte or EKG abnormalities in a low-weight client could lead to imminent death in one client but not in another, as multiple additional factors may play a role. When deciding in which target a particular behavior falls, it is important to consider the function, lethality, imminence, degree of disability, complexity, and intentionality of the behavior for a particular individual, taking into account the behavior's history. For instance, ipecac abuse may be immediately life-threatening in a low-weight, bradycardic client (independent of the client's *intent* to die or harm herself; Target 1), or may constitute "therapy-interfering behavior" (Target 2, see below) if it occurred with a normal-weight client without electrolyte imbalances as a "legitimate" excuse for missing a group skills session. Finally, the same behavior could be a quality-of-life-interfering behavior (Target 3) in a client who infrequently abuses ipecac as means of inducing vomiting.

Given the difficulty of predicting risk and the fact that opinions will vary as to whether an ED behavior is life-threatening, it is important that these decisions are made on an individual basis and that they adhere to the behavioral definition of this class of behaviors (i.e., imminent risk of death). Consultation with medical professionals will often be required to determine whether a particular behavior is indeed an imminently lethal behavior within the context of relevant laboratory results and findings. That a particular behavior *may* be lethal or *has been* lethal to another individual is insufficient justification to label the behavior a Target 1 behavior. Similarly, the clinician's or institution's tolerance of risk should not be considered a relevant factor in considering whether the behavior is a Stage 1 behavior.

Target 2: Therapy-Interfering Behaviors

Therapy-interfering behaviors that may occur within the context of treatment include but are not limited to not completing food diary cards, an inability to focus during the session due to a malnourished state, refusing to be weighed, falling below an agreed-upon outpatient weight range, engaging in behaviors to surreptitiously alter weight, exercising against medical advice, absence from treatment due to the need for medical intervention, and/or engaging in purging that interferes with medication efficacy.

Target 3: Quality-of-Life-Interfering Behaviors

ED and other quality-of-life-interfering behaviors such as substance abuse, domestic violence, and homelessness that are not associated with an imminent risk to life are classified as Target 3 "quality-of-life-interfering behaviors." Examples of specific ED behaviors include restricting, binge eating, vomiting, laxative use, diuretic use, diet pill use, excessive or compulsive exercise, and other eating-specific targets. The bulk of treatment for ED clients who are not suicidal or at imminent risk of death will fall within Targets 2 and 3.

For clients who have numerous quality-of-life-interfering behaviors across multiple classes of behavior (e.g., eating disorders, substance abuse, legal problems), it is important to determine the hierarchy of behavioral targets within this domain. Unless otherwise specified below, principles from standard DBT (Linehan, 1993a) should be applied, resulting in the following considerations:

1. The immediacy of the problem (no shelter or money for food is more immediate than objective binge eating).
2. The solvability of the problem (trying to solve the less difficult rather than the more difficult problems yields greater chances of reinforcing a client's use of skills and the likelihood of generalization).
3. The functional relationship of behaviors to higher priority targets (e.g., suicide crisis behaviors and nonsuicidal self-injurious behaviors; therapy-interfering behavior; suicide ideation and sense of "misery"; maintenance of treatment gains and other life goals)
4. The clients' goals.

Target 4: Increasing Behavioral Skills to Facilitate a Life Worth Living

The principles from standard DBT (Linehan, 1993a) should be applied.

Comprehensive DBT for Individuals with BPD and an ED

The model of DBT for individuals with BPD and an ED grew out of decades of work by Linehan and her colleagues at the University of Washington treating individuals with BPD who also had severe EDs, and a more recent small pilot study (Chen, O'Connor, & Linehan,

2004) focused on refining aspects of standard DBT for this comorbid population. Unlike the other models presented in this chapter, this model is essentially standard DBT, where a primary quality-of-life-interfering behavior is an eating disorder. In this manner, this model resembles the application of standard DBT originally developed for suicidal clients with BPD (Linehan, 1993a) to BPD clients with substance dependence. As in previous randomized controlled trials conducted by Linehan and colleagues at her research laboratory, individuals with schizophrenia, bipolar disorder, and/or another psychotic condition are excluded from participating because of the requirement that subjects be tapered off psychotropic medications (for research design purposes). Additionally, anorexic clients (e.g., those with a body mass of 19 or below) were excluded in this recent pilot study.

Targeting Quality-of-Life-Interfering Behaviors

As previously mentioned, individuals with BPD and EDs typically present with a multitude of quality-of-life-interfering behaviors. We initially considered creating a separate target hierarchy for the ED behaviors, as was done in Linehan's initial adaptation of DBT for substance-dependent individuals with BPD (Linehan et al., 1991, and manual of DBT-SUD; see Chapter 6) and later applied to the DBT for binge-eating and bulimia model described later in this chapter. We ultimately returned to the principles from standard DBT described above, as we discovered that it is more effective to treat other non-eating-disorder-specific quality-of-life-interfering behaviors first. Consider the client who, for example, engaged in binge eating, but also had a hoarding problem resulting in an apartment so full of belongings that it was difficult to move from one room to the next. The hoarding was a more immediate problem than the binge eating because the client found it difficult to eat at the table. Although the hoarding was a more extensive and difficult problem to solve, it was more functionally related to higher order targets. Specifically, the client felt more suicidal and miserable about the state of her home than about her binge eating. Also, the binge eating was not functionally related to suicidal ideation, nor was it lethal or imminently dangerous. The client did not recognize her binge eating as a problem, but did view the state of her apartment as a significant problem and thus as an important goal of therapy. Initially, the binge eating (our initial priority, imposed on her) was prioritized over the hoarding behavior (her priority). The client, not surprisingly, quit therapy. It was then that we realized that we had veered away from the principles set forth in standard DBT (Linehan, 1993a). Once we discovered our error and resumed application of standard DBT principles and we prioritized the hoarding behavior over the binge-eating behavior, the client remained in treatment and both behaviors significantly improved over time.

Assessment at pretreatment as well as assessment over time are invaluable in determining the organization of quality-of-life targets. Useful questions to consider include:

- If your binge eating increased or decreased, what would happen to being suicidal? To the frequency of self-harm? To drug or alcohol abuse?
- How would you rank these targets in getting a life worth living?
- If you quit binge eating, what would happen to your suicidal urges and, feeling miserable?
- If you had a cleaner house (in reference to the above clinical vignette), what would happen to you feeling suicidal, you feeling miserable?
- Which is most important to you (again in reference to the above clinical vignette), stopping binge eating, getting work, or stopping your hoarding?

One of the quality-of-life targets most likely to arise in the treatment of clients with BPD with BED or BN is weight loss. Initially, we deemphasized weight loss as a quality-of-life target because the focus of the research study was on the reduction of binge-eating behavior. However, this did not fit clients' goals, so weight loss was added as a quality-of-life target. In adding this goal, we also needed to address realistic expectations about weight loss. For instance, weight loss is more achievable in the short term, but is extremely difficult to maintain over time. Additionally, weight loss goals portrayed by the media or the diet industry are unrealistic. For example, most people believe that obese people need to lose a great deal of weight in order to be healthy (i.e., become a size 8), when in fact losing 5–10% of one's body weight is enough to make significant health improvements (e.g., decreasing diabetes risk and the risk of hypertension) (Wadden, Brownell, & Foster, 2002). Weight loss maintenance can also take much more than a year and is best viewed as involving a lifelong lifestyle change. Sometimes the goal of not gaining weight might be a more realistic one for a client who is noticing rapid, consistent weight gain.

While losing weight may be the goal, it says little about what needs to change behaviorally in order for the client to achieve the goal. With that in mind, the first step is to behaviorally define the problem or problems that are interfering with attaining the goal. Specifically, what behaviors need to be *increased or decreased* in order to attain this goal? Are there *cues or stimuli* that need to be better managed? Frequently, when the goal is translated into these behaviors, the following behaviors are identified:

1. Reduce binge eating.
   - Remove high-risk binge food from the house.
   - Reduce going to restaurants with "high-risk binge food" (e.g., a Mexican restaurant with chips and salsa).
   - Attend an ancillary self-help program (e.g., Weight Watchers, going to the gym, a joining walking club).
2. Increase exercise.

Program Structure

The optimal structure for clients with BPD and BN or BED adheres to the standard DBT structure for comprehensive DBT treatment. The decision to apply comprehensive DBT, based on standard DBT, was derived from the following theory: given the empirical evidence, standard DBT is the treatment of choice for clients with BPD; individual psychotherapy ensures that clients can discuss crises that arise that otherwise may be iatrogenic to discuss in group; and group allows clients to learn new skills without the interruption of crises. In our recent pilot study, we experimented with incorporating the chain analysis procedure used in DBT for binge eating and bulimia (detailed below) into the skills training group. These attempts were ultimately unsuccessful because discussion of the content of the chain analysis (i.e., suicidal behavior) functioned as a trigger for other clients who subsequently engaged in their dysfunctional target behavior. Our experience is consistent with Linehan's (1993a, 1993b) early discussions of not discussing suicidal and non-suicidal self-injurious behaviors in group with suicidal clients with BPD due to the potential contagion effect upon other Stage 1 clients.

Prior to the start of treatment, potential clients are screened to be sure that their needs and interests fit the treatment program. This is accomplished at the University of Washington (UW) setting by way of an assessment battery administered by the intake/assessment personnel. During this intake assessment, a diagnostic interview is performed and client history is recorded. Additionally, the intake staff provides a high-level orientation to the clinic, clinic procedures, and treatment. At the initial assessment, clients are asked to make an appointment with their own physician or nurse practitioner for a general physical exam and any necessary tests (e.g., blood work, electrocardiogram) to screen for electrolyte imbalances in clients with BN or medical problems associated with obesity (e.g., Type II diabetes) in overweight clients.

Individual DBT Sessions

As with standard DBT, clients beginning DBT are oriented to the structure of treatment such as the use of a consultation team of therapists, the 24-hour paging system, and that missing four consecutive scheduled group or individual sessions constitutes dropping out from the treatment program. The clients for whom weight loss is a goal of treatment are encouraged to consider other ancillary supports or treatment for weight loss.

In the initial sessions (Table 7.3), therapists teach Linehan's (1993b) crisis survival skills from the distress tolerance module to stop dysfunctional behaviors including self-harm, binge eating, and drug use to help clients change their behavior as soon as possible. They review 10 skills that a client can use in the case of urges: (1) Distract with Wise Mind ACCEPTS skills, (2) IMPROVE the moment, (3) self-soothe skills, (4) surfing the urge, (5) pros and cons of engaging in the dysfunctional behavior, (6) taking a cold shower, (7) rehearsing in one's mind effective ways of changing dysfunctional impulsive behaviors, (8) reviewing exercises from Linehan's (1993b) skills training manual, (9) calling someone, and (10) using these skills one-mindfully.

After the initial sessions devoted to gaining a commitment from the client to participate in treatment and orienting the client to DBT, individual psychotherapy generally entails the following structure. Immediately prior to an individual therapy session, in order to track weight change for study purposes, all clients (BPD with BN or BED) are weighed in a separate room by the individual therapist, with the client being made aware of her or his weight. In clinical practice, weekly weighing of clients with anorexia nervosa or clients who are overweight or obese is suggested. It is important in the case of clients with anorexia nervosa that the individual therapist is aware of the client's weight, so that he or she can act quickly to provide more intense treatment if the client loses weight dramatically. This may be conducted by an ancillary treater, but only with adherence to the consultation-to-the-client rule (e.g., if the client agrees to having the ancillary treater fax in the weight before the session each week). With regards to normal-weight clients with EDs, weighing in clinical practice may not be so important. However, many clients with EDs have weight concerns and either avoid weighing themselves or weigh themselves too frequently. Weighing provides exposure to the number on the scale and together with psychoeducation about how weight fluctuates regularly can be particularly helpful for clients who avoid weighing themselves. For clients with EDs who are at normal weight but who check their weight frequently, learning to weigh only once a week or not at all as opposed to daily (i.e., opposite action with urges to weigh that is associated with anxiety about weight) can be useful.

At the start of the session, therapists ask clients to rate their urge to commit suicide, to quit therapy, to use drugs (if applicable), or to binge eat (see diary card). The therapist then reviews the diary card to establish and prioritize targets and to set, with the client, an agenda for that individual session. Chain analyses are conducted on dysfunctional behaviors occurring since the last session, with attention to higher targeted behaviors

TABLE 7.3. Covered Topics in Pretreatment (First Four Sessions or When the Client Makes a Commitment to Cease Dysfunctional Behaviors)

1. What brings you here?
2. Client's goals in treatment.
3. History of suicidal behaviors and assessment of current risk.
4. Crisis plan to deal with suicidal behavior.
5. Description of therapist's credentials, training, and experience.
6. Assessment of current eating disorder behavior—e.g., objective binge eating; subjective binge eating; restriction; vomiting, laxative, diuretic, and diet pill abuse; overexercise.
   a. Frequency.
   b. With whom and where.
   c. Prompting events, e.g., urges, emotions.
   d. Vulnerability factors.
   e. Consequences.
   f. Weight (measured).
   g. Menstrual history.
7. Eating disorder history.
   a. First time, prompting event, vulnerability factors, and consequences?
   b. History of attempts to stop behavior—what worked and what did not work? What is different this time?
8. Current drug and alcohol abuse or dependence.
   a. Define behavior, prompting event, vulnerability factors, consequences.
9. Drug and alcohol history (see eating disorder history questions).
10. Other quality-of-life problems?
   a. Define behavior, prompting event, vulnerability factors, consequences.
11. History of other quality-of-life problems.
12. Other relevant history: medical, psychological, family, and friends and work?
13. Commitment to ceasing dysfunctional behaviors.
14. Treatment agreement, e.g., four-miss rule; agreement to tape; agreement to either have the client weigh herself or to gather weekly weigh-in data.
15. Application of crisis survival skills to dysfunctional behaviors—e.g., pros and cons of "Saying NO" to various dysfunctional behaviors that the client wishes to change.
16. Establishing what are the cues for dysfunctional behaviors. Explaining how exposure to these cues but using skills instead of engaging in dysfunctional behaviors leads to adaptive brain changes.
17. Explanation of the diary card.
18. Explanation of the target hierarchy.
19. Explanation of the biosocial theory.
20. Explanation of "What is DBT" (e.g., structure of treatment)?
21. Explaining the concept of dialectics.

first. The session is audio- or digitally recorded for the client to review during the course of the week to facilitate skills generalization.

Group Skills Training

Group skills training involves the three standard skills training modules, along with the core mindfulness training that precedes each module. There are no modules devoted entirely to eating disorders. Instead, discussion about the treatment of eating disorders, related issues, and experiences is woven throughout the teaching of the DBT modules. Groups may be highly heterogeneous, including BPD clients with and without EDs, clients with BPD with a primary problem of substance dependence, and clients ranging in body size from underweight to obese. As described by Linehan (1993b), the trick to conducting skills training groups with a heterogeneous group of clients is to focus on the shared problem of emotion dysregulation that precipitates a number of impulsive, out-of-control behaviors.

Minor adaptations have been made to the group skills program. The use of skills is modeled using binge eating as an example (e.g., using an example of doing pros and cons with urges to binge eat). Discussion of binge eating, unlike discussion of suicidal behavior, does not appear to have a negative contagion effect upon clients. With emotion regulation PLEASE skills and crisis survival distract (ACCEPTS) skills, those who restrict their exercise or who overexercise are asked to use more adaptive alternatives. In applying crisis survival distract skills to stop binge eating, clients are asked to find alternatives incompatible with binge eating, such as crocheting or knitting. Mindfulness exercises around eating and body awareness, including the raisin exercise described by Kabat-Zinn (1990), have also been added. A client favorite is mindfulness with chocolate. This exercise teaches one to observe and describe the taste and texture of a piece of chocolate as it melts in one's mouth (no chewing). If the client notices that judgmental thoughts arise (e.g., chocolate is sinful, bad, wicked, fattening, unhealthy), she or he is asked to notice this and gently bring her or his mind back to the exercise.

Groups at the UW are typically held from 5:30 P.M. to 8:00 P.M. to encourage and accommodate employment during the day. Because group coincides with dinner time, clients are permitted to bring along dinner (e.g., a sandwich) and snacks, if they wish. Healthy snacks (e.g., fruit, vegetables, crackers) are also provided. Additionally, clients are also told in advance that a potluck will be held at group on the night of a member's graduation from group in her honor. No foods are "banned" at any time from group, as the presence of diverse foods and exposure to foods that clients may typically avoid allows members to increase their capacity to learn to skillfully manage cues associated with binge eating.

DBT Consultation Team

There are no differences in the function or structure of the DBT consultation team that is providing services to clients with an ED. Given that the DBT team consults to the DBT therapist in how best to treat an individual DBT client, it is imperative, however, that all members of the team have expertise in assessing and treating clients with EDs and knowledge regarding weight and obesity. This standard is important whether there is only one client or many clients with an ED or if all clients have EDs. When members of the consultation team lack the requisite competency in EDs, it is highly recommended that they receive the necessary training or find appropriate consultation. Basic knowledge about how to make healthy food choices, regulate food portions, and engage in healthy activities can be helpful for an individual therapist in treating clients with ED because they often seek guidance on these concerns. However, this is where having the client seek guidance from an ancillary dietician can also be helpful. At the UW, experts in EDs and obesity provided training to the other team members without this expertise in a series of trainings that occurred before the weekly team meeting.

With regard to outside consultation, it is part of a therapist's agreement in standard DBT to obtain consultation when needed. Where there may not be an eating disorder and/or obesity specialist available to lecture or consult on cases, therapists can be trained by inviting a consultant to provide a series of talks, either in person or by teleconferencing. Suggestions for finding a consultant include contacting the Academy for Eating Disorders, the National Eating Disorders Association, the American Obesity Association, or a behaviorally oriented graduate training program in clinical psychology. A less costly alternative would include conducting a journal club during the training hour devoted to the reading and presentation of articles on eating disorders and obesity. Table 7.4 lists topics that might be reviewed and published materials for reading.

Telephone Consultation

Phone coaching follows the same principles and protocol as defined by Linehan (1993a) for standard comprehensive DBT. The most significant modification involves the 24-hour rule. In contrast to standard DBT, where the 24-hour rule applies only to Target 1 life-threatening behaviors, this rule is also applied to eating disorders behaviors. The idea is that most dysfunctional behaviors serve to "solve" problems related to emotion dysregulation. The point of contacting the therapist is to gain help in skillfully solving problems related to emotion dysregulation in the "real world."

In addition to this modification of the 24-hour rule, we have also adapted, as needed, the *actual length or time interval* for the 24-hour rule. The reason for this modification involved the high-frequency nature of criterion eating-disordered behaviors. Consider the client, for example, who binges and purges five times a day and has done so for many years. Without modifying the time interval, there will never be an occasion for her to receive coaching in the context of her environment to facilitate skills generalization (a primary function of phone consultation). And without skills generalization, there is little chance that her target behavior will actually change. The key here is to remember that the 24-hour rule does not exist to be excessively punitive. Instead, it is intended to shape the

TABLE 7.4. Relevant References for EDs and Obesity Topics

ED behaviors	Chapter and reference
1. Definitions of eating disorder behaviors including restriction and overexercising	Garner and Garfinkel (1997), Chapters 3 and 9
2. Definitions of healthy eating and healthy activity for any weight	CDC web site,[a] FNIC web site[b]
3. Definitions of the Body Mass Index (BMI), and BMI cutoffs for obesity, normal healthy weight, and AN	Garner and Garfinkel (1997), Chapter 3; Brownell and Fairburn (2002), Chapter 68; CDC web site[a]
4. Height and weight charts for adults and children	CDC web site[a]
5. Medical and psychosocial consequences of eating-disordered behaviors and weight regulation	Garner and Garfinkel (1997), Chapter 8; Brownell and Fairburn (2002), Chapters 76 and 84
8. Expected weight gain during AN treatment (different in inpatient and outpatient settings)	Garner and Garfinkel (1997), Chapter 19
9. The medical and psychosocial consequences including discrimination experienced by overweight and obese people	Brownell and Fairburn (2002), Chapters 20, 76, and 84
10. Minimum weight loss to have improved medical outcomes	Brownell and Fairburn (2002), Chapter 91

[a] *www.cdc.gov/page.do/id/0900f3ec80112422*
[b] *www.nal.usda.gov/fnic/*

client to call before, rather than after, a crisis, and to prevent the potential reinforcement of the dysfunctional behavior by increasing contact with the therapist immediately following the dysfunctional behavior (assuming the therapist is a reinforcer for the client).

The question, then, is how to determine the appropriate time interval and when to introduce it to the client so as not to inadvertently reinforce dysfunctional behavior by providing more therapy following dysfunctional behavior. The important point is that discussion and agreement as to how long the time interval is before she can page after engaging in binge eating is agreed upon with the client beforehand, and not, for instance, during the event of a client paging after a binge. We do this differently for each client dependent on the result of an initial chain analysis, assessment of frequency of her binge eating, to what degree contact with the therapist after binge eating has reinforcing qualities, and to what both the client and the therapist agree upon as feasible and helpful in generalizing behavior. Take a client who binge eats five times a day, for whom there is little reinforcement from speaking to a therapist but who agrees with the therapist that telephone coaching is important for reduction in binge eating. In this case the 24-hour rule may be shifted to a "2-hour rule." If it is a circumstance in which a client is reinforced by therapist contact, this time may be lengthened (say to a "4-hour rule"). If the binge-eating behavior is not as frequent (say twice per day), the 24-hour rule would be reduced accordingly (say to a "6-hour rule"). The length of time may also change over the course of treatment as binge-eating frequency reduces or as new information regarding the reinforcing properties of paging is gathered. However, the most important thing here is careful in-session assessment and orientation of the client to these changes before she uses telephone consultation outside the session.

Consistent with standard DBT, clients are encouraged to use crisis survival strategies when intense urges arise to engage in dysfunctional behaviors before contacting their individual therapist. Dependent on the client's skill level, the individual therapist may specify the number of skills to try before contacting the individual therapist. Once the client calls and the specific reason for the call is identified, the individual therapist should ask, "What skills have you tried to prevent binge eating?" or "What help do you need to use skills to not binge eat?" Sometimes it is difficult to assess whether problem-solving or change-based skills (e.g., crisis survival strategies) are required, or if acceptance-based strategies would be more beneficial, like mindful eating. It is often difficult to eat mindfully when one's urges to binge are very high, or the emotion experienced is very intense—often situations like this are experienced as a crisis. In such instances, therapists should suggest skills that will change a person's emotions quickly by changing her physiology or behavior (e.g., taking a swift aerobic walk, perform progressive muscle relaxation). Sometimes clients who are new to DBT do not like calling their therapist during the week for help. In such cases, phone calls are assigned as homework and practiced in order to increase the probability that the client will call during an actual crisis situation.

Ancillary Treatments

Ancillary treatments are important in treating eating disorders because the most lethal problems associated with BED and BN are ones that medical professionals, not psychologists, are qualified to assess and monitor. For this reason, we require clients with EDs in the DBT program to have a full medical workup before they start treatment and to submit to ongoing monitoring by medical professionals over the course of treatment (e.g., regular assessment of electrolytes). Attendance at these appointments is monitored by the DBT individual therapist. Nonattendance is targeted as therapy-interfering behavior.

In addition to the use of ancillary treatments to monitor the health status of clients with EDs, other common ancillary programs utilized by our clients with EDs are those for weight management or related medical issues (e.g., consulting with a dietician or a personal trainer, attending Weight Watchers or a gym, and consulting with chronic pain specialists or diabetes specialists) or for other psychological treatment (e.g., attending Narcotics Anonymous, tapering off psychotropic medications with a pharmacotherapist). Allowing clients to see ancillary treaters keeps the DBT program focused on teaching skills to manage emotions and the behaviors resulting from these emotions. As described earlier, it is important that the individual therapist has some knowledge of the relative efficacy of interventions for obesity (e.g., the efficacy of behavioral weight loss, Weight Watchers, medication, or surgery) in order to provide clients with guidance in choices of weight management programs. However, typically clients have tried numerous weight and exercise programs but have had limited benefit or discontinued them due to difficulty regulating their emotions (e.g., frustration, anger, and anxiety) and negotiating the interpersonal difficulties that may arise. So coaching clients how to make the most of these programs is often addressed in treatment.

Most clients with EDs and those who treat them are accustomed to the use of a multidisciplinary approach that involves many treatment professionals and a variety of "self-help" programs. It is important that the DBT therapist orient both the client and the treatment network to the DBT approach, including the consultation to the client (vs. environmental intervention strategies) as well as the general treatment model (e.g., biosocial theory, stages and targets of treatment).

Family Treatment

Family involvement is very important for adolescent clients with AN or BN and BPD. Standard DBT includes guidelines for working with family members of an individual client receiving DBT. These guidelines and special considerations can be adapted for adolescent clients with EDs and BPD, as described in Chapter 1.

Therapist Dialectical Strategies

Dialectical Abstinence

Dialectical abstinence particularly focuses upon targeting objective binge eating, that is, eating more than the average person would in the given situation while feeling a loss of control. Dialectical abstinence from objective binge eating refers to simultaneously committing in the moment to both quitting binge eating forever and to reducing binge eating when it occurs. Making the commitment of being abstinent from objective binge eating makes it more likely that people will maintain the commitment, but is more difficult to sustain when the commitment has been broken. On the other hand, making the commitment to reducing objective binge eating is easier to adhere to when objective binge eating occurs, but is a weaker commitment than quitting completely, making it more likely that a client will lapse. The synthesis of this, that is, dialectical abstinence, is committing to being completely abstinent from objective binge eating while simultaneously having in one's mind that if an objective binge does occur, then the goal is to return to abstinence from objective binge eating (this is covered in greater detail in the DBT for binge eating and bulimia section). Dialectical abstinence from objective binge eating is different from dialectical abstinence from substance abuse in that the aim of the latter is to stop all use of substances while the aim of the former cannot be the cessation of eating (see Chapter 6 for thorough description of dialectical abstinence and its application to substance-dependent clients with BPD).

Dialectical Dilemmas for BPD and BED or BN

Relating a client's goals to secondary targets and dialectical dilemmas can be a helpful introduction to the notion of dialectics (see Figure 7.1). A key dialectical dilemma for clients with EDs is "overcontrolled eating" versus "out-of-control objective binge eating," which describes clients' vacillation between extreme dieting and eating larger-than-healthy amounts and feeling out of control. The synthesis is the balance of the two extremes. This allows for eating more than usual at special social occasions without experiencing a loss of control. Dialectical dilemmas are also useful to discuss in the context of clients who are trying to lose weight using the dialectic of "no activity" versus "overexercise," with the synthesis being healthy regular activity. These concepts are highlighted throughout treatment, beginning with the pretreatment phase where such discussions naturally occur in learning about the client's problems and teaching the client about the treatment philosophy.

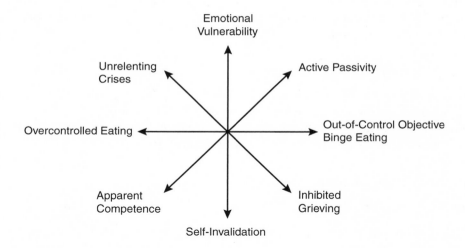

DBT for BPD and BED or BN Secondary Targets

Increase	Decrease
1. Emotional Modulation	1. Emotional Reactivity
2. Self-Validation	2. Self-Invalidation
3. Realistic Judgment	3. Crises-Generating Behaviors
4. Emotional Experiencing	4. Grief Inhibition
5. Active Problem Solving	5. Active-Passivity
6. Accurate Expression	6. Apparent-Only Competence
7. Flexible Eating	7. Overcontrolled Eating
8. Mindful Eating	8. Out-of-Control Objective Binge Eating

FIGURE 7.1. Dialectical dilemmas for BPD and BED or BN.

Future work needs to be undertaken to understand what aspects of these dilemmas pose particular problems for different subgroups of clients. For instance, older, more socially isolated clients with BPD and BED with comorbid obesity may enter treatment struggling with inhibited grief and younger BPD clients with BN who are normal weight may enter treatment in a state of unrelenting crises.

Core Therapist Strategies

Diary Card and Chain Analyses

The diary card instructions (see Figure 7.2) and diary card (see Figure 7.3) for the DBT program for Stage 1 clients with out-of-control behaviors and meeting BPD and BED or BN criteria covers ED behaviors, substance use, and suicidal and self-injurious behaviors. It is based on the diary cards used for clients with BPD and substance dependence or for highly suicidal BPD.

The DBT therapist and client may choose to add other behaviors being monitored by ancillary providers to the diary card. For instance, the dietician may recommend that the client monitor number of meals and snacks in a day or insulin use in the case of diabetes. This can be added to the blank column on this existing card. Alternatively, a food diary consisting of time of day when food/liquid is consumed, quantity, and description of the food and liquid consumed can be made to gather this additional information. This can be useful in the individual DBT context as long as the therapist is knowledgeable about its use.

DBT for Serious, Complex, and Treatment-Resistant EDs

The Cleveland Center for Eating Disorders (CCED), an independent eating disorder program near Cleveland, Ohio, offers partial hospital (PHP) and intensive outpatient (IOP) programs. Clients generally present to this program with moderate to severe eating disorders, significant medical and psychiatric comorbidity, and previously failed treatment attempts. Diagnoses treated include BN, AN, BED, and EDNOS.

In late 2000, when this eating disorder treatment program was being developed, the author (L. W.) and her colleagues were keenly aware both of the large empirical literature supporting the use of CBT to successfully treat the EDs, as well as the limits to these data described earlier in this chapter. DBT was considered a treatment option for clients with EDs because of its evidence base with other complex, multidiagnostic patient populations with problems arising from emotion dyscontrol, as well as data from Stanford University (described below) suggesting that DBT could be used successfully with clients with EDs. Given the populations served at CCED, however, it was problematic that the DBT for binge eating and bulimia model did not address clients with AN, the full range of clients presenting with EDNOS, and those presenting with significant medical and psychiatric comorbidity. These more complicated clients are traditionally those who, as treatment failures, present to a specialty care facility. CCED had as its goal to develop an eating disorder treatment program to meet the needs of a broad and difficult-to-treat population with EDs.

Because the patients treated by CCED were Stage 1 clients, standard DBT (Linehan, 1993a) was chosen as the foundation of the treatment model (as opposed to DBT for binge eating and bulimia, geared more to Stage 3 clients). It is important to note that given the potential symptom severity of the targeted population, with many clients dan-

How to Complete the Diary Card: Instructions for Therapists and Clients

- *Initials/ID #*: The client's initials are the first letter of the first name and the first letter of the last name. The client's ID# is a unique 6-digit randomly generated number.

- *Filled out in session?:* If the client filled the card out during the session, circle Y. Otherwise, circle N.

- *How often did you fill out this side?*: In the past week, did the client fill out the card daily, 2–3 times, 4–6 times, or once?

- *Started*: Note the first date the card was started, including year (e.g., 07/01/04).

- *Urges to commit suicide (0–5)*: The client rates the intensity with which he or she experienced urges to commit suicide on a scale from 0 (no urges at all) to 5 (the strongest, most intense urges possible). High scores may indicate either an intense or a pervasive occurrence of urges to commit suicide. The client rates the *most intense* or *highest* urges experienced on that particular day. For example, if the client experienced several instances of urges rated 3/5, but one instance of urges rated 5/5, he or she would put a "5" in the column for Urges to Commit Suicide.

- *Urges to self-harm (0–5)*: The client rates the highest intensity with which he or she experienced urges to self-harm on a scale from 0 (no urges at all) to 5 (the strongest, most intense urges possible) on that particular day.

- *Urges to binge (0–5)*: For the urge to binge, rate 0–5 according to intensity where 0 indicates no urge and 5 the strongest urge to binge. Rate your greatest urge in the day.

- *Urges to use drugs (0–5)*: The client rates the intensity with which he or she experienced urges to use drugs (this includes alcohol, over-the-counter meds, prescription meds, and street/illicit drugs) on a scale from 0 (no urges at all) to 5 (the strongest, most intense urges possible). High scores may indicate either an intense or a pervasive occurrence of urges to use drugs. The client rates the *most intense* or *highest* urges experienced on that particular day. For example, if the client experienced several instances of urges rated 3/5, but one instance of urges rated 5/5, he or she would put a "5" in the column for Urges to Use Drugs.

- *Emotional misery*: Emotional misery refers to a subjective emotional state experienced by the client as misery. Emotional misery may involve a conglomeration of several different unpleasant emotional experiences, such as sadness, despair, depression, fear, and so on. The client rates the intensity with which he or she experiences emotional misery on a scale from 0 (no experience of the emotion at all) to 5 (the strongest, most intense experience of the emotion possible).

- *Physical misery*: Physical misery refers to a physical state experienced by the client as misery. Physical misery may involve intense or prolonged pain, aches, cramps, symptoms of short- or long-term physical illnesses (e.g., a cold, the flu), acute injuries, and so on.

- *Joy (0–5)*: Rate the intensity of joy from 0–5.

- *Eating disorder behavior*:
  - **Objective binges.** Write in the number of objective binge episodes that occurred in the day. An objective binge involves eating an unusually large amount of food for a situation very quickly (2 hours maximum) with a sense of loss of control (e.g., eating a quart of ice cream very quickly alone).
  - *Subjective binges.* Write in the number of subjective binge episodes that occurred in the day. A subjective binge involves eating an average-size or less-than-average-size meal but feeling a loss of control (e.g., eating a sandwich at lunch but feeling a loss of control).
  - *Vomiting.* Write in the number of vomiting episodes in response to bingeing that occurred in the day.
  - *Laxatives (L), diuretics (D), or diet pills (DP).* Write in whether or not you used any of these pills for the purpose of getting rid of food. Write in the # of pills in the day.

(continued)

FIGURE 7.2. University of Washington instructions for filling out skills diary card.

- *Dieting.* Describe whether fasting or restriction occurred in the day. Fasting (F) is no eating outside the times of an objective binge and not eating 8 waking hours or more; restriction (R) is either eating infrequently or only eating low-calorie foods but eating less than 1200 kcal per day outside the times when one objectively binges.
- *Note for overexercising.* If a client compensates for bingeing by overexercising, place this in the blank column at the end of the table. Write in the type of exercise and the number of times in the day and for how long it occurred.

- *Drugs/Medications*:
  - *"#".* The number of drugs (as described in the specify column) used on this date (e.g., "3" for three beers).
  - *What?* For **alcohol**, specify the type of drink (e.g., beer, cocktails, mixed drinks, whiskey, wine). For **illicit drugs**, specify the type of illicit drug (e.g., Valium, marijuana, heroin, methadone, methamphetamine, cocaine). In the case of prescription drugs, it's acceptable to write "ditto" in subsequent specify boxes, to indicate daily use.
  - *Meds as prescribed.* Write Y (Yes) or N (No) to indicate whether prescribed medications were taken as prescribed.
  - *PRN/over-the-counter.* Under the # column, write down the number of prn drugs that were taken on that particular day. Under the **What** column, write down the name of the prn drug(s) that was/were taken that day.
  - You can use horizontal lines through rows and vertical lines through columns to indicate no use (e.g., if the client didn't use any prescription meds this week, lines down the #, specify, and 0 columns under prescription meds are okay. Or, if the client didn't use alcohol, over-the-counter meds, or prescription meds on Wednesday, then a horizontal line may be drawn through the corresponding boxes for Wednesday).

- *Actions*
  - *Self-harm.* The client writes Y (Yes) or N (No) to indicate whether he or she has engaged in any self-harm behavior. Self-harm here is the same as "parasuicidal behavior," or any overt, acute, self-injurious act that, without outside intervention, would result in tissue damage, illness, or death. The act of self-harm must be *intentional*: the client intended to inflict tissue damage, illness, or death.
  - *Reinforce.* The client places a checkmark in this column to indicate that he or she actively reinforced him- or herself, or successfully got others in his or her social environment to provide reinforcement. The reinforcement should be for effective behavior (e.g., skillful behavior, not bingeings, not self-harming).

- *Blank column*: This column may be used to keep a record of any additional behavior.

- *Used skills*: The client circles the number that best corresponds to his or her experience of using/not using skills.

- *Urge to*: Quit therapy, binge, commit suicide before and after session. The client rates the intensity of his or her *current* urges to engage in these behaviors, at the beginning of the session, on a scale from 0 (no urges at all) to 5 (the strongest, most intense urges possible).

- *Ability to self-regulate/self-control: emotions, actions, thoughts:* The client rates the extent to which he or she feels capable of regulating his or her emotions, behaviors (actions), or thoughts at the beginning of the session, on a scale from 0 (no ability to regulate at all; absolutely no control over thoughts, behaviors, or emotions) to 5 (totally and completely able to regulate thoughts, behaviors, or emotions).

- *Chain analysis notes:* In this section, the therapist jots down any important notes based on a chain analysis conducted during the session.

- *Med changes/other:* The client writes down any changes in prescribed medications. These changes may consist of modifications in the dosage (increase or decrease) of the medications (e.g., increase from 5mg to 10mg; a decrease from 20mg to 10mg), the dropping of a medication, or the addition of a new medication.

FIGURE 7.2. *(continued)*

Dialectical Behavior Therapy Skills Diary Card	Initials ID #	Filled out in Session? Y N (Circle)	How often did you fill out this side? ___ Daily ___ 2–3× ___ 4–6× ___ Once	Started: Date __/__/__

Circle Start Day	Highest Urge To:				Highest Daily Rating			Eating Disorder Behavior						Drugs/Medications							Actions			
Day of Week	Commit suicide	Self-harm	Binge	Use drugs	Emotion. misery	Physical misery	Joy	Obj. binge	Subj. binge	Vomit	Lax., diur, diet pills		Dieting:	Alcohol		Illicit drugs		Meds. as prescrib	PRN/over the counter		Self-harm	Skills	Reinforce	
	0–5	0–5	0–5	0–5	0–5	0–5	0–5	#	#	#	y/n	#	Fast or Restrict	#	What	#	What	Y/N	#	What	Y/N	0–7	✓	
MON																								
TUE																								
WED																								
THUR																								
FRI																								
SAT																								
SUN																								

Chain Analysis Notes

Med Changes/Other:

* USED SKILLS:

0 = Not thought about or used
1 = Thought about, not used, didn't want to
2 = Thought about, not used, wanted to
3 = Tried but couldn't use them
4 = Tried, could do them, but they didn't help
5 = Tried, could use them, helped
6 = Didn't try, used them, didn't help
7 = Didn't try, used them, helped

Urge to:	Before Session (0–5)	After Session (0–5)	Ability to self-regulate/self-control:	Before Session (0–5)	After Session (0–5)
Quit therapy			Emotions:		
Obj. binge			Action:		
Commit suicide			Thoughts:		

(continued)

FIGURE 7.3. University of Washington skills diary card. Copyright by the Behavioral Research and Therapy Clinic, University of Washington. Reprinted by permission.

DBT Skills Diary Card	Filled out this side? ___ Daily ___ 2–3× ___ 4–6× ___ Once ___ In session ___						
Homework:	Check Skill (if more than one) and Circle days skill was practiced						
1. Wise mind	MON	TUE	WED	THUR	FRI	SAT	SUN
2. Observe: just notice	MON	TUE	WED	THUR	FRI	SAT	SUN
3. Describe: put words on, just the facts	MON	TUE	WED	THUR	FRI	SAT	SUN
4. Participate: enter into the experience	MON	TUE	WED	THUR	FRI	SAT	SUN
5. Nonjudgmental stance	MON	TUE	WED	THUR	FRI	SAT	SUN
6. One-mindfully: present moment	MON	TUE	WED	THUR	FRI	SAT	SUN
7. Effectiveness: focus on what works	MON	TUE	WED	THUR	FRI	SAT	SUN
8. Describe ___ Express ___ Assert ___ Reinforce ___ **DEAR**	MON	TUE	WED	THUR	FRI	SAT	SUN
9. Mindful: Broken record ___ Ignore attacks ___ **MAN**	MON	TUE	WED	THUR	FRI	SAT	SUN
10. Appear confident ___ Negotiate ___	MON	TUE	WED	THUR	FRI	SAT	SUN
11. Gentle ___ Interested ___ Validate ___ Easy manner ___ **GIVE**	MON	TUE	WED	THUR	FRI	SAT	SUN
12. Fair ___ no-Apologies ___ Stick to values ___ Truthful ___ **FAST**	MON	TUE	WED	THUR	FRI	SAT	SUN
13. Attend to relationships	MON	TUE	WED	THUR	FRI	SAT	SUN
14. Figure out interpersonal goals and priorities	MON	TUE	WED	THUR	FRI	SAT	SUN
15. Opposite-to-emotion action	MON	TUE	WED	THUR	FRI	SAT	SUN
16. Temperature ___ Intense exercise ___ Progressive relaxation ___ **TIP**	MON	TUE	WED	THUR	FRI	SAT	SUN
17. Mindfulness of current emotion	MON	TUE	WED	THUR	FRI	SAT	SUN
18. Problem-solve	MON	TUE	WED	THUR	FRI	SAT	SUN
19. Accumulate positives ___ Build mastery ___ Cope ahead ___ **ABC**	MON	TUE	WED	THUR	FRI	SAT	SUN
20. Care: PhysicaL Ills ___ Eating ___ Avoid drugs ___ Sleep ___ Exercise ___ **PLEASE**	MON	TUE	WED	THUR	FRI	SAT	SUN
21. Mindful of current thoughts, ___ Challenge thinking ___ **PREVENT**	MON	TUE	WED	THUR	FRI	SAT	SUN
22. Distract	MON	TUE	WED	THUR	FRI	SAT	SUN
23. Self-soothe **CRISIS**	MON	TUE	WED	THUR	FRI	SAT	SUN
24. Improve the moment **SURVIVAL**	MON	TUE	WED	THUR	FRI	SAT	SUN
25. Pros and cons	MON	TUE	WED	THUR	FRI	SAT	SUN
26. Radical acceptance	MON	TUE	WED	THUR	FRI	SAT	SUN

FIGURE 7.3. (continued)

gerously underweight, the author did not feel comfortable with entirely dropping the empirically supported CBT treatments known to be helpful to clients with EDs (e.g., meal planning, self-monitoring of intake, ED psychoeducation). Hence, a decision was made to integrate DBT into existing cognitive-behavioral approaches to the treatment of EDs. This integrated approach, called "DBT-enhanced cognitive-behavioral therapy," or "DBT–CBT," is described in this section, and will be of particular interest to clinicians versed in traditional CBT approaches to EDs who wish to incorporate DBT into their CBT treatments.

The incorporation of standard DBT into the current model of CBT treatment for EDs made intuitive sense since DBT draws heavily from cognitive-behavioral theory and treatment approaches. In fact, cognitive-behavioral treatment is the basis or foundation of DBT and provides a treatment frame in which to integrate other treatment protocols for Axis I problems. Acceptance-based components of DBT that are not cognitive-behavioral in origin can be considered complimentary and could potentially enhance traditional ED treatments. For example, many CBT approaches focus mainly upon strategies for change, while DBT focuses equally on strategies to promote *acceptance* as well as change. It was hoped that the acceptance-based strategies could be particularly useful for clients diagnosed with EDs since by definition clients with EDs do not accept themselves or their bodies. Furthermore, clients with AN, in particular, often have difficulty staying in the treatment they need, making DBT's motivation and commitment strategies attractive.

The DBT–CBT model that is described here may be used with any adult client with an ED. Given the success of standard CBT, however, the reader may wonder when and with whom should a therapist use DBT–CBT. This is a question that has yet to be addressed empirically. However, some related literature may provide guidance. Data suggest that response to a CBT for ED will be evident within the first six sessions (Mitchell et al., 2002). Treatment failures for standard CBT may therefore be identified fairly quickly. The addition of DBT may be considered for clients who fail to progress in CBT or IPT and who also exhibit problems in emotion regulation, motivation, or commitment, all three of which are addressed directly within the DBT model.

It should also be noted here that the CCED program has two treatment tracks: an adult program (described here) and a child and adolescent program. Although the child and adolescent program does include many of the components that are described below, the model includes a family therapy component that, although it is informed by DBT, is not DBT-driven in philosophy. The CCED program attempts to provide treatment that is evidence-based, and there are no published data to date on the use of DBT with adolescent clients with EDs.

Stages and Target Hierarchy

All potential clients to the CCED program attend an initial assessment to evaluate the appropriate level of care, given the severity of the disorder and the degree of functional impairment. The client participates in a semistructured clinical interview designed to assess eating pathology as well as other comorbidities. Using the level-of-care criteria outlined in the *Practice Guidelines for the Treatment of Patients with Eating Disorders* (American Psychiatric Association, 2000), the treatment team meets in order to recommend an appropriate level of care for each client. The American Psychiatric Association (APA) guidelines suggest the use of a multiaxial evaluation that includes weight, the presence of bingeing and/or purging, and access to treatment in order to determine level of care. At CCED, clients meeting criteria for inpatient or residential treatment are given a referral and are helped to transition to these settings. Clients who meet criteria for IOP/PHP are offered treatment within the appropriate format. These clients have generally failed other treatments, have severe ED behavioral problems (e.g., purging several times/day; body weight = 75% of ideal), and may also carry significant psychiatric and medical comorbidity. Although the CCED program does accept clients who engage in self-harm behaviors, those clients who are *acutely suicidal* may first be referred to a general DBT program in order to effectively target suicidal behaviors. Once a client is no longer imminently suicidal, she may then be admitted to the CCED program. Clients in this program range from those who have ED behaviors that are imminently life-threatening (Stage 1) to those who have ED behaviors that interfere only with quality of life (Stage 3). The CCED program utilizes the same target hierarchy that was described earlier in this chapter.

What will be described below is the DBT–CBT treatment offered in the IOP and PHP settings at CCED. Length of stay in the CCED program is determined individually by change in client behaviors. However, clients in the IOP engage in 9 hours/week of treatment over 3 days, and stay in treatment for approximately 5 weeks, while the clients in the PHP engage in 30 hours/week of treatment over 5 days and stay for approximately 3–4 weeks. Clients may move between these two levels of care, depending on their severity of behaviors. For example, as a PHP client improves, she may be transitioned to the IOP before moving to individual therapy alone. Likewise, a client whose symptoms are not responding to the IOP level of care may be moved to the PHP setting for increased structure and accountability. On the rare occasion that an individual in PHP is not making progress or whose symptoms increase while in treatment, a recommendation for inpatient or residential care may be given. The practice of moving clients among the various levels of care is always conducted with full awareness of the behavioral principles at work. Specifically, the treatment team attempts to remain aware of instances in which it is reinforcing to give more treatment when a client is not doing well and consider that decision within the context of severity of behavioral symptoms as well as medical stability.

Treatment Structure

By definition, IOP and PHP programming, with multiple hours/week of treatment, is carried out in group format. In addition, clients from all ED populations are treated in the same group. This is successfully managed by requiring that clients refrain from talking about numbers of any kind (e.g., current/desired weight, calories, amount of food eaten) and any self-harm or suicidal behavior. This requirement appears to dampen the tendency toward social comparison that is inherent in group treatment for eating disorders.

With respect to skills, DBT skills groups are conducted 2 days each week (e.g., Monday and Thursday), with the homework from Monday's skill reviewed on Thursday and vice versa. All skills from all four modules (i.e., core mindfulness, interpersonal effectiveness, emotion regulation, distress tolerance) are taught. Clients can enter the group at any time and therefore may enter in the middle of a module. We recommend that clients stay in treatment a minimum of 6 weeks in order to receive all needed skills at least one time. In order to best prepare clients to begin learning DBT skills in our environment given this format, core mindfulness skills are reviewed during an orientation meeting prior to starting treatment. A CBT group is taught once each week. This group focuses on standard CBT for ED issues such as cognitive restructuring, identifying ineffective thoughts, and understanding how thoughts affect behavior. As described below, a behavior chaining group is also conducted weekly.

Nutrition and meal planning groups are each provided by a nutritionist in the DBT-CBT program once per week. During these groups, clients are taught specific skills to promote balanced eating. These include basic nutrition education and meal planning skills, as well as how to complete their CCED diary card. The goal of this group is to educate (or reeducate) clients with EDs about topics such as portion size, meal planning, metabolism, the function of a varied diet, and the effects of food restriction and compensatory behaviors on weight control and mood. Other topics of this group include myths about dieting, advertising and cultural reinforcers for dieting behavior, psychoeducation regarding eating disorders, weight regulation, and medical issues. These topics were chosen because they are typically addressed in the cognitive-behavioral treatment of EDs. Within a DBT conceptualization, this group may be considered teaching self-management skills.

Another integral component of the CCED treatment is the therapeutic meal. During these meals, one staff member and approximately five to seven clients eat together. Clients bring foods that meet the requirements designated by the meal plan they created with a nutritionist. In an effort to give clients an opportunity to interact more naturally around meal time, talk is conversational and not food- or eating-focused. Suggested meal topics include movies, music, and current events. The meal context functions as an exposure for many clients, who often prefer to eat alone and/or in secret. Moreover, since the therapeutic meal gives the staff member *in vivo* observation of client behavior, interventions can be designed in the moment for a particular client while the group has the opportunity to provide support to the client as well. For example, a client who excessively cuts up her food can be asked by a staff member to use a specific DBT skill appropriate to the client, the behavior, and the context to stop this behavior in the moment (e.g., act opposite to emotion, practice pros and cons, urge surf). A client who is having difficulty finishing her meal may receive cheerleading and suggestions of skill use from the other group members. Of note, staff members are asked to eat a well-balanced meal. The therapist's meal choice and eating behavior can serve to model effective behavior for clients.

Note that with respect to the use of mindful eating during therapeutic meals, the CCED experience is that some clients can benefit from a mindful approach to eating with a focus on awareness of hunger and satiety cues. Specifically, clients are encouraged to begin to monitor their hunger and fullness at the start of treatment, since by definition our clients do not respond to these cues (e.g., they do not eat although hungry, or they do not stop eating although full). Using a dialectical approach, we take the stand that clients must learn to attend effectively to hunger and satiety since "food is medicine" *and* that eating according to the meal plan must occur regardless of hunger or fullness at the start of treatment, as these systems are often disrupted in our clients (e.g., see Wisniewski et al., 1997). Therefore, early in treatment clients are often encouraged to act opposite or to use distractions during therapeutic meals. Over time, when clients show mastery over the act of eating per se, they are encouraged to approach the therapeutic meal more mindfully.

Providing all of the DBT treatment components within a group framework was a logistical struggle. While the CCED program could easily offer DBT skills groups, provide telephone consultation, and conduct a weekly consultation team (see below), we were limited in our ability to also offer true individual therapy as clients are only with us for several weeks. In our system, the program leader (i.e., the IOP leader or the PHP leader) takes on many of the roles of the individual therapist, however. For example, it is the program leader's job to treat self-harm and suicidal ideation if it occurs during ED treatment. It is also the program leader ultimately who reviews diary cards and BCAs completed by a particular client. The program leader meets with clients for several brief meetings over the course of a week to accomplish these goals. In addition, given that the prime goals of individual therapy in DBT are to enhance motivation and to promote skill generalization (Linehan, 1993a), two groups were developed to meet these aims. The *motivation/commitment group* focuses on helping clients stay motivated for treatment and to identify and problem-solve factors that hinder motivation/commitment. The *DBT in action* group attempts to aid clients in identifying and discussing ways in which they are/are not able to use skills outside of treatment. Again, clients who bring up issues of self-harm during these groups are referred back to their program leader to specifically address these episodes.

Telephone Consultation

The ED program at CCED provides telephone coaching (see, e.g., Wisniewski & Ben Porath, 2005) to all IOP and PHP clients. Like the UW program, we too discovered that the application of the 24-hour rule was problematic for use with targeting ED behaviors. Since food, eating, weight, and shape stimuli are omnipresent in many environments, we felt it important to be able to provide telephone coaching to clients with EDs for managing urges related to targeted ED behaviors. The standard 24-hour rule would make it extremely unlikely for a client to be able to use the telephone consultation if she engaged in any ED behavior at all! We therefore decided to adopt the next meal/snack rule (NM/S rule) for use with ED behaviors (Wisniewski & Ben-Porath, 2005). The NM/S rule states that a client should call for consultation prior to engaging in a targeted ED behavior. If the client does engage in a targeted ED behavior, however, she may call for coaching at the *next scheduled meal or snack*. If the client purges at lunch, for example, she may (and is expected to) call for coaching for her afternoon snack, if there is a problem. The focus of that afternoon call, however, is only on the *current* episode (i.e., urges to restrict the afternoon snack). It should be noted that in our experience, clients with EDs frequently have difficulty initiating calls and are often placed on "mandatory paging" (i.e., clients are asked to call at a certain time, whether or not they have engaged in a behavior) in order to shape the behavior initially.

Of note is how calls are managed from an administrative perspective. Due to the size of this program (10–25 adult clients in treatment at any one time), the CCED program rotates weekly which staff member carries the pager to take calls from clients. Although this can be somewhat distressing to clients initially (e.g., an IOP patient may call for coaching and get a PHP leader, whom she does not know well), this is framed to clients as an opportunity to get coaching and to use interpersonal effectiveness skills from a variety of professionals on the treatment team. In order to ensure effective communication, the staff member on call sends out an email at the end of each day with a brief synopsis of the calls received. In this way, the team leader can follow up with the client the next day.

DBT Consultation Team

Two weekly meetings are attended by all CCED staff on the PHP and IOP programs. The first of these meetings (multidisciplinary rounds) focuses on a chart review of the patients' progress and is not considered a component of DBT. The second is focused specifically on enhancing treatment providers' motivation and capability to work with our patients—the specific functions of a DBT consultation team. While the multidisciplinary rounds meeting is attended by all treatment staff—therapists, psychiatrist, nutritionist, nurse, and so on—involved in the patients' care on the unit, the DBT consultation team is attended only by those members of the unit applying DBT. The DBT consultation team meeting lasts approximately 90 minutes and follows the standard functions and structure described by Linehan (1993a) and in Chapter 1 of this book.

Preparing for the Next Generation: Staff Training

Providing adequate training to staff is a monumental task. Staff needs to be trained in DBT as well as in CBT for eating disorders and be in agreement that they will adhere to the governing treatment manuals. Toward this goal, new staff are required not only to read primary DBT and CBT sources, but also to observe and cofacilitate the above groups led by experienced DBT–CBT clinicians before leading the groups themselves. All applicants for positions within CCED are fully oriented to this expectation during the interview process and are asked explicitly if they are willing to do the necessary reading and learning should they be offered the job. They are also asked explicitly if they agree to using the DBT–CBT protocols. The purpose of this orienting and commitment of new staff is to increase the probability that the CCED treatment team will successfully apply the intended treatment.

Therapists' Dialectical Strategies

Effective Eating

Clients are encouraged to find the dialectical synthesis between the extremes of over-controlled/rigid eating and absence of an eating plan (Wisniewski & Kelly, 2003). This synthesis is discussed within a framework of "effective eating." Effective eating can be described as eating when hungry, stopping when full, and using a variety of foods to achieve these goals. Discussing eating within the DBT concept of effectiveness can help a client become unstuck from whether or not a particular food, or even eating in and of itself, is "good or bad." An example of this is the client who eats a high-calorie, fast-food lunch and so skips dinner because she feels that she has "eaten too much already." This client may then become hungry in the evening, setting her up for a binge-eating episode. Eating a fast-food lunch and skipping dinner, therefore, may be viewed as ineffective with helping the client to meet her goal of stopping binge eating. The therapist and client might jointly come up with a more effective plan that includes a moderate lunch so that the client feels able to eat dinner as well. Note that the language of effectiveness can help the client stay away from stating that she was "bad" or that the food she ate was "bad" or fattening.

Core Therapist Strategies

Diary Cards

In standard DBT, as well as in CBT for clients with EDs, self-monitoring is considered an essential component of treatment. In DBT–CBT, the standard DBT diary card (see Figures 7.4 and 7.5) has been broadened in order to meet the particular needs of clients with EDs. The diary card includes standard DBT components of self-monitoring target behaviors (modified to reflect ED behaviors) and monitoring skill use. It also includes an important component of traditional ED treatment: recording dietary intake. The recording of intake reflects the CBT tradition of meal planning and expects that following a regular pattern

The Correct Method of Completing a Diary Card (Cleveland Center for Eating Disorders)
*In order for diary cards to be an effective component of your treatment,
diary cards must be filled out daily!*

- NAME: Your name.
- DAY/DATE: Day, month, and year. Ex. 01/05/04.
- TIME: The time the meal/snack was eaten.
- PLAN: What number of each exchange does your current meal plan require as designed by you dietitian? This may change frequently, so you will need to update as each change occurs.
- ACTUAL (ACT): This is the actual amount of each exchange that you consumed at that meal/ snack. For example, if you ate 3 protein exchanges, but your meal plan required 2, you still write 3.
- EMPTY–NEUTRAL–STUFFED: Shade in where your sense of hunger was when you began your meal and where your sense of hunger was once you completed your meal.
- FOOD INTAKE: Describe the approximate quantity and description of food consumed. Ex., 1 cup (8 oz.) of 2% milk, 1 oz. of turkey bacon, 2 slices of wheat bread. Give as much detail as possible regarding size and quality of the food.
- LOCATION: Describe where you were when you consumed the food. If in group, indicate PHP, IOP, etc. If at another location indicate where you were. Ex., in the kitchen, in the living room, in the car, etc.
- FLUID INTAKE: Indicate how much fluid was consumed during the meal/snack in either cups or ounces. If you drank any fluids immediately before eating, indicate that amount also.
- URGES TO ENGAGE IN A TARGET BEHAVIOR (TB): This includes the urge to binge, purge, use pills, restrict, exercise, or any other behavior that is identified by you or your treatment team as a "TB." **If you engage in a "TB," mark that column with an *. If you had an urge, but did not engage in the behavior, use the 0–5 scale to rate the intensity of your urge. 0 indicates no urge to engage in the behavior, while 5 indicates the strongest urge to engage in the behavior. Note: If you do not meet all your exchanges in a meal/snack, you would put a star (*) in the restriction column.** If you engage in a level of exercise that is above and beyond what your treatment team has prescribed, then you would put a star in the exercise column. You **do not** need to put a star if your level of exercise was within your treatment limits. **It is important that each column has a 0–5 rating or an * in it.**
- EMOTION: Indicate any emotions you may have been experiencing during your meal/snack. **You must indicate any emotion experienced at every meal.** Examples of emotions include calm, anxious, sad, angry, guilty, and overwhelmed. Also indicate any body image issues that may be occurring during this time.
- SKILL(S) USED: Indicate any skills you used during the meal/snack, even if you engage in a "TB." You may circle any DBT skills you used on the back of the diary card, but also indicate these skills in the column for that meal. If you are not familiar with any/many of the DBT skills, indicate what you did to help you through that meal (watched TV, called a friend, used the paging service, etc.).

Place your diary card and this handout somewhere in plain view in order to remind yourself to fill it out at each meal.

FIGURE 7.4. CCED directions for filling out diary card.

CCED ☼

DIARY CARD

Eating Disorder Program

Name: _____ Day/Date: _____

Time	PLAN	ACT	MEALS	Food Intake W0—Include approximate quantity and description of food — Hunger Scale—Graph hunger level from start to end of meal										Location	Fluid Intake (cups/czs.)	BINGE PURGE	PURGE LAXATIVES	RESTRICT EXERCISE	Emotion	Skill Used
				empty	2	3	4	neutral	6	7	8	9	stuffed						Mark (*) if you engaged in behavior. Rate (0–5) if you had an urge but did not engage in behavior.	
			BREAKFAST																	
			Protein																	
			Vegetable																	
			Grain																	
			Lipid Nutr.																	
			Fruit																	
			Dairy																	
			SNACK																	
			LUNCH	empty	2	3	4	neutral	6	7	8	9	stuffed							
			Protein																	
			Vegetable																	
			Grain																	
			Lipid Nutr.																	
			Fruit																	
			Dairy																	
			SNACK																	
			DINNER	empty	2	3	4	neutral	6	7	8	9	stuffed							
			Protein																	
			Vegetable																	
			Grain																	
			Lipid Nutr.																	
			Fruit																	
			Dairy																	
			SNACK																	
			VITAMINS																	

Please describe what was important to you today:

(continued)

FIGURE 7.5. CCED diary card and skills diary card.

Skills Diary Card

(Circle the days you practiced each skill)

CORE MINDFULNESS SKLLS

Wise Mind	Mon	Tues	Wed	Thurs	Fri	Sat	Sun
Observe: just notice	Mon	Tues	Wed	Thurs	Fri	Sat	Sun
Describe: put words on	Mon	Tues	Wed	Thurs	Fri	Sat	Sun
Nonjudgmental stance	Mon	Tues	Wed	Thurs	Fri	Sat	Sun
One-mindfully: in the moment	Mon	Tues	Wed	Thurs	Fri	Sat	Sun
Effectiveness: focus on what works	Mon	Tues	Wed	Thurs	Fri	Sat	Sun

INTERPERSONAL EFFECTIVENESS SKILLS

Objective Effectiveness: DEAR MAN	Mon	Tues	Wed	Thurs	Fri	Sat	Sun
Relationship Effectivness: GIVE	Mon	Tues	Wed	Thurs	Fri	Sat	Sun
Self-Respect Effectiveness: FAST	Mon	Tues	Wed	Thurs	Fri	Sat	Sun

EMOTION REGULATION SKILLS

Reduce Vulnerability: PLEASE	Mon	Tues	Wed	Thurs	Fri	Sat	Sun
Build MASTERy	Mon	Tues	Wed	Thurs	Fri	Sat	Sun
Build Positive Experiences	Mon	Tues	Wed	Thurs	Fri	Sat	Sun
Opposite to emotion action	Mon	Tues	Wed	Thurs	Fri	Sat	Sun

DISTRESS TOLERANCE SKILLS

Distract	Mon	Tues	Wed	Thurs	Fri	Sat	Sun
Self-Soothe	Mon	Tues	Wed	Thurs	Fri	Sat	Sun
IMPROVE the moment	Mon	Tues	Wed	Thurs	Fri	Sat	Sun
Pros and Cons	Mon	Tues	Wed	Thurs	Fri	Sat	Sun
Radical Acceptance	Mon	Tues	Wed	Thurs	Fri	Sat	Sun
	Mon	Tues	Wed	Thurs	Fri	Sat	Sun
	Mon	Tues	Wed	Thurs	Fri	Sat	Sun

FIGURE 7.5. (continued)

of eating will help decrease ED and other targeted behaviors. For example, a client who follows a prescribed pattern of eating three meals and two snacks per day will likely be less hungry and feel less deprived, decreasing the likelihood of heightened feelings of hunger and deprivation leading to a binge. In addition, both meal planning and self-monitoring of intake are essential when treating a client with low body weight, as weight gain is a primary goal of treatment. It is important to note that this particular diary card assumes that the client has received a meal plan as a result of a meeting with a dietician who understands EDs. The meal plan is designed to help the client to eat normally and effectively and may reflect the goal of the client gaining or maintaining weight. This monitoring allows the client and the therapist to become aware of what the client is able to eat and in what context.

Application of Chain Analysis

In contrast to the model of DBT for individuals with BPD and an ED, chain analyses are taught and conducted within the group setting. In should be noted here that in a review of the relevant literature and consistent with our clinical experience, we could find no evidence of a contagion effect linked to talking about ED behaviors, as is seen with group discussions around suicidal behaviors (e.g., Linehan, 1993a, 1993b). We therefore felt quite comfortable conducting the BCAs within the group format. In a group entitled "Behavior Chaining," clients are encouraged to share their eating-disordered BCAs verbally, with a therapist facilitating this process using a white board. If a client volunteers to share her BCA with the group, she is not required to complete a written BCA for that particular event. It is expected that all other events have written BCAs to be turned in to the program leader. The program leader later reviews all written BCAs, gives written feedback on them, and then returns the completed BCA to the client on the next day of treatment. Sharing the BCA within a group with the therapist's help allows all group clients to improve their behavior analysis/solution analysis skills and for clients to get experience giving others suggestions for more effective behavior. In this group, clients are asked not to discuss self-harm or suicidal behavior, as these are to be addressed with their program leader.

DBT Adapted for the Treatment of BED and BN

DBT for binge eating and bulimia was developed to target Stage 3 clients whose primary focus of treatment is ED behavior (BED or BN) that interferes with quality of life. This model was developed for adult women who met criteria for BED, BN or partial BN (met DSM-IV criteria for BN except had objective binge episodes at a lower frequency—an average of one objective binge episode/week for 3 months). As a treatment developed specifically for Stage 3 clients, suicidal clients or clients with other out-of-control behaviors (e.g., substance abuse or dependence) are not appropriate for DBT for binge eating and bulimia. Indeed, these individuals were excluded from the original research on which this model is based. DBT for binge eating and bulimia involves a number of adaptations to standard DBT that reflect the patient population, their diagnosis, and level of disorder consistent with Stage 3 (and not Stage 1) of treatment. Additional published resources detailing the DBT for binge eating and bulimia model include an overview by Wiser and Telch (1999) and descriptive case reports by Telch (1997a) and Safer, Telch, and Agras

(2001a). Much of the content for this section is derived from the original, currently unpublished treatment manual (1997b) and is intended to provide the "nuts and bolts" of how to implement DBT for binge eating and bulimia.

DBT for binge eating and bulimia is currently the only adaptation of DBT for EDs supported through randomized trials. While the evidence base is limited, five studies to date (two randomized controlled studies, one uncontrolled study, and two case reports) have been reported (Telch et al., 2001; Telch et al., 2000; Telch, 1997a; Safer et al., 2001a; Safer, Telch, & Agras, 2001b). Preliminary results are promising. For example, in the randomized controlled trial of DBT for BED 16 of the 18 women (89%) who received DBT were abstinent at the end of the 20-week treatment compared to two of 16 (12.5%) wait-list controls (Telch et al., 2001). In another randomized controlled trial, DBT for bulimic symptoms was compared to a wait-list control. Abstinence rates at the end of 20 weeks of treatment were 28.6% (four of 14) compared with 0% (zero of 15) for the wait-list control (Safer et al., 2001b).

A Word before Getting Started

It is noteworthy that in the research conducted to date, DBT for BED was conducted in a group format and DBT for BN was conducted in the context of individual therapy alone. The rationale for this distinction is more an artifact of the research than for any clinical reasons. While the data collected to date is based on these varied formats, we know of no reason to anticipate that changing the delivery format (i.e., group or individual) would aversely affect clinical outcomes. Other than the original difference in the delivery format and specific disorder targeted by the treatment, there was no difference in DBT for BN and DBT for BED. Hence, while the present content focuses on DBT adapted for BED, it is fully transferable to DBT for BN.

Stages and Target Hierarchy

DBT for binge eating and bulimia targets Stage 3 clients with a primary treatment focus that includes problematic eating behaviors interfering with their quality of life. In the absence of data on applying the model for Stage 1 clients and the plethora of data on DBT's efficacy for Stage 1 clients, we strongly discourage application of the DBT for binge eating and bulimia model for Stage 1 clients. When Stage 1 clients wish to enroll in the Stanford program, they are instead referred to a Stage 1 treatment according to standards presented earlier in this chapter and in Koerner, Dimeff, and Swenson (Chapter 2, this volume).

Please refer to Figure 7.6 (a–e) for the Path to Mindful Eating target hierarchy used in DBT for binge eating and bulimia.

Treatment Structure

There are two distinct features of DBT for binge eating and bulimia that are different from the previously presented approaches for EDs and from standard DBT. First, the model combines elements of the functions of individual and group together. Specifically, where enhancing motivation is typically done in individual psychotherapy and acquiring/ strengthening new skills occurs within a skills training group in standard DBT, these functions are combined in DBT for binge eating and bulimia. Second, where standard DBT is typically provided in no less than a year, this model consists of 20 sessions. These

Treatment Goals: Stop problematic eating behaviors.

Goals of Skills Training: Learn and practice adaptive emotion regulation skills to replace maladaptive binge eating and other problem eating behaviors.

Treatment Targets:

1. Decrease life-interfering behaviors.*
2. Decrease behaviors that interfere with treatment.
3. Decrease quality-of-life-interfering behaviors.
    PATH TO MINDFUL EATING
    a. ED-specific examples include binge eating, purging, restrictive sating
    b. Eliminate mindless eating
    c. Decrease cravings, urges, preoccupation with food
    d. Decrease capitulating—that is, closing off options to not binge eat
    e. Decrease apparently irrelevant behaviors—for example, not weighing
4. Increase skillful emotion regulation behavior:
    mindfulness skills, emotion regulation skills; distress tolerance skills.

Following the Path to Mindful Eating will naturally lead to healthy weight regulation and an enhanced quality of life.

FIGURE 7.6. Goals of treatment, goals of skills training, and treatment targets. *In DBT for binge eating and bulimia, the Path-to-Mindful-Eating handout given to participants is focused on Targets 2 and 3 (e.g., 1. Decrease therapy-interfering behaviors; 2. Decrease binge eating; 3. Eliminate mindless eating; 4. Decrease cravings, urges, preoccupation with food, etc.). This is because the DBT for binge eating and bulimia model excludes participants with active Target 1 behaviors. However, though not explicitly delineated in DBT for binge eating and bulimia, decreasing any life-threatening behaviors takes precedence over the other targets (just as in standard DBT) if crises arise.

adaptations were made primarily for pragmatic purposes. For example, the other efficacious treatments for BED and BN against which DBT would be compared during the research trials, such as CBT and IPT, typically run no longer than 20 sessions. To add more sessions to the DBT treatment sequence or to increase the frequency of sessions was felt to make DBT a less competitive outpatient treatment option. In order to "fit" the content into 20 sessions, a decision was also made to reduce the number of modules taught to three, namely, core mindfulness, distress tolerance, and emotion regulation. This decision to remove interpersonal effectiveness was made primarily for research design purposes: to avoid criticism that the treatment was "powered" by this module, given that numerous studies have demonstrated that interpersonal therapy is efficacious (Wilfley et al., 1993; Wilfley et al., 2002). For clinicians and programs that are not limited by the constraints of time, resources, or research, there is no research-based reason not to add back the interpersonal effectiveness module—particularly given the data on IPT's efficacy with BED.

The covered modules, in sequence, are the mindfulness module (Sessions 3–5), emotion regulation module (Sessions 6–12), and distress tolerance module (Sessions 14–18). Sessions 1 and 2 are introductory (orientation to the treatment model and treatment targets, group rules and agreements, group commitment to stop binge eating), while Sessions 19 and 20 are devoted to review and relapse prevention. As described below, participation in group treatment is preceded by a pretreatment orientation visit.

Pretreatment Orientation Visit

An essential component of DBT for binge eating and bulimia is that every participant meets individually with one of the cotherapists (or, for BN, the individual therapist) for 30–45 minutes prior to beginning therapy. The major goals of this pretreatment visit involve orienting the participant to the DBT emotion regulation model of binge eating and the targets of treatment, describing the expectations of group members (e.g., regular timely attendance, listening to tapes of any missed sessions, completing homework assignments), and eliciting commitments from the client to stop binge eating and to address any treatment-interfering behaviors that may arise. Therapist and client agreements are reviewed and agreed upon during this visit. The list of client agreements and therapist agreements are listed in Figure 7.7.

The therapist conducts this session and obtains a commitment using the same strategies applied by the individual therapist in standard DBT. In addition to the standard DBT agreements (e.g., agreement to attend all sessions and do all homework, work with therapist on problems in the therapeutic relationship should they arise), a commitment is sought specifically to give up behaviors associated with their ED (e.g., binge eating).

Format of Skills Training Sessions

Like standard DBT, skills training groups are comprised of eight to ten members and are taught by two skills trainers: a leader and a coleader. The length of the group should be no less than 2 hours and no more than 2.5 hours (or 50 minutes, if skills training is conducted individually). The format is divided evenly into two halves, with a brief (5–10 minutes) break separating the two halves of the group (e.g., at least 2 hours) sessions. The first segment is devoted to homework review (skills strengthening) and includes discussion of client diary cards (see Figure 7.8), and chain analyses. The second half is devoted to teaching new content (skills acquisition) and practice of new skills. During the homework review, each group member will have between 5 and 10 minutes to report on her use of new skills in the past week and to describe specific successes or difficulties in applying the skills to replace the targeted problem eating behaviors. The length each member has varies based on the total length of group and the number in attendance so that sufficient time is available for everyone to share. Group members are encouraged to help one another identify solutions to problems encountered in using the skills and to "cheerlead" efforts made.

Therapeutic Pointers for Homework Review

It is important to assign group members the homework of filling out at least one chain analysis each week for at least the first 15 sessions. Even if they do not engage in binge eating, clients should use the chain to address another target behavior, either one targeted in the Path to Mindful Eating (see Figure 7.6, a–e) or to a problem behavior that is unique to them and associated with binge eating. If they have had absolutely no eating-related problem behaviors a particular week, they might describe a past binge or a non-eating-related problem behavior. The rationale for requiring that no less than one chain be conducted per week for the first 15 sessions is that clients must practice using the chain in order to understand it sufficiently to continue using it on their own once treatment ends. By Week 16, clients can begin to fill out chain analyses only as needed for any problem eating-related episodes.

Therapist's Treatment Agreements

1. I agree that I will keep confidential the information discussed, including the names of group members.
2. I agree not to form private relationships with other group members outside of group sessions.
3. I agree to arrive at group sessions on time.
4. I agree to attend group sessions each week and to stay for the entire 2 hour session.
5. I agree to inform the group if I will miss or be late for a session. If I miss a session I agree to listen to the audiotaped session.
6. I agree to practice the skills taught.
7. I agree to do my absolute best to deliver the best treatment that I can to help group members stop binge eating.

_____   _____
Therapist's signature   Date

Group Member's Treatment Agreements

1. I agree that I will keep confidential the information discussed during group sessions, including the names of other group members.
2. I agree not to form private relationships with other group members outside of the group sessions.
3. I agree to arrive at sessions on time.
4. I agree to attend sessions each week and to stay for the entire 2-hour session.
5. I agree to call ahead of time if I will miss or be late for a session. If I miss a session, I agree to come to the clinic to listen to the audiotaped session and to complete the skills practice and share this practice during the homework review.
6. I agree to practice the skills taught.
7. I agree to do my absolute best to stop binge eating and to help other group members to stop binge eating.
8. I agree to complete the homework assignments and bring them with me to each session.
9. I agree to complete the research questionnaires and interviews that are part of this treatment program.

_____   _____
Group Member's signature   Date

FIGURE 7.7. Therapist and client treatment agreements.

Because of the very limited time available, therapists encourage their clients to stay focused during the group. Clients are oriented to the importance of making maximal use of the allotted time by coming to sessions prepared to discuss their completed diary card, a chain analysis (including all relevant elements of the chain, especially where they might have intervened with a skillful alternative that would have eliminated the problem behavior), and specific skills homework sheets. This orientation is given briefly in Session 1, and in more detail in Session 2.

When discussing their chain analyses, group members are asked to focus on their highest order targets first, according to the Path to Mindful Eating (see Figure 7.6, a–e) treatment hierarchy (e.g., a binge episode rather than a mindless eating episode). Clients are asked to provide an overview of the chain, paying particular attention to the following elements:

- *Key location of the chain.* Where on the chain (i.e., a vulnerability factor, the prompting event, a particular link or series of links) could the client have the greatest probability of successfully intervening to avert the dysfunctional behavior?
- *Skill(s) identification.* What skill or skills could have been used (and will be used next time) to replace that dysfunctional link?

It is important to distinguish between "telling a story" and reporting from the chain. When storytelling occurs, the primary skills trainer should aid the client in focusing on the relevant elements. This can typically be done by asking the client to read directly from the chain analysis worksheet describing the links.

Occasionally, a group member will report not doing the homework or attempting it but having difficulty completing it or practicing her skills. Consistent with standard DBT, noncompletion of the homework is identified and addressed as therapy-interfering behavior. As in standard DBT, the skills trainer should behaviorally assess what interfered. For example, did the client hear what the homework was and remember the homework? Was the client unclear about some aspect of the skill that interfered with practice? Did emotions interfere with applying the skill, or did willfulness show up? Because the therapist's ability to treat the problem starts with understanding what the problem is, there is no substitution for this important first step.

Session 1: Obtaining the Group Commitment to Stop Binge Eating

A major task of Session 1 is to obtain a group commitment to stop binge eating. After initial introductions by each group member and the cotherapists, it is key that therapists create a groundswell of motivation and commitment from group members by flexibly utilizing the commitment strategies of standard DBT. Therapists might begin by using a devil's advocate strategy (Linehan, 1993a). In a somewhat puzzled and challenging manner, for example, they might say:

> "OK, we're assuming that you're all here because you want to gain control over your eating behavior. Specifically, we're assuming that you want to stop binge eating, right? We're also assuming that you want to enjoy your life—that is, you want a quality of life in which you enjoy your relationships, feel a sense of mastery, and feel good about yourself most of the time. And as we understand it, binge eating is a problem because it interferes with feeling good about yourself and having the quality

of life you desire. What isn't clear to us and what we'd like explained now is: Why can't you have a quality life *and* stay a binge eater? Why can't you do both? Explain that to us [Telch, 1997b]."

As Telch (1997b) further details, the point is for therapists to draw group members into arguing that it is imperative for them to stop binge eating in order to lead a quality life. Therapists must be sure to polarize the argument by describing the quality of life they believe the group members can attain as one that is deeply rewarding, one in which group members are fully alive and feel very *very* good about themselves—a seeming impossibility to many clients with BED. In other words, therapists must ensure that group members understand that by "quality of life" one is not referring to simply existing, getting through, or minimizing pain.

Therapists then use the group members' arguments as a starting point for eliciting the pros and cons of continuing life as a binge eater and list these on the board. Therapists might then assert:

> "OK, based on what we've just heard from you, there is absolutely no other choice than to stop binge eating. You've convinced us with your arguments. So let's face it and put this on the table before we get any further. Binge eating is over. Whenever you last binged, that was the last one. You simply can't have the kind of life you want to lead and continue binge eating and problem eating. So we're all in agreement, right? We're all committed, right [Telch, 1997b]?"

The intention is to obtain a verbal commitment from each group member. Some clients may fear committing because of worries that they will fail. The therapist might say:

> "Are you worried about binge eating in *this* moment or are you worried about the future? We're not talking about the future but about this one moment. Can you make a commitment to try your absolute hardest to never ever binge again in this one moment, right now [Telch, 1997b]?" [This is an example of Door in the Face.]

If a client insists "It's impossible" or that making a commitment would be a "set-up," the therapist might say:

> "Would it literally be impossible? I mean, it would likely be very, very difficult and scary—but are you saying that you think there is no way for you to physically survive unless you were binge eating?" [using a matter-of-fact tone, irreverence]

If the client concedes that it actually would be *possible*, the therapist can say:

> "So it sounds like you agree it might actually be possible to stop bingeing but you are very certain that you would fail in the attempt. Therefore it feels easier to tell yourself that stopping binge eating is more impossible than to try to stop. Because if you were to try your best but fail, you would have to feel awful about yourself not only for having binged but for failing in your attempt to stop. I can understand that kind of thinking [validation]. Yet we know from research on commitments that when people don't make a commitment or say they will accept less—when, right from the beginning they say there's no hope—the likelihood of success is very low [Telch, 1997b]."

Other tasks of Session 1, in addition to the group commitment to binge abstinence, is to orient group members to (1) the emotion regulation model of binge eating, (2) the treatment targets and group agreements, (3) the biosocial model including explanation of the invalidating environment (see adaptation of DBT's biosocial theory to EDs), and (4) the diary card (described below) and chain analysis.

Session 2: Explaining The Concept of Dialectical Abstinence

In session 2, therapists introduce clients to the concept of dialectical abstinence, a concept originally developed in DBT-SUD (Linehan & Dimeff, 1997) and discussed by McMain, Sayrs, Dimeff, and Linehan, Chapter 6, this volume).

Dialectical abstinence is a synthesis of a 100% commitment to abstinence and a 100% commitment to relapse management strategies. Before a client engages in problematic behaviors (e.g., binge eating), there is an unrelenting insistence on total abstinence. After a client has binged, however, the emphasis is on radical acceptance, nonjudgmental problem solving, and effective relapse prevention, followed by a quick return to the unrelenting insistence on abstinence (Linehan et al., 1999).

Therapists might introduce this concept with an explanation that a "dialectical view" recognizes that for every force or position there exists an opposing force or position: a thesis and an antithesis, yin and yang. A dialectical view searches for a synthesis that is more than the sum of the opposite parts. For example, the yin and yang symbol is black and white, yet the synthesis of these is not merely the color gray. A synthesis transcends both (modeling dialectical thinking).

This leads to discussion of a problem as well as its solution. On the one hand, group members have all made a 100% commitment to binge abstinence. Anything short of that would be failure. When faced with the urge to binge, one cannot have the idea that it is "OK" to binge and fail and to "just try again." Such thinking is undermining and will make it more likely one will decide to binge eat. On the opposite side, it is clear that in not anticipating and preparing for a slip clients will be less likely to handle such an event effectively, should it occur. This is the problem that therapists and group members are faced with and which is presented for discussion: How can one deal with these two opposing forces of success and failure?

Telch's metaphor of the Olympics becomes quite useful at this point (Telch, 1997b). The therapists suggest that group members are like Olympic athletes and the therapists like coaches. Clients are participating in an incredibly important event, improving their lives by stopping binge eating. It takes tremendous effort. Absolutely nothing is discussed before a race in the Olympics except winning, or "going for the gold." An Olympian cannot think "maybe a bronze would be OK" or consider what might happen if she falls down. Similarly, the only thing group members can possibly allow themselves to think about and discuss is absolute and total binge abstinence. Yet of course athletes and group members must be prepared for the possibility of failure. The key is to be prepared to fail well. The dialectical dilemma is that both success and failure exist. The dialectical abstinence solution involves 100% certainty that binge eating is out of the question and 100% confidence that one will never binge again. However, simultaneously, one keeps in mind ("Way, way back in the very farthest part so that it never interferes with your resolve") that if one slips, one will deal with it effectively by accepting it nonjudgmentally and picking oneself back up, knowing one will never slip again.

Unlike the DBT–SUD model, the DBT for binge eating and bulimia model does not include the "touchdown every time" concept (e.g., the understanding that clients only are making the commitment for as long as they know with absolute certainty that they can keep it). The commitment is discussed as a powerful skill in and of itself, even if the client is uncertain about her ability to keep it.

Sessions 3–5: Mindfulness Skills

The mindfulness skills are introduced in these three sessions and reviewed in session 12. These skills are the same as in standard DBT (e.g., Wise Mind, the "what" skills, the "how" skills) except for three: mindful eating, urge surfing, and alternate rebellion. Urge surfing and alternate rebellion were borrowed from DBT–SUD (Linehan & Dimeff, 1997), with urge surfing first described by Marlatt and Gordon (1985) in their relapse prevention treatment for substance abuse. These three, mentioned in earlier program descriptions, are discussed in more depth below.

Homework assignments for these consist of a definition of the skill along with space for the client to report on her experience practicing it.

Mindful Eating. Mindful eating, as opposed to mindless eating, is the experience of full participation in eating. It is eating with full awareness and attention (one-mindfully) but without self-consciousness or judgment. When the mindfulness "what" skills of observe, describe, and participate are applied to eating, this is labeled mindful eating.

Urge Surfing. Urge surfing involves mindful, nonattached observing of urges to binge or eat mindlessly. Mindfulness skills teach one to accept the reality that there are cues in the world that will trigger the urge to binge eat. Clients are educated about how urges and cravings are classically conditioned responses that have been associated with a particular cue. Mindful urge surfing involves awareness without engaging in impulsive mood-dependent behavior. One simply notices and then describes the ebb and flow of the urge. One is "letting go" or "detaching" from the object of the urge, being fully in the moment "riding the wave" of the urge. Though bearing similarities to mindfulness of the current emotion, urge surfing is a mindfulness skill that involves nonjudgmental observing and describing of urges, cravings, and food preoccupation.

Alternate Rebellion. This mindfulness skill involves using the "how" mindfulness skill of *effectively* to satisfy a wish to rebel without destroying one's overriding objective of stopping binge eating. The purpose is not to suppress or judge the rebellion but to find creative ways to rebel that do not involve "cutting off your nose to spite your face." Many clients with BED have described the desire to "get back" at society, friends, and/or family whom they perceive to be judgmental about their weight. For these clients, "getting back" can involve rebelling by consuming even more food, but in the process compromise achieving their own goals. Alternate rebellion involves finding effective ways to rebel in a fashion that does not compromise their long-term goals. One can encourage clients to observe the need to rebel, label it as such, and then, if they decide to act on the wish, to do so effectively. Group members can be creative in thinking up alternate rebellion strategies. For example, a client who feels judged by society for being obese might "rebel" by buying and wearing lacy lingerie.

Sessions 6–12: Emotion Regulation

These sessions cover the emotion regulation skills taught in standard DBT, without any specific adaptations for BED except as involves the focus on the problem eating treatment hierarchy. These skills involve observing and describing emotions, learning about the function of emotions, decreasing vulnerability to emotion mind, increasing positive events, and acting opposite to the current emotion.

Sessions 13–18: Distress Tolerance Skills

These sessions cover the distress tolerance skills of standard DBT. As described, one skill has been added: Burning Bridges. Like many of the other skills adapted for BED, it was borrowed from DBT–SUD (Linehan & Dimeff, 1997).

Burning Bridges. This skill involves accepting at the deepest and most radical level the idea that one is really not going to binge eat, or eat mindlessly, or abuse oneself with food ever again—thus, burning the bridge to those behaviors. One accepts that one will no longer block, deny, or avoid reality with binge eating. Instead, one makes a covenant from deep within to accept reality and one's experiences.

Sessions 19–20: Relapse Prevention

Session 19 begins with a review of mindfulness, emotion regulation, and distress tolerance. In addition, clients are asked to fill out a worksheet for Session 20 on which the following is asked:

1. Detail your specific plans for continuing to practice the skills taught.
2. Outline your specific plans for skillfully managing emotions in the future. Think of circumstances and emotions that previously set off binge eating. Outline your plans for dealing with the emotions that will prevent any problem eating behaviors. Write about at least three different emotions.
3. Write about what you need to do next in your life to continue building a satisfying and rewarding quality of life for yourself

Session 20 includes each group member reviewing their worksheet as well as final good-byes. Like standard DBT, many groups come up with rituals to mark the ending of treatment.

DBT Consultation Team

Therapists meet weekly with the treatment team to confer regarding the progress of treatment and adherence to DBT principles. However, these consultation teams lack the exchange between individual and skills therapist because, unlike standard DBT, clients are only treated in a group context. Because the DBT for binge eating and bulimia model was researched at a site where members of the treatment team were all highly familiar with eating disorders but not all were familiar with DBT (the opposite of the University of Washington consultation team experience), it was often useful to have an expert DBT therapist who was not identified as an eating disorder specialist as a member of the treatment team. Currently, the Stanford therapy consultation team includes the two co-therapists, the principal investigator of the research study, an expert DBT therapist, a senior psychiatrist with expertise in clinical trials, and a psychiatrist who specializes in eating disorders.

Telephone Consultation

Although clients are encouraged to call therapists if they have questions during the week (e.g., for clarification of a particular skill, for dealing with uncertainty of how to apply a skill in a particular situation), telephone coaching and/or paging as practiced by individual therapists in standard DBT is not used in DBT for binge eating and bulimia. Skills generalization is addressed during the first hour of the group treatment (with the focus on the diary cards and chain analyses) as well as with written feedback given by therapists on weekly homework. As with other components of DBT for binge eating and bulimia, this decision to not implement standard DBT telephone skills coaching was made for research purposes so that the treatment would be comparable to other short-term (e.g., 20-week) outpatient therapies for this population in terms of clinician time demands. Standard DBT telephone coaching might well be indicated in other settings.

Use of Irreverence with Stage 3 Clients with EDs

There are various issues around which clients and therapists become polarized. These are examples of such situations and of ways in which to address these problems using irreverence.

> CLIENT: My Wise Mind told me to binge.
>
> THERAPIST: (*laughing good-naturedly*) Come on! Wise Mind would never say that—you must have gotten Wise Mind confused with some other character! [irreverent reframe, confronting]
> *or*
> Bzzz. Wrong answer! Try again! [irreverent reframe, confronting]
>
> CLIENT: Nothing has changed. This isn't working. [Note: client has not been practicing skills.]
>
> THERAPIST: (*gently teasing tone*) What a mystery! I can't imagine why everything isn't totally different for you, since you're doing everything exactly the same! [irreverence]
>
> CLIENT: I couldn't keep practicing the skills because they were taking too much time.
>
> THERAPIST: (*with a humorous tone*) Ah—I get it. Practicing the skills took up too much time . . . but you *were* able to fit in time for a binge. [irreverent, confronting]
> *or*
> If you had time to binge, you had time to practice the skills. [speaking directly and to the point]
>
> CLIENT: The skills just aren't strong enough to help me stop binge eating!
>
> THERAPIST: Oh, I've certainly heard that one before. You're going to have to come up with something way more original and creative than that if you want to demoralize me! [irreverent reframe]

Diary Card and Chain Analyses

DBT strategies are used per the treatment manual (Linehan, 1993a) without modification with the exception of the diary cards (see Figures 7.8 and 7.9) and the modification to the target hierarchy with the Path to Mindful Eating (see Figure 7.6, a–e). In other words, the

Instructions for Completing Your Diary Card

Completing your diary card on a daily basis is an essential component of your treatment. "Mindful" completion of the diary card (i.e., paying attention *without* judging) increases awareness of what is going on for you. Therefore, completing the diary card is a skillful behavior. You will derive the greatest benefit if you complete the diary card on a daily basis. We suggest that you complete it at the end of each day, but if another time is more convenient for you, that is fine. Here's how you complete the card:

Initials: Write in your initials.

ID#: Do not write in this space. We will complete this.

How Often Did You Fill Out This Side?: Place a check mark to indicate how frequently you filled in the diary card during the past week.

Day and Date: Write in the calendar date (month/day/year) under each day of the week.

Urge to Binge: Refer to the legend and choose the number from the scale (0–6) that best represents your highest rating for the day. The key characteristics of the urge to consider when making your rating are intensity (how strongly you felt the urge) and duration (how long the urge lasted).

Binge Episodes: Write the number of binge episodes you had each day. A "binge" refers to an eating episode in which you felt a loss of control during the eating.

Mindless Eating: Write in the number of "mindless" eating episodes that you had each day. "Mindless eating" refers to not paying attention to what you are eating, although you do not feel the sense of loss of control that you do during binge episodes. A typical example of mindless eating would be sitting in front of the TV and eating a bag of microwave popcorn without any awareness of the eating (i.e., somehow the popcorn was gone and you were only vaguely aware of having eaten it). Again, however, you didn't feel a sense of being out of control during the eating.

Apparently Irrelevant Behaviors (AIBs) : Circle either "Yes" or "No" depending on whether you did or did not have any AIBs that day. If you did, briefly describe the AIB in the place provided or on another sheet of paper. An "AIB" refers to behaviors that, upon first glance, do not seem relevant to binge eating and purging but which actually are important in the behavior chain leading to these behaviors. You may convince yourself that the behavior doesn't matter or really won't affect your goal to stop bingeing and purging when, in fact, the behavior matters a great deal. A typical AIB might be buying several boxes of your favorite Girl Scout cookies because you wanted to help out a neighbor's daughter (of course, you could buy the cookies and donate them to the neighbor).

Capitulating: Refer to the legend and choose the number from the scale (0–6) that best represents your highest rating for the day. The key characteristics to consider when making your rating are intensity (strength of the capitulating) and duration (how long it lasted). "Capitulating" refers to giving up on your goals to stop binge eating and to skillfully cope with emotions. Instead, you capitulate or surrender to bingeing, acting as if there is no other option or way to cope than with food.

Food Preoccupation: Refer to the legend and choose the number from the scale (0–6) that best represents your highest rating for the day. "Food preoccupation" refers to your thoughts or attention being absorbed or focused on food. For example, your thoughts about a upcoming dinner party and the presence of your favorite foods may absorb your attention so much that you have trouble concentrating at work.

Emotion Columns: Refer to the legend and choose the number from the scale (0–6) that best represents your highest rating for the day. The key characteristics to consider when making your rating are intensity (strength of the emotion) and duration (how long it lasted).

(continued)

FIGURE 7.8. Stanford University instructions for filling out diary card.

Used Skills: Refer to the legend and choose the number from the scale (0–6) that best represents your attempts to use the skills each day. When making your rating, consider whether or not you thought about using any of the skills that day, whether or not you actually used any of the skills, and whether or not the skills helped.

Weight: Weigh yourself once each week and record your weight in pounds in the space provided. Please write in the date you weighed. It is best if you choose the same day each week to weigh. Many women find that arriving a few minutes early to the session and weighing at the clinic is a good way to remember to weigh.

Urge to Quit Therapy: Indicate your urge to quit therapy before the session and after the session each week. Both of these ratings should be made for the same session as the one in which you received the diary card. It is best to make both of these ratings as soon as possible following that day's session. Use a 0–6 scale of intensity of the urge, with 0 indicating no urge to quit and a 6 indicating the strongest urge to quit.

Completing the Skills Side of the Diary Card:

How Often Did You Fill Out This Side? Place a check mark to indicate how frequently you filled out the skills side of the diary card during the week.

Skills Practice: Go down the column for each day of the week and circle each skill that you practiced/used that day. If you did not practice or use any of the skills that particular day, then circle that day on the last line, which states, "Did not practice/use any skills."

FIGURE 7.8. *(continued)*

chain analyses are those used in standard DBT (Linehan, 1993a) with maladaptive eating behavior (e.g., binge eating, mindless eating) as the targeted problem behavior for these Stage 3 clients.

Summary

This chapter presents three models of DBT as adapted for the treatment of eating disorders. Each model was developed independently and was influenced by its target client population and treatment setting. Comprehensive DBT for BPD and ED, for example, was specifically developed for clients with EDs and comorbid BPD. An advantage of this model is its appropriateness for clients who are suicidal and/or engaging in self-harm and/ or engaging in substance abuse in conjunction with their ED. This program requires a setting with a suitable infrastructure that can provide standard DBT components such as group and individual DBT, a consultation team for therapists, and a 24-hour on-call system. The model of DBT for serious, complex, and treatment-resistant EDs, which utilizes the intensive outpatient and partial hospital settings, has the advantage of being designed to treat all the ED diagnoses (AN, BN, BED, and EDNOS) as well as clients with psychiatric and medical comorbidity. This model uses a DBT framework (with some alterations) as well as components of standard CBT. This affords the DBT for serious, complex, and treatment-resistant EDs model with the advantage of building upon and enhancing a therapeutic model, CBT, that is already well validated for the treatment of EDs. The last model presented, DBT for binge eating and bulimia, was specifically designed for clients with BED and BN in an outpatient clinic setting. Elements of standard DBT, such as weekly individual sessions and weekly skills training groups, were combined into a single format (e.g., 20 sessions of 2-hour weekly group therapy for BED). DBT for binge eating and bulimia has the advantage of having the most empirical

Diary Card Initials _____ ID # _____

How often did you fill out this side?
___ Daily ___ 4–6× ___ 2–3× ___ Once

Day and Date	Urge[1] to binge (0–6)	Binge episodes # OBE lg	Binge episodes # SBE sm	Mindless eating # episodes	AIB[2] Circle one	Capitulating[1] (0–6)	Food[1] craving (0–6)	Food[1] preoccupation (0–6)	Anger[1] (0–6)	Sadness[1] (0–6)	Fear[1] (0–6)	Shame[1] (0–6)	Pride[1] (0–6)	Happiness[1] (0–6)	Used[3] (0–7)
Mon					yes / no										
Tues					yes / no										
Wed					yes / no										
Thurs					yes / no										
Fri					yes / no										
Sat					yes / no										
Sun					yes / no										

[1] Use the following scale to indicate the highest rating for the day:

0 = urge/thought/feeling not experienced

1 = urge/thought/feeling experienced slightly and briefly

2 = urge/thought/feeling experienced moderately and briefly

3 = urge/thought/feeling experienced intensely and briefly

4 = urge/thought/feeling experienced slightly and endured

5 = urge/thought/feeling experienced moderately and endured

6 = urge/thought/feeling experienced intensely and endured

[2] Describe Apparently Irrelevant Behaviors (AIBs): _____

[3] USED SKILLS:

0 = Not thought about or used

1 = Thought about, not used, didn't want to

2 = Thought about, not used, wanted to

3 = Tried but couldn't use them

4 = Tried, could do them, but they didn't help

5 = Tried, could use them, helped

6 = Didn't try, used them, didn't help

7 = Didn't try, used them, helped

Weight _____ Date Weighed _____

Urge to quit therapy (0–5): Before therapy session: ___ After therapy session: ___

NIMH 1997–2000
ER BED TELCH

(continued)

FIGURE 7.9. Stanford University diary card and skills diary card.

SKILLS DIARY CARD	Instructions: Circle the days you worked on each skill.							How often did you fill out this side? Daily ___ 4–6x ___ 2–3x ___ Once ___
1. Diaphragmatic breathing	Mon	Tues	Wed	Thurs	Fri	Sat	Sun	
2. Wise Mind	Mon	Tues	Wed	Thurs	Fri	Sat	Sun	
3. Observe: just notice	Mon	Tues	Wed	Thurs	Fri	Sat	Sun	
4. Describe: put words on	Mon	Tues	Wed	Thurs	Fri	Sat	Sun	
5. Participate: enter into the experience	Mon	Tues	Wed	Thurs	Fri	Sat	Sun	
6. Mindful eating	Mon	Tues	Wed	Thurs	Fri	Sat	Sun	
7. Nonjudgmental stance	Mon	Tues	Wed	Thurs	Fri	Sat	Sun	
8. One-mindfully: in-the-moment	Mon	Tues	Wed	Thurs	Fri	Sat	Sun	
9. Effectiveness: focus on what works	Mon	Tues	Wed	Thurs	Fri	Sat	Sun	
10. Urge surfing	Mon	Tues	Wed	Thurs	Fri	Sat	Sun	
11. Alternate rebellion	Mon	Tues	Wed	Thurs	Fri	Sat	Sun	
12. Mindful of current emotion	Mon	Tues	Wed	Thurs	Fri	Sat	Sun	
13. Loving your emotions	Mon	Tues	Wed	Thurs	Fri	Sat	Sun	
14. Reduce vulnerability: PLEASE	Mon	Tues	Wed	Thurs	Fri	Sat	Sun	
15. Build MASTERy	Mon	Tues	Wed	Thurs	Fri	Sat	Sun	
16. Build positive experiences	Mon	Tues	Wed	Thurs	Fri	Sat	Sun	
17. Mindful of positive experiences	Mon	Tues	Wed	Thurs	Fri	Sat	Sun	
18. Opposite-to-emotion action	Mon	Tues	Wed	Thurs	Fri	Sat	Sun	
19. Observing your breath	Mon	Tues	Wed	Thurs	Fri	Sat	Sun	
20. Half-smiling	Mon	Tues	Wed	Thurs	Fri	Sat	Sun	
21. Awareness exercises	Mon	Tues	Wed	Thurs	Fri	Sat	Sun	
22. Radical acceptance	Mon	Tues	Wed	Thurs	Fri	Sat	Sun	
23. Turning the mind	Mon	Tues	Wed	Thurs	Fri	Sat	Sun	
24. Willingness	Mon	Tues	Wed	Thurs	Fri	Sat	Sun	
25. Burning your bridges	Mon	Tues	Wed	Thurs	Fri	Sat	Sun	
26. Distract	Mon	Tues	Wed	Thurs	Fri	Sat	Sun	
27. Self-soothe	Mon	Tues	Wed	Thurs	Fri	Sat	Sun	
28. Improve the moment	Mon	Tues	Wed	Thurs	Fri	Sat	Sun	
29. Pros and cons	Mon	Tues	Wed	Thurs	Fri	Sat	Sun	
30. Commitment	Mon	Tues	Wed	Thurs	Fri	Sat	Sun	
30. Did not practice any skills	Mon	Tues	Wed	Thurs	Fri	Sat	Sun	

FIGURE 7.9. (continued)

support at present. By using the information provided in this chapter as a foundation, readers should gain greater clarity in implementing ED-specific adaptations suitable for other treatment settings and target client populations.

REFERENCES

American Psychiatric Association. (1994). *Diagnostic and statistical manual of mental disorders* (4th ed.). Washington, DC: Author.

American Psychiatric Association. (2000). *Practice guidelines for the treatment of patients with eating disorders.* Washington, DC: Author.

Brownell, K. D., & Fairburn, C. G. (Eds.). (2002). *Eating disorders and obesity: A comprehensive handbook* (2nd ed.). New York: Guilford Press.

Chen, E. Y., & Linehan, M. M. (in press). DBT and eating disorders. In A. Freeman (Ed.), *Encyclopedia of CBT.*

Chen, E., O'Connor, & Linehan, M. M. (2004, November). *Dialectical behavior therapy and cognitive-behavioral therapy for borderline personality disorders and eating disorders.* Paper presented at the meeting of the Eating Disorders Research Society, Amsterdam.

Dulit, R. A., Fyer, M. R., Leon, A. C., Brodsky, B. S., & Frances, A. J. (1994). Clinical correlates of self-mutilation in borderline personality disorder. *American Journal of Psychiatry, 151,* 1305–1311.

Fairburn, C. G. (1997). Interpersonal psychotherapy for bulimia nervosa. In D. M. Garner & P. E. Garfinkel (Eds.), *Handbook of treatment for eating disorders* (pp. 278–294). New York: Guilford Press.

Fairburn, C. G., Doll, H. A., Welch, S. L., Hay, P. J., Davies, B. A., & O'Connor, M. E. (1998). Risk factors for binge eating disorder: A community-based, case–control study. *Archives of General Psychiatry, 55,* 425–432.

Fairburn, C. G., & Harrison, P. J. (2003). Eating disorders. *Lancet, 361*(9355), 407–416.

Fairburn, C. G., Marcus, M. D., & Wilson, G. T. (1993). Cognitive-behavioral therapy for binge eating and bulimia nervosa: A comprehensive treatment manual. In C. G. Fairburn & G. T. Wilson (Eds.), *Binge-eating: Nature, assessment and treatment* (pp. 361–405). New York: Guilford Press.

Garner, D. M., & Garfinkel, P. E. (Eds.). (1997). *Handbook of treatment for eating disorders.* New York: Guilford Press.

Greeno, C. G., Wing, R. R., & Shiffman, S. (2000). Binge antecedents in obese women with and without binge eating disorder. *Journal of Consulting and Clinical Psychology, 68,* 95–102.

Grilo, C. M., Masheb, R. M., & Berman, R. M. (2001). Subtyping women with bulimia nervosa along dietary and negative affect dimensions: A replication in a treatment-seeking sample. *Eating and Weight Disorders, 6,* 53–58.

Hayaki, J., Friedman, M. A., Whisman, M. A., Delinsky, S. S., & Brownell, K. D. (2003). Sociotropy and bulimic symptoms in clinical and nonclinical samples. *International Journal of Eating Disorders, 34,* 172–176.

Heatherton, T. F., & Baumeister, R. F. (1991). Binge eating as escape from self-awareness. *Psychological Bulletin, 110*(1), 86–108.

Herzog, D. B., Greenwood, D. N., Dorer, D. J., Flores, A. T., Ekeblad, E. R., Richards, A., et al. (2000). Mortality in eating disorders: A descriptive study. *International Journal of Eating Disorders, 28,* 20–26.

Herzog, D. B., Keller, M. B., Sacks, N. R., Yeh, C. J., & Lavori, P. W. (1992). Psychiatric comorbidity in treatment-seeking anorexics and bulimics. *Journal of the American Academy of Child and Adolescent Psychiatry, 31,* 810–818.

Kabat-Zinn, J. (1990). *Full-catastrophe living.* New York: Delta.

Keel, P. K., Dorer, D. J., Eddy, K. T., Franko, D., Charatan, D. L., & Herzog, D. B. (2003). Predictors of mortality in eating disorders. *Archives of General Psychiatry, 60,* 179–183.

Lieb, K., Zanarini, M. C., Schmahl, C., Linehan, M. M., & Bohus, M. (2004). Borderline personality disorder. *Lancet, 364*(9432), 453–461.

Linehan, M. M. (1993a). *Cognitive-behavioral treatment of borderline personality disorder.* New York: Guilford Press.

Linehan, M. M. (l993b). *Skills training manual for treating borderline personality disorder.* New York: Guilford Press.

Linehan, M. M., Comtois, K. A., Brown, M., Reynold, S., Welch, S., Sayrs, J. H. R., et al. (2002, November). DBT versus nonbehavioral treatment-by-experts in the community: Clinical outcomes. In S. Reynolds (Chair), *The University of Washington Treatment Study of Borderline Personality Disorder: DBT vs. non behavioral treatments by experts in the community.* Symposium conducted at the 36th annual association for Advancement of Behavior Therapy Convention, Reno, NV.

Linehan, M. M., & Dimeff, L. A. (1997). *Dialectical behavior therapy manual of treatment interventions for drug abusers with borderline personality disorder.* Seattle: University of Washington.

Linehan, M. M., Schmidt, H., Dimeff, L. A., Craft, C. C., Kanter, J., & Comtois, K. A. (1999). Dialectical behavior therapy for patients with borderline personality disorder and drug-dependence. *American Journal on Addictions, 8,* 279–292.

Marlatt, G. A., & Gordon, J. R. (1985). *Relapse prevention and maintenance strategies in the treatment of addictive behaviours.* New York: Guilford Press.

McCabe, E. B., La Via, M. C., & Marcus, M. D. (2004). Dialectical behavior therapy for eating disorders. In J. K. Thompson (Ed.), *Handbook of eating disorders and obesity.* New York: Wiley.

Pike, K. M., & Rodin, J. (1991). Mothers, daughters, and disordered eating. *Journal of Abnormal Psychology, 100,* 198–204.

Rizvi, S. L., & Linehan, M. M. (2005). *Treatment of shame in borderline personality disorder: A pilot study.* Manuscript submitted for review.

Safer, D. L., Telch, C. F., & Agras W. S. (2001a). Dialectical behavior therapy for bulimia nervosa: A case study. *International Journal of Eating Disorders, 30,* 101–106.

Safer, D. L., Telch, C. F., & Agras, W. S. (2001b). Dialectical behavior therapy for bulimia nervosa. *American Journal of Psychiatry, 158,* 632–634.

Sanftner, J. L., & Crowther, J. H. (1998). Variability in self-esteem, moods, shame, and guilt in women who binge. *International Journal of Eating Disorders, 23*(4), 391–397.

Steinhausen, H. C. (2002). The outcome of anorexia nervosa in the 20th century. *American Journal of Psychiatry, 159,* 1284–1293.

Stice, E., & Agras, W. S. (1999). Subtyping bulimic women along dietary restraint and negative affect dimensions. *Journal of Consulting and Clinical Psychology, 67,* 460–469.

Stice, E., Agras, W. S., Telch, C. F., Halmi, K. A., Mitchell, J. E., & Wilson, T. (2001). Subtyping binge-eating disordered women along dieting and negative affect dimensions. *International Journal of Eating Disorders, 30,* 11–27.

Striegel-Moore, R. H., Dohm, F., Pike, K. M., Wilfley, D. E., & Fairburn, C.G. (2002). Abuse, bullying, and discrimination as risk factors for binge eating disorder. *American Journal of Psychiatry, 159*(11), 1902–1907.

Telch, C. F. (1997a). Skills training treatment for adaptive affect regulation in a woman with binge-eating disorder. *International Journal of Eating Disorders, 22,* 77–81.

Telch, C. F. (1997b). *Emotion regulation skills training treatment for binge eating disorder: Therapist manual.* Unpublished manuscript.

Telch, C. F., Agras, W. S., & Linehan, M. M. (2000). Group dialectical behavior therapy for binge-eating disorder: A preliminary, uncontrolled trial. *Behavior Therapy, 31,* 569–582.

Telch, C. F., Agras, W. S., & Linehan, M. M. (2001). Dialectical behavior therapy for binge eating disorder. *Journal of Consulting and Clinical Psychology, 69,* 1061–1065.

Wadden, T. A., Brownell, K. D., Foster, G. D. (2002). Obesity: Responding to the global epidemic. *Journal of Consulting and Clinical Psychology, 70*(3), 510–525.

Waller, G. (2003). The psychological factors in a functional analysis of binge eating. In C. G. Fairburn & K. D. Brownell (Eds.), *Eating disorders and obesity: A comprehensive handbook* (2nd ed.). New York: Guilford Press.

Wilfley, D. E., Agras, W. S., Telch, C. F., Rossiter, E. M., Schneider, J. A., Cole, A. G., et al. (1993). Group cognitive-behavioral therapy and group interpersonal psychotherapy for the non-purging bulimic individual: A controlled comparison. *Journal of Consulting and Clinical Psychology, 61*, 296–305.

Wilfley, D. E., & Cohen, L. R. (1997). Psychological treatment of bulimia nervosa and binge eating disorder. *Psychopharmacology Bulletin, 33*, 437–454.

Wilfley, D. E., Friedman, M. A., Dounchis, J. Z., Stein, R. I., Welch, R. R., & Ball, S. A. (2000). Comorbid psychopathology in binge eating disorder: Relation to eating disorder severity at baseline and following treatment. *Journal of Consulting and Clinical Psychology, 68*(4), 641–649.

Wilfley, D. E., Welch, R. R., Stein, R. I., Spurrell, E. B., Cohen, L. R., Saelens, B. E., et al. (2002). A randomized comparison of group cognitive-behavioral therapy and group interpersonal therapy for the treatment of overweight individuals with binge eating disorder. *Archives of General Psychiatry, 59*, 713–721.

Wilson, G. T., Fairburn, C. G., & Agras, W. S. (1997). Cognitive-behavioral therapy for bulimia nervosa. In D. M. Garner & P. E. Garfinkel (Eds.), *Handbook of treatment for eating disorders* (pp. 67–93). New York: Guilford Press.

Wiser, S., & Telch, C. F. (1999). Dialectical behavior therapy for binge eating disorder. *Journal of Clinical Psychology, 55*, 755–768.

Wisniewski, L., & Ben-Porath, D. (2005). Telephone skill-coaching with eating disordered clients: Clinical guidelines using a DBT framework. *European Eating Disorder Review, 13*, 344–350.

Wisniewski, L., Epstein, L. H., Marcus, M. D., & Kaye, W. (1997). Differences in salivary habituation to palatable foods in bulimia nervosa patients and controls. *Psychosomatic Medicine, 4*, 427–433.

Wisniewski, L., & Kelly, E. (2003). The application of dialectical behavior therapy to the treatment of eating disorders. *Cognitive and Behavioral Practice, 10*, 131–138.

World Health Organization. (1998). *International classification of diseases, 10th revision, clinical modification*. Geneva, Switzerland: Author.

CHAPTER 8

Dialectical Behavior Therapy with Families

Alan E. Fruzzetti, Daniel A. Santisteban, *and* Perry D. Hoffman

Dialectical behavior therapy (DBT; Linehan, 1993a) is founded on a transactional or biosocial model of borderline personality disorder (BPD) and related disorders that maintains a dialectical position: severe psychopathology is the result of an emotionally vulnerable person transacting with others in an invalidating environment. However, most targets and strategies employed in DBT are designed to help individuals regulate their own emotions. Direct intervention in the family and social environment is not highly emphasized. Yet there are several reasons to consider using family interventions to complement individual ones in DBT:

1. There is a substantial literature supporting the efficacy of augmenting individual treatments for severe psychopathology with family interventions (cf. Fruzzetti, 1996; Fruzzetti & Boulanger, 2005).
2. Theoretically, the transactional or biosocial model maintains a central role for the social and family environments in the development, maintenance, relapse, and/or remediation of problems associated with severe and chronic emotion dysregulation (Fruzzetti & Fruzzetti, 2003; Fruzzetti, Shenk, & Hoffman, 2005).
3. Data suggest that family DBT outcomes are quite promising (e.g., Fruzzetti, 2006; Fruzzetti & Mosco, 2006; Hoffman et al., 2005), as are other family interventions when used to augment individual DBT (e.g., Santisteban, Coatsworth, et al., 2003).

Comprehensive DBT, of course, includes five functions (Linehan, 1993a): (1) client skill acquisition, (2) skill generalization, (3) enhancement of client motivation, (4) skill and motivation enhancement of therapists, and (5) structuring the environment to promote (or, at least, not to interfere with) client progress. Many family interventions typically include skill acquisition (in both individual and family DBT skills). Practicing skills in a family context provides opportunities for generalization. Family interventions that address problematic behaviors of family members or problematic family interactions (antecedents or consequences) that contribute to patient target behaviors therefore also address patient motivation. And, of course, intervening with families necessarily involves "environmental intervention." Thus, family interventions are efficient, and ideally are a highly integrated part of DBT.

Although the role of the family is highlighted in most models of the development of BPD (cf. Fruzzetti et al., 2005), very little prospective research has been conducted on the families of people with BPD. Family members are often blamed, criticized, and maligned for their putative role in the development of BPD, and people with BPD are frequently blamed for the difficulties and burden that their families experience. Interventions will be most useful when all parties (e.g., patients, family members, professionals) eliminate or at least significantly minimize blaming behaviors.

For our purposes, we will assume that families with a member with BPD (or significant BPD features) are heterogeneous. In our clinics, we have found many family members to be competent, caring, loving, devoted, and willing to work very hard to do anything that might help their child or partner with BPD. We also have found many family members who are quite distressed themselves, often needing treatment, and/or blaming the patient identified with BPD for a host of individual and family difficulties. Because we are adapting and extending DBT, we find it useful not to blame anyone. The transactional model that is the foundation of DBT (Fruzzetti et al., 2005; Linehan, 1993a) tells us that it does not really matter whether the family member with BPD started out with an extreme temperament or was quite normative, or whether the family was disengaged or abusive early on or loving and caring. Consistent with other applications of DBT, a nonpejorative way to understand families is essential to being effective when trying to engage family members and facilitate important changes in the family.

This chapter addresses a number of issues and problems relevant to family interventions associated with the delivery of DBT for adults and adolescents. We (1) discuss program issues germane to family participation in treatment; (2) describe family DBT skills to complement individual DBT skills; (3) describe multifamily skill groups; (4) summarize the use of individual and family DBT skills in the Family Connections program (groups for family members, led by family members); (5) explicate the steps involved in doing brief family interventions to augment outcomes in individual DBT; and (6) give an example of how to utilize non-DBT family therapy in the service of good outcomes for DBT patients (or, integrating traditional family therapy into DBT), particularly for adolescent substance abusers with BPD features. Relevant data in support of these family interventions is highlighted throughout our discussion.

Program Issues in Family Interventions in DBT

A number of issues are important to consider when offering family interventions. This section includes discussions about which therapist should work with a family, what modes of family intervention might be offered, how to structure groups (e.g., homogeneity vs. heterogeneity), and how to facilitate participation among family members.

Who Should Be the Family Therapist?

DBT programs have several alternative ways to provide or facilitate the delivery of family interventions: (1) individual therapists can also provide family interventions for their own clients and their families (i.e., same DBT therapist for both patient and family); (2) therapists can treat families of clients who are seen individually by other DBT therapists in the program (different therapist for patient and family, but both are on the DBT consultation team); (3) the DBT program can develop a separate family DBT team with its own consultation group, who provide family interventions for the program; or (4) the program can refer family work to "DBT-friendly" family therapists.

There are pros and cons to each of these arrangements. For example, treatment situations in which the individual DBT therapist also provides family interventions allow the therapist to be very aware of the patient's patterns, his or her "chains" (factors that are related to treatment target behaviors such as self-injurious behavior, aggression, and substance use). However, having the therapist do double duty as both individual and family therapist could make it difficult for him or her to remain neutral, and for other family members to perceive him or her that way. The perception of a biased alliance with the patient could reduce family members' motivation to participate fully in family interventions.

In contrast, utilizing another therapist to provide family interventions may help to establish an alliance with the whole family, but this other therapist may be less sensitized to the details and patterns of the patient and the patient may perceive him or her as siding with other members of the family. With both of these options it is important to consider that some teams do not have members with substantial family therapy training.

Although having an entire DBT team dedicated solely to family treatment (with concomitant family therapy training and experience) would provide wonderful treatment options and expertise, this option requires a significant investment of time and resources. For example, family therapists would need at least some minimal training to work within the DBT model.

Finally, referring families out to community family therapists is relatively easy and requires no resources on the part of the program, but in many communities few family therapists are well acquainted with DBT or the myriad problems of BPD, and it is possible that some models of family therapy would employ intervention strategies at odds with DBT principles, resulting in confusion and possibly poorer outcomes for the patient. Regardless of which course a program chooses, team members should try to prevent or mitigate potential problems associated with the particular structure they use.

Modes of Family Intervention

Programs must decide what mode(s) of family intervention to offer. Family interventions can be delivered in a traditional, one-family-at-a-time mode (traditional family therapy), or may be delivered in a group mode, with multiple families present. With groups, there is the additional choice of whether to have more heterogeneous groups (e.g., mixing parents, partners, siblings, and children of patients) or more homogeneous groups (e.g., a group just for parents, a group just for couples). Again, resources may dictate the answer: a small program may have very few families to treat at a given time, so it may need to see them individually, whereas a larger program might efficiently use a heterogeneous or homogeneous multifamily group. This can vary with the age of the patient and the program's focus. For example, a DBT program for adolescents might find having a parent group very helpful, and a larger program might have enough families wanting treatment at any given time to warrant separate groups for parents and partners.

The advantage to offering heterogeneous groups is high efficiency (every family member in treatment can participate in the same group), but that same heterogeneity may mean some family members feel left out because the group can easily become dominated by the problems of one particular type of family constellation. For example, if most members are parents of adolescents, the problems of others, such as spouses, could be marginalized (or vice versa). Thus, if there are sufficient family members available, it may be preferable for parents to be in groups with other parents, partners with other partners, and so on.

Structuring Family Groups

With multifamily groups, there is also the question of whether to include the patient in the group or to limit the group to family members of the patient. Programs with family components deal with this issue quite successfully in both ways. In part, the answer may depend on the targets of the group. For example, in a DBT program for adolescents, the target may be for parents to learn individual DBT skills in order to be able to support and coach their child in self-management skills. With this target, including the adolescent patient and parent(s) in the same group would likely afford the best outcome. However, if the goal is to provide psychoeducation, improve parent self-management, and strengthen parenting skills, having the parents meet separately, without their children, would likely be preferable. The presence of the child may inhibit accurate assessment, demonstrations of strong support for the parent (others may fear offending the child or eliciting a negative reaction in the youngster), and strong advocacy for change and improvement (others may fear "criticizing" the parent in front of the child, thereby giving the youngster "ammunition" in conflict situations). Similar issues are present with spouses, partners, and other family members: the nature of the targets of the program may influence the modes of family intervention offered.

Enhancing Participation among Family Members

With any type of family intervention, there may be difficulties getting family members to participate. Parents and partners are often stressed themselves, may feel "burned out" by their family member or by previous therapy experiences, may have been blamed for myriad problems by previous therapists or others in mental health, and may not see the value in expending the time and money required to participate in any form of family intervention. Of course, ordinary DBT commitment strategies are a useful place to start. In addition, it is important to highlight how essential it is to listen and to understand (assess) what might block active participation in whatever intervention mode you want to provide. Then it is possible to collaborate right from the beginning with the family—even in trying to decide whether family interventions make sense at that time. Clearly, validating their experiences is essential, as is highlighting the "no blame" component of any DBT intervention (individual or family). Similarly, doing a thorough "pros and cons" of treatment can be very helpful in identifying targets to validate, and to understanding family member goals of treatment.

For very reluctant family members, it may be helpful to provide a clear sense of what would be expected, and perhaps to orient them toward brief intervention (at least initially). We often find that family members think they are being asked to participate in ongoing (even interminable) therapy, which they cannot afford (in terms of money and/or time). However, when offered brief interventions (e.g., three sessions of family therapy, or a six-session parent group), these same family members may agree. Of course, further interventions may be offered later on, if needed. Thus, beginning with a very brief commitment may be a good "door in the face" strategy.

Similarly, some burned-out family members may state that they have done all they can (or they are willing to do) for their child or partner with BPD. It may be useful to note (dialectically) that family interventions are also designed to help family members, not only the patient. In fact, family interventions can be designed primarily to benefit family members. Similarly, the transactional model suggests that anything one family member can do to help another family member function more effectively will make his or her own life (and relationship with that person) a bit better.

Some family members have a style that is more logical or cognitive. For these family members, it may be useful to appeal to the data. Hundreds of studies document the salutary effects of family involvement in treatment for a variety of disorders. Data concerning family interventions for individuals with BPD, although quite limited, are consistent with the larger body of data for other disorders. Other family members may have a more emotional style (sometimes are similar to that of their child or partner in individual DBT for BPD). In these cases it is important to identify their emotions, assess the origins of their strong feelings, and provide validation before discussing how joining treatment may help improve these situations and/or ameliorate their negative emotions. Regardless of their style, being clear and honest about the rationale for treatment, therapist expectations for participation, and minimizing blame, while validating concerns the family members may have, will maximize the chances of successful participation.

DBT Family Skills

Several individual DBT skills have been adapted specifically for use with families, and several new family skill modules have also been developed (Fruzzetti, 1997/2004; Fruzzetti, 2006; Fruzzetti & Fruzzetti, 2003; Fruzzetti & Iverson, 2006). Below we describe briefly these new adaptations and developments. They are relevant to multiple DBT intervention modalities with families.

Mindfulness, of course, is the "core skill" in DBT. Although it is essential for family members to learn basic mindfulness, the specific application of mindfulness to relationships is particularly important. Thus, the "relationship mindfulness" skills module includes awareness of oneself (especially emotions and desires) and awareness of one's partner, child, or other family member. In addition, the ability to stay grounded in long-term goals in the face of rising reactivity is a focus (e.g., "This is my child/partner, a person I love"—which of course comes out of "Wise Mind"). Special attention is placed on letting go of judgments, and transforming anger into other more primary emotions (e.g., sadness, disappointment, fear, dislike), given how corrosive both judgments and strong anger are in relationships. Finally, practice in bringing attention to everyday activities and interactions with loved ones ("being together when you are together") and "relationship activation" complete the module. These relationship mindfulness skills are designed in part to help reduce negative reactivity, which in turn helps to reduce aversive conflict, both of which are hallmarks of problematic relationships (Fruzzetti, 1996). Both mindfulness and relationship mindfulness also therefore contribute to a reduction in invalidating statements and interactions.

Communication skills are also central in family DBT skills training. The transactional model of the development and maintenance of emotion dysregulation posits a reciprocal relationship between high emotional arousal (including secondary emotions), judgments, and inaccurate self-disclosure and invalidation as a core problematic *invalidating* transaction (Fruzzetti, 2006; Fruzzetti & Iverson, 2004a; Fruzzetti et al., 2005). Figure 8.1 shows this transaction. A healthy relationship, in contrast, would include the identification of the primary emotion(s), accurate self-disclosure or expression, and validating responses (and vice versa), as shown in Figure 8.2. Thus, this module includes (1) identifying primary emotions and letting go of high anger in close relationships, (2) accurate expression, and (3) validation. Because of its emphasis on validation, this is often called the "validation" module.

Validation skills (Fruzzetti, 1997/2004; Fruzzetti, in press; Fruzzetti & Fruzzetti, 2003; Fruzzetti & Iverson, 2006; Linehan, 1997) focus on how to understand the other person, communicate that understanding genuinely, and reinforce accurate expression. One might think of this skill module as beginning with the "V" in the DBT GIVE skills (Linehan, 1993b) and building it out into a whole set of skills relevant to families. Validation skills require relationship mindfulness (nonjudgmental awareness of another), which is also a very basic validating response (paying attention, listening, and communicating interest and acceptance). Of course, listening mindfully in turn requires the ability to stay focused on the other person and not respond with a lot of negative emotion that would interfere with listening, understanding, and ultimately validating. Family members must also learn what to validate (targets) and how to validate.

Just as there are many ways to validate in psychotherapy (e.g., Linehan, 1997), there are many ways to validate in family relationships (e.g., Fruzzetti, 2006; Fruzzetti & Iverson, 2004a, 2006). Although therapist validating responses and those of family members overlap, there are important differences. Family validation may take many forms:

1. Maintaining nonjudgmental attention and active listening.
2. Understanding and reflecting back (acknowledging) the other person's emotions, wants, or other disclosures.

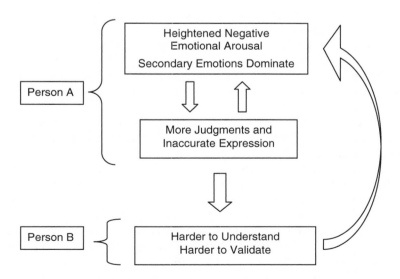

FIGURE 8.1. Invalidating transaction. Data from Fruzzetti (2006).

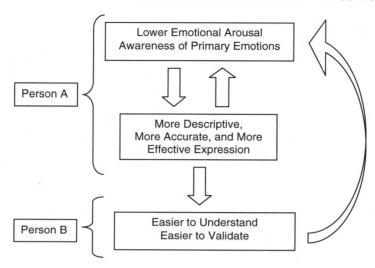

FIGURE 8.2. Validating transaction. Data from Fruzzetti (2006).

3. Engaging in behaviors that uncover more depth and accuracy in the other's expression (especially if it is a different experience than you might have in a similar situation), or asking questions to facilitate understanding what has not been articulated.
4. In the face of child or partner "problem" behaviors, putting his or her behavior in context to lessen its negative valence (i.e., understanding the behavior given the other's history or current level of functioning, or remembering other less problematic behaviors and including these as "context" to reduce invalidation).
5. "Normalizing" normative behavior (e.g., "I'd feel that way too—anyone would").
6. Treating the family member with BPD as an equal human being, not as fragile (taking into account, of course, a child's developmental abilities).
7. Expressing reciprocal vulnerability, often by reciprocating self-disclosures of vulnerability (e.g., "I'm sad we haven't been getting along too").

Thus, this module includes teaching not only *how to* validate, but also *what to* validate, when to do so, how to build motivation to validate, and how to recover from invalidation.

In fact, understanding *invalidation* is also an important part of letting go of invalidating responses and increasing skills at validating (Fruzzetti, 2006). Invalidation can be obvious (e.g., hostile, angry tone or severe criticism), but also can be quite subtle. The distinction between validation and invalidation is based less on the form of the behavior than on its function. For example, gently supporting a family member in choosing not to go to school or work could be invalidating (e.g., By saying "Yes, I can see how tired you are. Of course you're too tired to go" even though one knows the person was out really late drinking or up until 3:00 A.M. surfing on the Internet). In this example, acknowledging the person's fears, tiredness, sadness, and the like, and helping the child or partner to skillfully get on with his or her day could be much more validating, although it might appear more "pushy" and less warm (e.g., "Yes, I can see how tired you are. Still, if you sleep all day, you're likely to be up all night again, and then have the urge to stay home again tomorrow and be miserable. Let's take it one step at a time. How about you get up and get in the shower, and I'll get you a little breakfast. We can take it from there.").

Of course, in a different context, accepting the partner's or child's limitations and supporting him or her in staying home might also be validating. For example, he or she may have the flu and self-invalidate ("I should go to work anyway. Most people don't stay home just because they're sick to their stomach and have a low fever."). In this case, blocking the self-invalidation and supporting the person in going back to bed would probably be much more validating (e.g., "No, most people *do* stay home when they have a fever and the flu. Come on, you look like you feel awful. Listen to your body. It probably makes sense to go back to bed. I can make you some tea and bring it to you there."). The various types of validating and invalidating behavior that we look at in couple and parent–child interactions are summarized in Table 8.1.

TABLE 8.1. Validating and Invalidating Behaviors

Validating responses	Invalidating responses
1. Basic attention, listening, ordinary nonverbals; behaviors that communicate attention, listening, openness.	1. Not paying attention, distractable, changes subject, anxious to leave or to end the conversation.
2. Reflecting or acknowledging the other's disclosures; what he or she is thinking/feeling/wanting; or functionally responding to him or her by answering or problem solving.	2. Not participating actively, missing needed minimal conversational validation opportunities, not providing evidence of tracking the other person; functionally unresponsive.
3. Articulating/offering ideas about what the other might want/feel/think, etc., in an empathic (not insistent) way; helping the other to clarify; asking questions to help clarify.	3. Telling the other person what he or she *does* feel/think/want, etc. (or insisting) even when the other provides contradictory statements; or telling what he or she *should* feel/etc.
4. Recontextualizing the other's behavior (including feelings/desires/thoughts); putting more understanding "spin" on it; acceptance because of history; reducing the negative valence.	4. Agreeing with other person's self-invalidation when behavior makes sense in terms of history (almost always) and could be spun differently; increasing its negative valence; "kicking when he or she's down"; includes making judgments about the other's problematic behavior (public or private).
5. Normalizing other's behavior (any type) given present circumstances; e.g., "Anyone [or I] would feel the same way in this situation" or "Of course, you would feel/think/want that."	5. Pathologizing/criticizing other's behavior when it is reasonable or normative in present circumstances (remember: self-descriptions of private behaviors are assumed to be accurate unless evidenced otherwise); taking specific (may be valid) criticism and globalizing it, or overgeneralizing it; also includes making judgments about normative behaviors (public or private).
6. Empathy, acceptance of the person in general; acting from balance about the relationship; not treating the other as fragile or incompetent, but rather as equal and competent.	6. Patronizing, condescending, and/or contemptuous behavior toward the other; treating the other as not equal (less than), as fragile, or incompetent; character assaults/overgeneralizing negatives.
7. Reciprocal (or matched) vulnerability/self-disclosure in context of the other's vulnerability, and the focus stays on the other person.	7. Leaving the other person hanging out to dry: not responding to (validating) his or her vulnerable self-disclosures, thereby assuming a more powerful position.

Note. Data from Fruzzetti (2004) and Fruzzetti et al. (2006).

In addition, many families lack skills in solving or managing problems. For these families, a *problem management* module is available (Fruzzetti, 1997/2004; see also Fruzzetti, in press). This includes basic instruction in describing and defining problems accurately (without judgment), how to look at intersecting "chain analyses" (in which two family members' "chains" intersect in a problematic way), solution generation, contracting, and follow-up. For example, Figure 8.3 shows a schematic "chain analysis" of two people interacting. This is similar to an ordinary chain analysis that is standard in DBT, except that the shaded "links" show public behaviors that are immediately relevant to both people (such as verbal statements or observable facial expression and relevant body movements), and the open links show the participants' private behaviors (wants, thoughts, urges, emotions, etc.). Going over this chain can be helpful not only to identify change targets (what skills each person could have used to facilitate a more effective outcome), but also to demonstrate how one person's behaviors influence another's, and to help each family member (and the therapist) begin to understand and validate the other's feelings and desires along the chain, thereby increasing mutual understanding and communication.

Although similar to many forms of couple and family problem solving (e.g., Jacobson & Margolin, 1979), the module builds in practice opportunities for the other family skills already learned (relationship mindfulness, accurate expression, validation), and recognizes that some problems cannot easily (or, perhaps ever) be solved, and therefore must be accepted and managed.

Closeness skills provide couples and parent–child dyads opportunities to transform conflictual interactions into understanding and connection. They were designed to help resolve the intimacy–independence polarity common in distressed couples and the dependence–autonomy polarity common among distressed adolescents and their parents. This skill module includes three steps, which build to some extent from "radical accep-

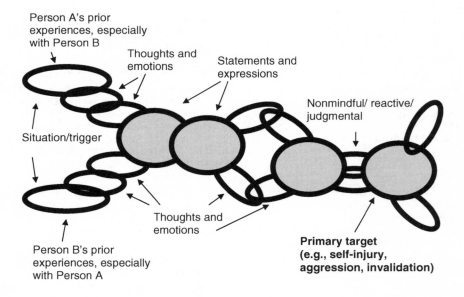

FIGURE 8.3. Double chain for understanding sequences of family interactions. Data from Fruzzetti (2006).

tance" in the DBT skill manual (Linehan, 1993b) and extend these skills to close relationships (Fruzzetti, in press; Fruzzetti & Iverson, 2006):

1. Behavioral tolerance (stopping nagging, no longer putting energy into changing the other person).
2. Pattern awareness (becoming mindful of the consequences of conflict and the exclusive focus on the other person changing).
3. Letting go of suffering and focusing on connection (or recontextualization, in which previously problematic behaviors are reconditioned or understood in a different context, leading to less conflictual, more genuine, and validating responses).

Parenting skills can be extremely beneficial for both parents of adolescent DBT clients and for parents who are themselves DBT clients. DBT parenting skills (Fruzzetti, 1997/2004) are tailored for the age of the child, and may include (1) attending to child safety, (2) education about healthy child development across multiple domains, (3) relationship mindfulness, (4) reducing negative reactivity, (5) validation skills, (6) synthesizing parenting polarities, (7) building a positive parent–child relationship, (8) effective limits, (9) transforming conflict into understanding and validation; and (10) facilitating child competencies.

These skills can be used with individual families or in multifamily groups, and can be offered alone (via skill groups) or as part of couple or family therapy. Preliminary studies have shown DBT family therapy to be effective with couple and with parent–child relationships. For example, in a six-session treatment utilizing DBT family skills, partners demonstrated significantly increased validating and decreased invalidating responses (coded by unbiased observers), and reported significant reductions in individual distress and improvements in relationship satisfaction (Fruzzetti & Mosco, 2006). In a pilot study of DBT parenting skills, parents reported reduced distress and their adolescent children (who did not participate in the intervention) reported increased individual and relationship satisfaction and significant reductions on various measures of distress and psychopathology (Shenk & Fruzzetti, 2005). Similarly, the Family Connections program described later in this chapter, which uses these skills as the core part of its curriculum, has been shown to help family members reduce grief, depression, and burden, while increasing mastery (Hoffman et al., 2005). Of course, significantly more research is needed to understand the effectiveness of DBT family skills training interventions in general.

Heterogeneous Multifamily Groups

DBT–Family Skills Training

In this section a model of a multifamily group, including clients and their family members, is presented. This multifamily model includes traditional skills training, group support, and an additional emphasis on family psychoeducation.

The treatment mode that historically has received the most recognition with psychiatric disorders (but not with BPD) is family psychoeducation (Hoffman & Fruzzetti, 2005). Focusing on the key components of education and coping skills, the initial intention of the family psychoeducation model was to improve patient well-being. Additional points of interest that developed later are the well-being or functioning of the family and the well-being of nonpatient family members. Although family psychoeducation is still not widely available, the value of psychoeducation for both client and family members is now well acknowledged (cf. Hoffman & Fruzzetti, 2005).

Multifamily groups may serve six to eight (or more) families at one time (and thus may include up to 20 participants in each group session). The information distributed includes facts about a variety of topics relevant to BPD, such as identifying the behaviors associated with the disorder, its etiology, treatment options, medication issues, BPD's impact on family members, and community resources. The program also includes a set of strategies to improve communication and problem solving.

Dialectical behavior therapy–family skills training (DBT-FST) is based largely on, and is compatible with, the theories and philosophy of the family psychoeducation model. This modality includes as a "family member" anyone the client chooses to invite over the age of 18. DBT-FST teaches DBT skills to family members and clients alike and targets emotional, cognitive/attitudinal, and behavior change for all participants. DBT-FST was developed in the early 1990s and was first reported in the original DBT skills training manual (Linehan, 1993b, p. 37). Details of the program have been published separately (Hoffman, Fruzzetti, & Swenson, 1999). Although the multifamily group was originally developed to be offered concurrently with individual DBT treatment, it may also be considered even when the individual with BPD is not in active treatment.

Theory and Targets

The conceptualization of the DBT-FST modality grew from two basic hypotheses, one about patients and one about family members:

1. Increasing skill application for DBT patients in a setting with their family members offers a unique opportunity for skill generalization (and structuring the environment) in the context of what is often one of their most stressful environments (the patients' families).
2. Both distress and skill deficits in family members can be ameliorated with DBT individual and family skills.

Consequently, two overarching goals of DBT-FST were established: (1) to provide family members and patients an opportunity to learn about BPD and (2) to teach specific self and relational skills to benefit each individual and to benefit family relationships.

Three of the central functions of standard DBT—skill acquisition, skill generalization, and structuring the family environment—are the foundation of the program. Skill acquisition and generalization are achieved through skill lectures and skill rehearsal along with the generalization of skills through in-session family problem solving among group members and practice between sessions. These standard DBT components are augmented by attention to structuring the family environment, in which changes among family members that may help reinforce skillful behaviors of the BPD patient are facilitated. This added component provides a unique opportunity to put skill acquisition and skill generalization practice directly into the family environment. Similar to standard DBT, "coaching" provides clients in-the-moment support to address a particular situation in their family environment. The group may provide coaching concurrently to several family members. Group members work together on their own and relationship targets. The ultimate aim is to find a balance (synthesis) between what works (is desired and effective) for each individual and for the relationship.

There are four primary goals or targets of DBT-FST.

1. Provide information and education on the disorder: the diagnosis, its criteria, and accompanying behaviors are outlined and discussed as well as the etiological theory on which DBT is formulated.
2. Teach a new approach to and language for communication (based on mindfulness) that replaces judgments with description.
3. Create a no-blame environment. Often participants enter the group ready to express their feelings of blame toward themselves and other members in their family. A nonjudgmental atmosphere is essential, along with a "no-blame" tenet.
4. Establish an effective forum that promotes discussion, accurate expression, validating responses, family problem solving, and conflict resolution.

Format

DBT-FST typically is conducted weekly for 6 months, but shorter or longer programs could be useful. Participants have the option to repeat the curriculum on an individual basis. However, a longer commitment might be a deterrent to family members participating, and 24 weeks allows for a full explication of skills. Led by two professionals who follow the semistructured manual, the class is divided into two 45-minute units. The first 45 minutes is didactic with lectures based on standard DBT skills or family DBT skills. The second unit, called "Consultation Hour," is based in part on the DBT team consultation concept, described below. The weekly lectures include many of the skills traditionally taught in individual DBT treatment (Linehan, 1993b), but the context in which they are presented is the family itself. For example, "emotion mind" is expanded into the concept of an "emotion family." The richness that evolves from such extensions offers dialogue that is nonpejorative, less provocative, and less antagonistic. In addition, DBT family skills such as accurate expression and validation (described earlier) are also presented (Fruzzetti, 1997/2004; Fruzzetti, in press), which build on the skills and language of traditional DBT skills.

The curriculum consists of:

Orientation
DBT Phases of Treatment
Core Mindfulness and Relational Mindfulness Skills
Interpersonal Effectiveness Skills
Emotion Regulation Skills
Distress Tolerance Skills
Accurate Expression
Validation
Consultation to the Family (Problem Solving/Problem Management)

All lectures include suggested practice assignments that participants are encouraged to complete between sessions. These assignments are reviewed at the next class.

The second component, the Consultation Hour provides multiple opportunities for skill application and problem solving/management. Using skills, individual families work on problems specific to them. Both leaders and other group members provide coaching and input with the dual focus of skill implementation and conflict resolution. Because family members have many common issues, all group participants can benefit from this process. Topics include financial issues, relationship responsibilities, family friction and communication, self-injury, fears of suicide, recovery from conflict, family roles, and observing limits.

The process in the Consultation Hour resembles that of a DBT consultation team and/or behavioral family therapy, and includes attention to sharing consultation time, keeping a dual focus on skill enhancement and support/validation, staying nonjudgmental, use of chain analysis, a role-playing or practice component, and opportunities for input from everyone in the group. The group leaders work to establish a group "culture" that is supportive and noncompetitive. For example, because many others in the group share problems that come up with one family, the leaders try to provide validating responses to all and link solutions in one family to those in another. Thus, multiple family consultations can sometimes be addressed in one role play or demonstration, and all group members can practice solutions separately as homework. This enhances the efficiency of the group and reduces stress due to time constraints.

DBT-FST has been very well received by both DBT clients and their relatives. For example, family members report their satisfaction level to be at a "5" (on a 1–5 scale), the drop rate is low, and half of the participants request to continue after completing the 6-month cycle. However, controlled research is required to evaluate the effectiveness of DBT-FST and to learn what effects should be attributed to FST versus concurrent individual treatment.

Family Connections

The effectiveness of professionally led patient and family psychoeducation has been demonstrated across a variety of disorders (cf. Hoffman & Fruzzetti, 2005). However, despite considerable research showing that psychoeducation provided by professionals helps patients with major mental illnesses (e.g., schizophrenia, bipolar disorder), relatively few families actually participate in available programs because such programs are often not available. Consequently, the actual number of participating families reported is less than 10% of those likely to benefit from this type of program (Lehman, 1998). Barriers to implementation include the limited number of clinicians interested in and trained to provide patient and family psychoeducation, the resources required (e.g., space, time), and the fact that third-party reimbursement rates are low, when available at all (Dixon, McFarlane, & Lefley, 2001). To address the above concerns, a variant of psychoeducation, family education (sometimes referred to as "family psychoeducation"), was created (Solomon, 1996).

Unlike patient psychoeducation, the focus of family education is primarily to address the needs of family members, rather than those of patients. Of course, patients are expected to benefit indirectly. Family education programs are typically conducted by trained family members, are generally housed in community settings, and do not charge fees. Such programs typically are shorter in duration than professional psychoeducation programs and are not associated with the individual treatment of the patient. Rather, they are stand-alone programs and the relative identified with the disorder does not attend. The model's goals are to educate participating family members (defined broadly) about psychological disorders, to teach them coping skills to enhance their own well-being, and to provide a network of family support. The most well known is the Family-to-Family program conducted under the auspices of the National Alliance for the Mentally Ill (NAMI). The Family-to-Family course focuses on family members who have a relative with an Axis I disorder.

Family Connections (FC) is also based on the family education model but focuses on families with a relative with BPD. FC is a 12-week family education program conducted in community settings (Fruzzetti & Hoffman, 2004), led by family members (and sometimes by professionals or a combination of professionals and family members) who have been trained to teach the course curriculum. The overall goals include psychoeducation, learning individual and family skills relevant to having a family member with BPD (reducing "quality-of-life-interfering behaviors"), and creating a social support network, starting in the group. The targets include directly increasing the participating family member's well-being directly and indirectly enhancing outcomes for the person with BPD.

Format

FC has many similarities to DBT-FST. However, there are certain limitations that must be understood in an FC group: It is not family or individual therapy, and no matter how skilled its leaders are, they are not trained therapists. Thus, the emphasis is appropriately placed on education, skills, and social support. The FC program follows a clear curriculum. The group typically runs for 2 hours each week. The group typically begins with homework review, then turns its attention to an education segment (a lecture or a presentation on skills), and finally shifts to discussion and consultation. More time is devoted here than in DBT-FST to promoting the development of an ongoing support network (discussion and consultation); thus the group meeting time is 30 minutes longer than in DBT-FST.

Content

The course content is organized around six different curriculum modules. There is no specified length of time dedicated to each module; rather, time allotment is flexible and is left to the discretion of the group leaders, based on the composition and specific needs of each group. Some groups require more time for support and discussion; other groups are more focused on the skills and are less interactive. The modules are:

1. Introduction
2. Education about BPD
3. Relationship Mindfulness and Emotion Self-Management
4. Family Environments
5. Validation
6. Problem Management

Practice assignments are given each week. Handouts are used and group leaders have "teaching notes" to guide them and to help provide consistency from one location to another.

Group leaders must complete a FC group (or an equivalent workshop) themselves, and then complete extensive group leader training provided by the National Education Alliance for Borderline Personality Disorder (NEA-BPD). Experienced group leaders assist in the development of the program and in training and coaching new group leaders.

There is no cost to group participants to attend an FC group, nor is there any charge for group leader training, in order to maximize access to these important resources.

For many people entering the program, FC is the first place where they have been together with other families that share common situations and problems associated with BPD. The fears of participating in a group quickly dissipate when members hear each other's experiences. Immediate connections are made among the participants. Often, the first group is quite emotional, with people drawn to each other in part because of the understanding and compassion they experience from each other.

The first two modules provide information about BPD and summarize the most current research available. Materials are updated regularly, in particular via presentations at the annual Family Perspectives Conference on Borderline Personality Disorder, also sponsored by the NEA-BPD. In addition, FC participants are invited to request specific articles on topics of interest to them, which are provided by NEA-BPD staff.

Next is the first direct skill module, Relationship Mindfulness and Emotion Self-Management, in which the DBT "what" and "how" mindfulness skills are taught, framed in the context of relationships. Awareness of oneself, awareness of the other, adopting a nonjudgmental approach, and managing one's own emotions effectively are the central themes of these skills. The next two modules, Family Environments and Validation, build on prior skills, striving first toward the establishment of a no-blame environment and then teaching skills that promote a healthy family environment. Radical acceptance ends the module, which can include viewing a segment of one of Linehan's videotapes (e.g., *From Suffering to Freedom: Practicing Reality Acceptance: Alleviating Suffering Through Accepting the World as It Is*, the segment titled "Radical Acceptance"). Validation skills focus first on accurate expression and communication awareness, then on both validating another person and validating oneself. The final module, Problem Management, borrows standard problem-solving steps from behavioral couple and family therapy, but also includes more options for acceptance of problems that are difficult or impossible to solve.

FC has been evaluated both in an initial study (Hoffman et al., 2005) and in a replication study (Hoffman, Fruzzetti, & Buteau, 2007). Participants' levels of grief and burden and distress/depression were reduced significantly from pre- to postgroup, while a sense of mastery was increased overall. These improvements were maintained at a 3-month follow-up assessment, suggesting that the FC program may provide significant and perhaps enduring benefits to family members. Further research is needed, in particular to understand whether these improvements among participating family members have any salutary effect on the family member with BPD.

Conclusions

Family members of those with BPD experience their own levels of distress. Education alone is not enough to provide relief (Hoffman, Buteau, Hooley, Fruzzetti, & Bruce, 2003). Whether led by a professional or a trained family member, programs that provide information, skill building, and a support network offer family members of individuals with BPD the opportunity to learn to manage their own "emotional roller-coaster" more effectively. As data show, high levels of emotional involvement are beneficial to persons with BPD (Hooley & Hoffman, 1998), but skills are required to achieve constructive, supportive, and sustained validating emotional involvement. DBT-FST and FC provide two promising vehicles to promote a healthy and validating family environment.

Brief DBT Family Interventions to Augment Individual DBT Outcomes in Stage 1

When individual DBT therapists repeatedly find that the actions of family members, or patient–family member interactions, are an integral part of the patient's chain of dysfunctional behavior(s) in Stage 1, bringing the family in for direct family intervention has many advantages. First, family assessment provides an efficient way to assess the importance of family behaviors vis-à-vis patient target behaviors. In addition, if relevant family behaviors are identified, brief family interventions can be used to augment individual treatment and help to create safety and stability for the patient. In a series of difficult cases, even a few family intervention sessions have been shown to have a potent effect on reducing Stage 1 target behaviors (Fruzzetti, 2006). Details of this approach may be found elsewhere (e.g., Fruzzetti, 2006; Fruzzetti & Fruzzetti, 2003), but the targets for brief intervention are described below.

Target Safety

Unfortunately, many clients in DBT are victims of intimate partner violence or domestic abuse and often are involved in ongoing aggressive and violent interactions with parents, partners, or children. We consider these behaviors (physical and sexual aggression and violence) to be life-threatening. They are therefore among the highest order targets in DBT, along with suicidal and self-injurious behaviors. When DBT clients are victims of battering or other domestic abuse, safety must be the first concern of any family intervention. Similarly, when the DBT client is engaging in aggressive and violent behaviors, these actions must be targeted immediately (see Fruzzetti & Levensky, 2000, for details concerning treating aggression and violence in DBT). Thus, the first target for any family intervention is ensuring safety, which demands a thorough safety assessment and safety plan.

Family Assessment and Intervention

Good assessment of aggression and violence may be accomplished efficiently via the use of a combination of self-report (e.g., the use of the Conflict Tactics Scale—II; Straus, Hamby, Boney-McCoy, & Sugarman, 1996) and follow-up interview. Any self-reports should be administered in person, with partners or parents and children completing the forms in separate rooms to maximize the accuracy of the information collected and to minimize threats and coercion. Any aggressive or violent items that are endorsed by anyone in the family should then be followed up in an individual interview to understand the frequency and danger of these behaviors, the level of fear or perceived threat experienced, as well as the relevant controlling variables (via chain analysis). If any safety-related behaviors are identified, they should be the first treatment target.

The next assessment target is to identify any behaviors of family members that promote dysfunctional, especial suicidal and self-injurious, behaviors. Typically, a chain analysis already performed with the family member in individual DBT will identify some of the important links to be addressed. However, it may be useful to perform a "family" chain analysis in order to identify how one person's chain actually influences the other's, and vice versa. This process was described earlier and shown in Figure 8.3.

There are four common problematic family consequences of out-of-control patient behaviors to consider:

1. *Positively reinforcing dysfunctional behaviors* (providing warmth and caring following dysfunctional behavior)
2. *Negatively reinforcing dysfunctional behaviors* (stopping criticism, threats, or other negative behaviors after increased patient suicidality)
3. *Failing to reinforce self-management or skillful behaviors* (ignoring successful self-management)
4. *Punishing skillful behaviors* (criticizing nascent skill development, immediately increasing expectations of the patient following early success)

We have found that parents and partners frequently, and often unwittingly, engage in these behaviors, and that changing these consequences can be essential to reducing and eliminating out-of-control behaviors of the patient.

For example, it is common for family members to feel burned out and to become detached from the patient, only to move in closer and soothe the patient (thereby likely reinforcing dysfunction) following an escalation of suicidality (increased suicidal thoughts, urges, or actions) or other crisis behavior. In these cases, it is important to "move" rather than "remove" the warm, soothing, solicitous behavior. That is, if the patient is receiving very little nurturance, it is important to have the family member(s) provide at least that amount, but either on a fixed, regular basis (*x* minutes every day) or contingent on the patient *not* engaging in dysfunctional behaviors. These interventions require the use of quick skill training, teaching whatever individual or family skill is needed on that chain, along with all of the usual DBT intervention strategies (see Fruzzetti & Fruzzetti, 2003, for a more detailed explanation of this strategy).

Similarly, family members sometimes act in a highly aversive way toward the patient and only reduce those aversive behaviors when the patient responds with increasing suicidal behavior or other negative escalating behavior. For example, we have encountered many examples in which women are battered until they become self-injurious or suicidal, etc., at which time their partners stop battering and even become warm, soothing, and solicitous.

Less dramatically, but not necessarily less importantly, verbal criticism and invalidation are common antecedents of patient dysfunctional behaviors. Suicidal and parasuicidal behaviors can function to escape from aversive, invalidating interactions. In such cases, the treatment target is the reduction or elimination of those destructive behaviors of the family member. It is important here to "remove" as many aversive behaviors as possible from the chain. This may require a lot of attention to helping family members increase their skillfulness in a variety of domains in order to reduce judgments and negative emotional reactions and increase mindfulness of their goals and the needs of their family member with BPD. These efforts are more likely to be effective, of course, if the family member with BPD reinforces the change (i.e., does not respond to a less aversive environment by increasing his or her own aversive responding).

Increasing validating responses of family members can be effective on the antecedent side of a patient's dysfunctional behaviors: (1) validating wants and emotions may reduce negative arousal, making individual skills more likely to work in reducing arousal further, and (2) validating skill use may reinforce skill use, independent of the other effects of being skillful (in contrast to using previously learned, dysfunctional responses). Thus, validating the use of skills can be an important, if transient, source of reinforcement for skillful behavior, especially while the patient is learning the skills and these skills are still not very effective (the patient may not benefit much from skill use until he or she is skillful at it). Also, when a person is just beginning to learn a new skill, trying out the new behavior may surprise family members, who might respond by noticing the awkwardness or ineffectiveness of the skill, rather than the attempt to be skillful, and may punish the attempt. Consequently, it is important for family members to be alert to the emergence of newer, skillful behaviors and to greet these new behaviors in a validating way. Practicing in the family session can help prevent family members from inadvertently punishing nascent skill use. It also provides an opportunity for the therapist to model validation as an alternative, if necessary.

Utilizing Non-DBT Family Therapy

Despite the tremendous growth in the number of DBT therapists, the availability of family therapists who are also DBT therapists is very limited. Moreover, therapists who provide specific DBT family interventions are not yet widely available. Thus it may be useful to consider what kinds of family therapy can be used to complement individual DBT to result in successful outcomes. In this section, some general principles for collaborating with non-DBT family therapists are provided, and a new integration of systemic family therapy and DBT is described.

Family Systems Family Therapy

There are many different types of family therapy, each coming from its own background and theoretical orientation. Perhaps most common among the nonbehavioral family therapies are those that are considered "systemic." These types of family interventions share a theory of the family as a "system" or unit in which one family member affects another, and vice versa. Thus, "reciprocal causality" is a cornerstone of family systems theory. This idea should not be a new one to modern behaviorists or DBT therapists, who share this idea, albeit using different terminology (e.g., transactional model vs. systems theory). Indeed, there is considerable overlap between modern behavioral and family systems theories, and this makes systems-oriented family therapy potentially quite compatible with DBT. Moreover, family therapists are often used to using a consultation team to balance the therapy, and the dialectical communication style found in DBT (balancing radical genuineness with irreverence) is quite common in family therapy from a systemic perspective.

However, there are many subtypes of family therapy based on family systems theory. Although many are quite compatible with DBT, some may not be. For example, structural family therapy (Minuchin, 1974; Minuchin & Fishman, 1981) looks at the strengths and weaknesses of different relationships in the family (e.g., family structure) and tries to help the family achieve a healthy or balanced pattern of interacting. Many of the interventions found in this approach are also found in behavioral approaches, though under a different name. Moreover, the therapist coaches family members directly and genuinely on needed behavior changes. Thus, this approach would seem to be compatible with DBT. In contrast, strategic family therapy, although it employs some of the same theory, often tries to use the assumed "resistance" in the family to provoke changes, and sometimes even "prescribes the symptom" in the form of a paradoxical directive (intervention) given to a particular family member. Interventions such as paradoxical directives are quite different from DBT interventions that are irreverent or "enter the paradox" (increasing understanding from a dialectical perspective). Thus, they would be unlikely to be employed in DBT because they are much less genuine (e.g., asking someone to do more of something when you really want him or her to do less), and rely on a quite incompatible unconscious model of motivation.

The therapist's knowledge about BPD in general, and DBT in particular, is important to consider. If the family therapist has a strong background in DBT and sees no conflicts with DBT, it may be well worth considering a referral. Alternatively, you can consider inviting one or more local family therapists to sit in on your DBT training or your ongoing DBT consultation team, and discuss areas of similarity or potential conflict. The bottom line is not to contribute to patient or family distress by having multiple therapists work at cross-purposes.

Integrative Borderline Adolescent Family Therapy

A new integration of DBT and systems-oriented family therapy—integrative borderline adolescent family therapy (I-BAFT)—has recently been developed and evaluated specifically for use with drug-abusing adolescents with BPD or significant borderline features and their families. This treatment has shown promising results, (e.g., Santisteban, Muir, et al., 2003), and will be highlighted here.

Structure

I-BAFT seeks to bring about the fundamental "contextual changes" (e.g., improved parenting practices, validation) in the family that are efficient ways to change adolescent behavior (Santisteban, Muir, Mena, & Mitrani, 2003). I-BAFT is an outpatient treatment model that integrates structural family therapy (Minuchin & Fishman, 1981), DBT-informed individual therapy, and DBT skills training. I-BAFT is designed to be an intensive intervention program, requiring a significant commitment of time and energy: it includes three sessions per week for the adolescent (family therapy, skills training, and individual session) for a 6–8 month period. Consistent with standard DBT, separate therapists and skills trainers are recommended because it is extraordinarily difficult for one therapist to conduct skills training, which is highly structured, while postponing other urgent clinical issues typical of therapy sessions. The primary therapist conducts individual and family therapy sessions while the skills trainer focuses solely on the acquisition of new psychosocial skills. Although the therapist does not teach skills per se, he or she must promote the use of a new skill (skill strengthening or generalizing) in family therapy sessions as well as in other daily situations. In order to increase consistency across interventions, all I-BAFT therapists are trained to deliver family, individual treatment, and skills training.

Innovations

I-BAFT employs many of the ordinary targets and intervention strategies of DBT. However, I-BAFT also includes a number of innovations that may be important in working with drug-abusing adolescents and their families that are less common in DBT. For example, this model stresses helping adolescents establish goals across multiple domains (e.g., self, family, peers, school and career, and community) in order to facilitate commitment to treatment and to daily skill generalization. In addition, because this treatment targets drug-abusing adolescents, it also includes a module on HIV risk reduction, designed to address the life situations these adolescents confront.

Intervention Targets

Six targets of intervention for the family are emphasized:

1. *Developing the family members' understanding of the adolescent's vulnerability to emotion and dysregulation.* One of the important goals of I-BAFT family interventions is to create a new "frame," or way of understanding/perceiving the adolescent. Because of the often extreme behavior displayed by these adolescents, it is often difficult for the family to see the emotional distress experienced and to understand the adolescent's vulnerability to emotion dysregulation. This increased understanding of the adolescent's struggle can help family members stay more connected, be less invalidating, and more validating during difficult times.

2. *Making the problems systemic (transactional).* It is helpful for family members to accept a systemic view of family behaviors and an individual's problem behaviors. This is, of course, compatible with the transactional model utilized in DBT (e.g., Fruzzetti et al., 2005; Linehan, 1993a). Family members identify and understand how certain of their behaviors can inadvertently elicit, exacerbate, and/or reinforce the problematic behavior.

3. *Improving communication between the adolescent and other family members.* Adolescents with BPD features and their families have often become entrenched in maladaptive and invalidating communication patterns. One I-BAFT goal is to identify parent or adolescent behaviors that disrupt communication (e.g., shutting down, avoidance, or explosive reactions) and modify these interactions *in vivo*. In I-BAFT, the family therapist coaches family members to replace invalidating responses with responses that validate emotions and ideas even if they do not necessarily agree with them. Family interventions also seek to promote the adolescent's accurate expression of needs and the family's ability to validate them.

4. *Developing parenting skills needed with an adolescent with BPD features.* From one side of the transactional perspective, having an adolescent child with BPD features can make it difficult for parents to provide healthy family structures and responses (e.g., validating), even for parents who do provide them for other children in the family. Moreover, it is not easy for parents to change, particularly if they suffer from skill deficits or their own distress. Thus, I-BAFT has a strong focus on parenting, monitoring and blocking parents' tendencies toward becoming disengaged or inconsistent. In these cases, an important component of treatment is to attend to the parent's own difficulties and needs through direct interventions or referrals.

5. *Increasing the size of the supportive network around the adolescent.* Parents may sometimes lack the emotional resources needed to meet the adolescent's needs by themselves. One treatment strategy is to enhance outside support by promoting interactions with other empathic adult figures in the adolescent's life.

6. *Reducing aggressive and violent behaviors in family interactions.* Reducing aggression and violence is extremely important in this model, as it is in DBT. The critical transition point in the sequence toward violence must be identified and modified, just as one would do in DBT (using chain analysis and problem solving).

Preliminary Data on I-BAFT

Preliminary indicators of the feasibility/acceptability and impact of I-BAFT were very promising when tested with 13 adolescents who met full DSM-IV criteria for both BPD and drug abuse. For example, of 10 cases assigned to I-BAFT, seven (70%) were considered successfully engaged and retained in treatment (mean = 43 sessions), and both adolescents and parents reported high levels of satisfaction with the multiple treatment components (Santisteban, Muir, et al., 2003). The I-BAFT cases that were retained in treatment (70%) were more likely to meet criteria for reliable change (compared to a lower dosage I-BAFT treatment or treatment as usual) on BPD criteria, delinquency, and drug use (Santisteban, Mena, Muir, Mitrani, & Liu, 2007).

Summary and Conclusions

There are many reasons to consider providing family interventions as an ordinary part of any DBT program: outcomes may be improved, efficiency enhanced, and, theoretically, family factors play a central role (i.e., as an invalidating environment) in the transactional model on which DBT is founded. Family interventions may be successfully employed in multifamily groups or with individual families, and may utilize pure DBT principles and strategies or be integrated with common models of family therapy widely available in the community. This chapter has provided an overview of treatment targets and family skills, along with an overview of the emerging evidence that family interventions could be an important part of any DBT program.

REFERENCES

American Psychiatric Association. (1994). *Diagnostic and statistical manual of mental disorders* (4th ed.). Washington, DC: Author.

Dixon, L., McFarlane, W. R., & Lefley, H. (2001). Evidence-based practices for services to families of people with psychiatric disabilities. *Psychiatric Services, 52,* 903–910.

Fruzzetti, A. E. (1996). Causes and consequences: Individual distress in the context of couple interactions. *Journal of Consulting and Clinical Psychology, 64,* 1192–1201.

Fruzzetti, A. E. (1997/2004). *Family DBT skills.* Reno: University of Nevada.

Fruzzetti, A. E. (2004). *The Validating and Invalidating Behaviors Coding System: Understanding conflict and closeness processes in families and other relationships.* Reno: University of Nevada.

Fruzzetti, A. E. (2005). *DBT parenting skills.* Reno: University of Nevada.

Fruzzetti, A. E. (2007). *Dialectical behavior therapy with couples and families to augment outcomes in individual DBT: Procedures and pilot data.* Unpublished manuscript.

Fruzzetti, A. E. (2006). *The high conflict couple: A dialectical behavior therapy guide to finding peace, intimacy, and validation.* Oakland, CA: New Harbinger.

Fruzzetti, A. E., & Boulanger, J. L. (2005). Family involvement in treatment for borderline personality disorder. In J. G. Gunderson & P. D. Hoffman (Eds.), *Understanding and treating borderline personality disorder: A guide for professionals and families* (pp. 157–164). Washington, DC: American Psychiatric Publishing.

Fruzzetti, A. E., & Fruzzetti, A. R. (2003). Borderline personality disorder. In D. Snyder & M. A. Whisman (Eds.), *Treating difficult couples: Helping clients with coexisting mental and relationship disorders* (pp. 235–260). New York: Guilford Press.

Fruzzetti, A. E., & Hoffman, P. D. (2004). *Family Connections workbook and training manual.* Rye, NY: National Education Alliance for Borderline Personality Disorder.

Fruzzetti, A. E., & Iverson, K. M. (2004a). Mindfulness, acceptance, validation and "individual" psychopathology in couples. In S. C. Hayes, V. M. Follette, & M. M. Linehan (Eds.), *Mindfulness and acceptance: Expanding the cognitive-behavioral tradition* (pp. 168–191). New York: Guilford Press.

Fruzzetti, A. E., & Iverson, K. M. (2004b). Couples dialectical behavior therapy: An approach to both individual and relational distress. *Couples Research and Therapy, 10,* 8–13.

Fruzzetti, A. E., & Iverson, K. A. (2006). Intervening with couples and families to treat emotion dysregulation and psychopathology. In D. K. Snyder et al. (Eds.), *Emotion regulation in families.* Washington, DC: American Psychological Association.

Fruzzetti, A. E., & Levensky, E. R. (2000). Dialectical behavior therapy with batterers: Rationale and procedures. *Cognitive and Behavioral Practice, 7,* 435–447.

Fruzzetti, A. E., & Mosco, E. (2006). *Dialectical behavior therapy adapted for couples and families: A pilot group intervention for couples.* Manuscript submitted for publication.

Fruzzetti, A. E., Shenk, C., & Hoffman, P. D. (2005). Family interaction and the development of borderline personality disorder: A transactional model. *Development and Psychopathology, 17,* 1007–1030.

Fruzzetti, A. E., Shenk, C., Lowry, K., Mosco, E., & Iverson, K. A. (2006). *Reliability and validity of the Validating and Invalidating Behavior Coding System (VIBCS).* Manuscript submitted for publication.

Hoffman, P. D., Buteau, E., Hooley, J. M., Fruzzetti, A. E., & Bruce, M. L. (2003). Family members' knowledge about borderline personality disorder: Correspondence with their levels of depression, burden, distress, and expressed emotion. *Family Process, 42,* 469–478.

Hoffman, P. D., & Fruzzetti, A. E. (2005). Psychoeducation. In J. M. Oldham, A. Skodal, & D. Bender (Eds.), *Textbook of personality disorders* (pp. 375–385). Washington, DC: American Psychiatric Publishing.

Hoffman, P. D., Fruzzetti, A. E., & Buteau, E. (2007). Understanding and engaging families: An education, skills, and support program for relatives impacted by borderline personality disorder. *Journal of Mental Health, 16,* 68–92.

Hoffman, P. D., Fruzzetti, A. E., Buteau, E., Penney, D., Neiditch, E., Penney, D., et al. (2005). Family Connections: A program for relatives of persons with borderline personality disorder. *Family Process, 44,* 217–225.

Hoffman, P. D., Fruzzetti, A. E., & Swenson, C. R. (1999). Dialectical behavior therapy: Family skills training. *Family Process, 38,* 399–414.

Jacobson, N. S., & Margolin, G. (1979). *Marital therapy: Strategies based on social learning and behavior exchange principles.* New York: Brunner/Mazel.

Lehman, A. F. (1998). Public health policy, community services, and outcomes for patients with schizophrenia. *Psychiatric Clinics of North America, 21,* 221–231.

Linehan, M. (1993a). *Cognitive-behavioral treatment of borderline personality disorder.* New York: Guilford Press.

Linehan, M. (1993b). *Skills training manual for treating borderline personality disorder.* New York: Guilford Press.

Linehan, M. M. (1997). Validation and psychotherapy. In A. Bohart & L. S. Greenberg (Eds.), *Empathy and psychotherapy: New directions to theory, research, and practice* (pp. 353–392). Washington, DC: American Psychological Association.

Minuchin, S. (1974). *Families and family therapy.* Cambridge, MA: Harvard University Press.

Minuchin, S., & Fishman, H. C. (1981). *Family therapy techniques.* Cambridge, MA: Harvard University Press.

Santisteban, D. A., Coatsworth, D., Perez-Vidal, A., Kurtines, W. M., Schwartz, S. J., LaPerriere, A., et al. (2003). The efficacy of brief strategic/structural family therapy in modifying behavior problems and an exploration of the mediating role that family functioning plays in behavior change. *Journal of Family Psychology, 17*(1), 121–133.

Santisteban, D. A., Mena, M. P., Muir, J. A., Mitrani, V. B., & Liu, Y. (2007). *Integrated adolescent with BPD features family therapy: Preliminary indicators of treatment impact on adolescents meeting criteria for drug abuse and borderline personality disorder.* Manuscript submitted for publication.

Santisteban, D. A., Muir, J. A., Mena, M. P., & Mitrani, V. B. (2003). Integrated adolescent with BPD features family therapy: Meeting the challenges of treating adolescent with BPD features. *Psychotherapy: Theory/Research/ Practice/Training, 40*(4), 251–264.

Shenk, C., & Fruzzetti, A. E. (2005). *Mindfulness based interventions with parents and their distressed adolescent children: A pilot study.* Paper presented at the Fifth International Congress of Cognitive Psychotherapy, Göteborg, Sweden.

Solomon, P. (1996). Moving from psychoeducation to family education for families of adults with serious mental illness. *Psychiatric Services, 47*, 1364–1370.

Straus, M. A., Hamby, S. L., Boney-McCoy, S., & Sugarman, D. B. (1996). The revised Conflict Tactics Scales (CTS2): Development and preliminary psychometric data. *Journal of Family Issues, 17*, 283–316.

CHAPTER 9

Dialectical Behavior Therapy for Adolescents

Alec L. Miller, Jill H. Rathus, Anthony P. DuBose, Elizabeth T. Dexter-Mazza, *and* Arielle R. Goldklang

Historically, teens who experience repeated intentional self-injury or suicidal ideation are brought to emergency rooms and admitted to psychiatric inpatient units only to be rapidly discharged back to their traditional outpatient services which have done little to effectively help them. Dialectical behavior therapy (DBT), however, may be an effective alternative to treatment as usual for this population (Miller, Rathus, Linehan, Wetzler, & Leigh, 1997; Rathus & Miller, 2000; Miller, Glinski, Woodberry, Mitchell, & Indik, 2002; Miller, Rathus, & Linehan, 2007). In this chapter, we begin by discussing the rationale for considering DBT with adolescents. We then share what we have learned as we developed our own DBT programs for adolescents, focusing on the adaptations and particular emphases we consider important to the developmental level of this population. Throughout, we describe how to maintain the principles of DBT at the various decision points one encounters in developing an adolescent DBT program and we present vignettes to illustrate in detail how to use DBT with adolescents. We conclude with discussion of clinical and ethical issues that require special attention when working with chronically self-injuring and suicidal adolescents within a DBT frame.

Why Adopt DBT for Adolescents?

DBT makes sense for suicidal and self-injuring adolescent for two primary reasons. First, DBT is explicitly designed for individuals who are chronically suicidal or self-injuring and who have multiple serious mental health problems. DBT flexibly combines cognitive-behavioral protocols to treat problems characterized by emotional dysregulation and behavioral dyscontrol such as self-injury, behaviors that interfere with treatment, and multiple concurrent Axis I disorders (Linehan, 2000). This aspect of DBT offers an advantage over cognitive-behavioral therapy and interpersonal therapy for adolescents (Clarke, Rohde, Lewinsohn, Hops, & Seely, 1999; Mufson, Dorta, Moreau, & Weisman, 2004) that are designed to treat one problem at a time (e.g., depression, school avoidance, or interpersonal problems). In fact, research on these treatments has typically excluded teens with multiple problems (Miller et al., 1997). To date, there is not a single treatment with established efficacy[1] for suicidal multiproblem adolescents (Miller et al., 2007). In addition to directly targeting life-threatening behavior, DBT aggressively targets treatment noncompliance, an enormous problem among suicidal adolescents. For example, in one study 77% of adolescent suicide attempters who presented to an emergency room failed to attend or complete traditional outpatient treatment (Trautman, Stewart, & Morishima 1993).

Second, DBT is a multimodal approach. In addition to individual psychotherapy, consultation team for therapists, and as-needed phone consultation to patients, standard DBT includes group skills training, often an effective treatment modality for adolescents because peer relationships promote the development of social skills and identity formation (Brown et al., 1990). The flexibility of a multimodal approach also means that DBT adds family interventions as needed. (Both family skills training and family therapy will be discussed in subsequent sections.)

Research on DBT with Adolescents

Preliminary research to date suggests that the application of DBT for adolescents is quite promising. Although randomized clinical trials are not available, DBT programs in routine outpatient, inpatient, residential, and forensic settings for adolescents have been evaluated in quasi-experimental designs. For example, in a 12-week quasi-experimental investigation of an ethnic minority, suicidal, borderline personality-spectrum adolescent outpatient population, Rathus and Miller (2002) compared 29 subjects receiving DBT with 82 subjects receiving treatment as usual (TAU; in this case, supportive psychodynamic individual therapy and family therapy). At posttreatment, compared with subjects receiving TAU, those receiving DBT had significantly fewer psychiatric hospitalizations (DBT = 0% vs. TAU = 13%) during treatment and a significantly higher rate of outpatient treatment completion (DBT = 62% vs. TAU = 40%). Examining pre–post change within the DBT group (setting constraints prevented collection of self-report TAU data at posttreatment), there were significant reductions in suicidal ideation, general psychiatric symptoms, and symptoms of borderline personality disorder (BPD).

Using Miller et al.'s (1997) adaptation of DBT for adolescent outpatients, Fellows and her colleagues evaluated 23 patients who completed their 16-week outpatient program in New Hampshire. Patients in their DBT program showed significant reductions in three costly services: inpatient psychiatric days, emergency service contacts, and days of respite bed usage. Specifically, prior to treatment the group had 539 inpatient psychiatric days, compared to 40 days during DBT treatment and 11 days during the 6 months posttreatment (Fellows, personal communication, July 1999). In another study of outpatient adolescent DBT, Woodberry, Popenac, and Cook (2007) employed parental reports to help evaluate outcome at pre- and posttreatment. Parents corroborated their adolescents' self-reports of symptom reduction at posttreatment and, further, parents reported reduction in their own symptoms at posttreatment. Other researchers have obtained results that support the feasibility of applying DBT to suicidal adolescent inpatients.

Katz, Gunasekara, Cox, and Miller (2004) evaluated the feasibility of DBT implementation in a general child and adolescent psychiatry inpatient unit, comparing DBT to TAU. Sixty-two adolescents with a history of suicide attempts or suicidal ideation were admitted based upon bed availability at the time of the admission to one of two psychiatric inpatient units. One unit used a modified DBT protocol (Katz, Gunasekara, & Miller, 2002) in which the duration of treatment was changed to 2 weeks, DBT individual therapy was provided twice per week, and skills training groups were provided on a daily basis. The other unit employed TAU consisting of psychodynamically oriented milieu therapy. The patients were seen weekly for individual psychotherapy and attended daily psychotherapy groups. Results were that the DBT unit had significantly fewer behavioral incidents (these are mandated reporting of occurrences such as self-harm, suicidal behavior, aggression toward staff and property, etc.) on the unit during admission when compared to patients receiving TAU. Both groups demonstrated highly significant reductions in intentional self-injury, depressive symptoms, and suicidal ideation at 1-year follow-up. Although the effect sizes were larger in the DBT group (for depressive symptoms and suicidal ideation), they were not statistically significantly different between groups.

DBT has also been implemented within juvenile rehabilitation settings with promising findings (e.g., Trupin, Stewart, Beach, &Boesky, 2002; Washington State Institute for Public Policy, 2002).

These preliminary results suggest that, at a minimum, no harm was done to adolescents in DBT, and further that DBT may lead to better outcomes than TAU in reducing intentional self-injury and use of expensive psychiatric services, perhaps even reducing psychological symptoms of parents who choose to participate. DBT makes sense as an alternative to TAU because it explicitly treats the problems experienced by intentionally self-injuring adolescents, combines cognitive-behavioral methods and modes of therapy that are effective with adolescents, and has promising preliminary results. Given the lack of validated alternatives for this population and the promising preliminary data supporting the use of DBT for adolescents, we believe it is reasonable to develop DBT programs for multiproblem suicidal youth. In the absence of randomized controlled trials (the highest level of scientific proof of a treatment's efficacy), we would advise collecting data in your own setting (see Chapter 12, this volume). Because there is as yet no one particular model of using DBT with adolescents that has been shown to be effective in controlled research, there is no one prescribed model to follow. Therefore, it becomes essential for programs to evaluate the outcomes they obtain in their own setting. With this in mind, the particular models and parameters of DBT programs we present here are based on our own experience as well as from 12 adolescent DBT programs we surveyed. The programs were invited to participate in the survey based on our (the authors') familiarity with their programs or based on suggestions from other DBT providers and trainers. Of these programs we surveyed, seven were outpatient, one was inpatient, three were general residential programs, and one was a forensic residential program.

Deciding Whom You Will Treat with DBT: The Options

One of the first decisions in developing an adolescent DBT program has to do with inclusion and exclusion criteria for the program. One approach is to limit the DBT program to a relatively homogenous group (e.g., presence of BPD criteria and recent intentional self-injury) so that individuals in the program resemble the original group for whom DBT was shown to be efficacious (Linehan, Armstrong, Suarez, Allmon, & Heard, 1991; Linehan, 1993a). The resulting similarity of problems in a more homogenous group may create greater feelings of cohesion among youth in the program. On the other hand, the increasing evidence that DBT can be successfully adapted for a range of target behaviors (Linehan, 2000) makes it reasonable to consider mixed diagnostic groups that thereby serve more clients. As discussed throughout this volume, instead of limiting inclusion to those who meet criteria for BPD diagnosis, DBT may be offered to those who are at high risk to harm themselves or others, have a history of being unresponsive to past treatments, and have significant emotion regulation difficulties. The tradeoff as entry criteria broaden, however, is that individuals' needs (due to severity levels and differing treatment targets) also broaden, and these differences may mean that the program and group skills training in particular lose their focus.

In practice, outpatient adolescent DBT programs report differing inclusion criteria, yet, at a minimum, identify a unifying theme that brings group members together (e.g., emotion dysregulation). For example, one outpatient program's criteria are a suicide attempt within the past 16 weeks or current suicidal ideation plus at least three criteria of BPD. As a point of reference, youth selected for most DBT programs typically also have been given comorbid diagnoses including mood, anxiety, and disruptive behavior disorders.

The key principle to keep in mind regarding exclusion criteria is whether or not the patient is likely to benefit—exclude those for whom more appropriate evidence-based treatments are available and those who are not likely to benefit. For example, for an adolescent whose primary problems result from a thought disorder, DBT should not be the first-line treatment—other evidence-based treatments are more appropriate. However, one might consider DBT for an adolescent who is chronically suicidal and self-injuring and has psychotic features secondary to a major depression. Sometimes exclusion criteria have to do with how well a client will function in group skills training. For example, current mania or psychosis, severe substance abuse, mental retardation, and severe expressive or receptive language and reading disorders may interfere with the person's ability to learn and participate in group skills training. This may mean that admission to a DBT program is delayed until conditions are stabilized enough for the individual to benefit from group skills training or it may mean that skills training is delivered in an individual format that can accommodate factors that interfere with learning and participation. For example, youth with antisocial personality disorder or conduct disorder tend to fare *worse* in group formats because of the modeling and peer validation of antisocial behaviors that occurs (Dishion, McCord, & Poulin, 1999). Consequently, alternatives such as individual skills training may be needed to best meet their needs. Similarly, being legally mandated to treatment can interfere with the necessary voluntary nature of participation in DBT. In these cases, extra focus on commitment strategies and structuring the environment to create meaningful voluntary consent to treatment becomes important.

In practice, exclusion criteria across programs vary based on program resources, choices about homogeneous versus heterogeneous diagnostic groups, and program limits. Most outpatient DBT programs also exclude adolescents unwilling to (a) comply with the complete DBT program (i.e., attend individual and skills group) or (b) discontinue other non-DBT psychotherapy. These programmatic limits arise from the practical obstacles partial participation and dual, simultaneous therapy pose to treatment progress. For example, most teens are excluded from outpatient treatment when they are so behaviorally out of control (e.g., who are actively suicidal or homicidal, or who after extensive attempts to obtain commitment to safety still exhibit no capacity or willingness to commit to try to remain safe and use therapy to decrease suicidal/homicidal urges) that trying to maintain them in an outpatient setting would be dangerous to themselves or others (including family members). Again, the only a priori reasons to include/exclude have to do with how well DBT fits the patient's problems, minimal conditions needed for therapy to have a chance, and the availability of alternative treatments that are more appropriate.

Inclusion and exclusion criteria are typically less stringent in inpatient and residential DBT settings that often have the mandate to take all comers. For example, those we surveyed only require the teen to have been suicidal in the past 8 weeks to be included in the DBT program and include adolescents in DBT when they present with (1) severe and persistent self-injurious/suicidal behaviors and/or aggressive/assaultive behaviors toward others and (2) a diagnosis of BPD or borderline personality traits.

Like diagnostic criteria and presenting problems, age is another important inclusion criterion to specify. Adolescence is generally defined as ranging in age from 12 to 19 (e.g., Berk, 2004), and one must determine what age group(s) the DBT program will serve. The advantages to limiting treatment to particular age groups (early, middle, or late adolescence) within adolescence include increased homogeneity in terms of life issues, possibly leading to a greater connection to peers in group settings. However, constraints such as limited referrals or staff may necessitate a mixed-age program for adolescents. Again as a point of reference, most programs who responded to our survey accept patients ranging from 12 to 18 or 19 years of age, mixed together in skills groups.

Another factor to consider is gender and whether to admit both girls and boys, and then whether to include boys and girls together in groups. Some residential treatment settings are limited to treating one gender or else separate the genders into different residences. But most other settings admit boys and girls. Limiting skills group to a single gender allows for greater homogeneity of issues brought into group and perhaps greater comfort with self-disclosure. Further, it minimizes the degree of disruptive or distracted behavior due to factors such as heterosexual flirting or increased social anxiety due to the presence of the opposite sex. Yet combining males and females can make it possible to provide treatment for boys given the relatively lower percentage of male referrals (given the higher rate of intentional self-injury behavior in females). The presence of both genders can enhance development of skillful opposite-sex relationships.

What, If Any, Modifications to Standard DBT Should Be Considered with Adolescents?

In using DBT with adolescents, the functions of standard comprehensive DBT remain the same (see Chapter 1). Many problems and barriers encountered when adopting DBT for use with adolescents are related to the treatment setting more than to the age of the patients. Rather than repeat that information on treatment setting here, we instead focus on those aspects of implementation specific to adolescents as a group. The interested reader is referred to chapters on DBT in particular settings (outpatient, inpatient, forensic) and to Webster-Stratton and Taylor (1998) for technical assistance regarding the use of evidence-based treatments in general with adolescents. Nevertheless, we believe some problems and barriers that are specific to the age of clients justify modification of standard DBT or require emphases on certain strategies in DBT. We discuss family involvement, directly targeting common dialectical dilemmas of adolescents and families, and emphasis on DBT strategies tailored to enhance motivation, attention, and engagement.

The first modification we encourage is family involvement in skills training and family therapy sessions (Miller et al., 2002). In DBT, the etiology and maintenance of problems is conceptualized as a transactional process between an individual's vulnerability to emotion dysregulation and an invalidating environment. While there are instances where DBT therapists intervene in the environment on patients' behalf, the emphasis in DBT is on consulting to patients about how they themselves can effect changes in their own environment. In other words, rather than intervening on behalf of patients to effect changes or instructing others about how to deal with patients, DBT therapists emphasize that the patient him- or herself learn the requisite skills to independently manage and shape his or her social network on an ongoing basis. While a similar spirit pervades work with adolescents, direct environmental intervention may be particularly needed with this age group to decrease suicidal behavior and other important targets. Environmental intervention may be required because adolescents (particularly younger adolescents) often lack power to effect change in their environments (e.g., school administration, parents) and do not have the same degree of autonomy as adults, legally or otherwise, to make their own decisions. Further, because family relationships themselves are associated with the outcome and progress of adolescents' treatment, they are a logical focus of direct environmental intervention (Henggeler, Schoenwald, Rowland, & Cunningham, 2002). Consequently, family involvement may be needed to adequately treat primary targets and to structure the environment to ensure treatment progress. Similarly, cognitive and intellectual development often affect the rate at which an adolescent is able to assimilate and employ skills and problem solving. Thus, young patients often require additional support and assistance. Increased attention to generalization may be necessary with adolescents; family involvement can be helpful in this regard also. For these reasons, many adolescent DBT programs encourage parents to become as involved as possible and view parents as partners in the treatment team.

Should family participation be optional or mandatory for a youth to participate in a DBT program? Program evaluation data from an established adolescent DBT program suggest that more important than family members' actual participation in treatment is their "positive attitude" toward the treatment program (Halaby, 2004). It may be that as long as parents support the idea of therapy and encourage their teens to attend the DBT program, the adolescents will be more likely to continue in treatment and not drop out. In practice, based on responses to our survey, there is variability in how DBT programs involve parents, from little or no involvement to required caregiver attendance in weekly skills training and family therapy sessions. In part, such decisions are constrained by resources: Are there staff trained to conduct family therapy with families who usually exhibit high emotional intensity? Is there a large enough space to house a multifamily group and skills trainers comfortable managing a large mixed group of teens and adults? But such decisions should not be constrained only by resources. Instead, the guiding principle here is to consider whether each function of treatment is being accomplished to a sufficient level to make progress on therapy goals. It is our experience that, for multiproblem suicidal adolescents, adequate treatment of high-order targets requires direct attention to generalization and structuring the environment, and that this is most directly accomplished via caregiver involvement. While some adolescents with less severe or pervasive difficulties may not need as comprehensive treatment, for those who do, involvement of caretakers may make a tremendous difference. When practical obstacles arise to caregiver involvement, be creative. For example, sometimes family involvement is difficult because the family lives far from the DBT program (particularly for many residential and inpatient settings). Programs have creatively used the one family session that occurs during the initial intake to orient family members to DBT; they have scheduled weekly family sessions by phone; they have DBT program staff offer indirect support to families by coaching the adolescent patients to "teach" their parents the skills they learn. One program provides parents with a DBT skills manual as a method of orienting parents to the treatment. Our advice is to include caretakers—whether weekly, monthly, or as needed—to best address generalization and help structure the environment to enable treatment gains.

Many of the adolescents referred to a DBT program may be in foster care systems or dependents of the state. In other cases an adolescent may be interested in the therapy, but living with parents who are unwilling to engage in therapy with them. In these cases, decisions about who "counts" as family and whether the youth can participate without family arise. The key here is to be guided by the functions we are trying to accomplish via family involvement: assisting generalization and structuring the environment. With this in mind, selection of who will participate with the adolescent can be flexible. For example, an adolescent living in a group facility without a DBT orientation can invite one adult from the living situation to participate with him or her in DBT. Adolescents whose parents are unwilling or unable to attend the skills training class can identify a family friend or someone perceived as a mentor who is willing to attend the skills training class.

In one instance the case manager for a child who was the dependent of the state initiated DBT, and various additional caregivers participated in DBT with the youth. The teen had recently been removed from a foster mother, with whom he had lived for several years, after his violent behavior resulted in property destruction in the home. As a child he had suffered significant neglect and physical abuse and had been removed from his biological parents during his preschool years. When he first met the DBT individual therapist he stated his goal was to "stay out of trouble" so he could go back home (to his foster mother). In this case, a central treatment issue was how to assist the young man in generalizing skills to his environment. The treatment initially involved meeting with the various people responsible for his care including case managers, case aides, his previous foster mother, and his current foster parents. A plan was devised for the therapist to meet weekly with the young man, his previous foster mother, and his current foster parents for skills training. In addition, the young man met with the therapist weekly for individual therapy. The DBT therapists met monthly with the young man's community-based team to monitor progress, and to ensure that his multiple care providers were using the language of DBT skills in the multiple contexts of his life. As his behavior stabilized, he and the foster mother to whom he was so attached joined the multifamily skills training class, while he continued in individual therapy, and another therapist was specifically assigned to assist his foster mother during his transition back to her home. This illustrates a very intensive outpatient treatment protocol in which caregiver involvement was crucial to accomplish the generalization and structuring of the environment needed for the adolescent to make and sustain needed changes.

The Key Role of the Biosocial Theory

When involving family and caretakers, the biosocial theory plays a key role. Adults in the youth's life often view problem behavior as deliberately manipulative. Thus, caretakers may attempt to regain control of their adolescent's behavior via punishment and coercion strategies. The biosocial theory helps caretakers (and therapists) maintain a more compassionate, nonblaming stance toward their adolescent's behavior. This increases the likelihood that parents will feel less defensive about "failing" to control their child and will feel motivated to participate in their child's treatment.

When presenting the biosocial theory, the therapist faces the challenge of avoiding overemphasizing the teen's or the parents' role in problems, and staying true to the transactional nature of the theory. Pointers include practicing a nonjudgmental stance, stressing the transactional nature of the theory, staying dialectical, discussing the importance of not validating what is invalid, and focusing on specific behaviors rather than on the "global environment." Do not oversimplify the model by portraying the teen as being emotionally vulnerable and the parent as invalidating; instead, make the case that both can act out of high emotional vulnerability, and both can engage in invalidation. For example, below is a script that demonstrates the initial points of transaction, biological vulnerability, and invalidation of the biosocial theory.

> "DBT is a therapy that helps people regulate their emotions. It is based on the notion that the core of the problems that your family is experiencing is related to difficulty regulating emotions. Now, at the heart of this is the belief that some people come into the world with a basic level of vulnerability to things that provoke emotions that is higher than what it may be for others. For example, when something happens they may respond much more quickly, they may have a much more intense response than most people may have, and it may take a really long time to get over things. It's believed that this sensitivity is based in the biology of the brain. If there's anything that I hope you'll really remember from this session, it is that brains are different. [Writes the words 'Brains are different' on the board.] As a person who's worked in children's mental health, it's easy for me to believe that brains are different and that some people are born with more sensitivity to things than others. For example, I've had parents tell me that for some unexplained reason they could not get their child to stop crying when they were infants, or some parents have told me their child would act aggressively, long before the child could speak a word. So it's easy for me to be convinced that at the basic level of biology our brains are different and we respond differently to the emotional stimulation in the world. Now just think about this in your own family. Has there ever been a time when something has happened and for one person in the family it is a big thing? [Draws a horizontal continuum on the board and on the left side of the continuum writes 'A big deal.'] And then you noticed that for somebody else in your family the same event seems like no big deal. [Writes 'No big deal' on the right side of the continuum.] And then have you noticed that sometimes what happens is that the person for whom this is no big deal looks at the person for whom this is a really big deal and thinks, or maybe even says, 'You are overreacting.' [Writes 'Overreacting' on the left side of the continuum.] And the person for whom this is a really big deal looks at the person for whom this is no big deal, either thinks to themselves, or even says out loud to the other person, 'How can you be so insensitive?' or 'How can you be so cold?' [Writes the statements on the right hand of the continuum.] Now the point I'd like to make is that the reactions of these two people in your family are not necessarily because they are cold, or because they are overreacting, but rather that for some people it really is no big deal, and for other people it truly is a big deal, and that brains are different. Now, imagine you are a child for whom it is a big deal, and you are told, 'You're making too big deal out of this,' or 'Just ignore it,' or 'Stop crying, there's no reason to cry.' The person saying this to the child may actually have good intentions for saying these things, but as a

child you are left in the utter confusion of trying to figure why things are such a big deal for you when you are being told things are 'no big deal,' and you can't figure out your own emotional experience because the world's telling you that you're wrong. And what you're left with is the inability to trust your emotional experience. Should this happen repeatedly over time, then you're left with not really having a very strong sense of who you are as person. Now let me be clear, there are certain things that one does not want to validate. For example, if a child comes home and says, 'Oh, today I figured out how to kill somebody and not get caught,' this is not the time for parents to warmly reflect what their child has said to them, and respond, 'Good thinking!' It is not effective to validate what is invalid. But when one has strong emotional reactions, and one is repeatedly told that the reaction is inaccurate, then self-doubt sets in, along with the eventual inability to regulate that very intense experience. So what we want to help you do in this program is to understand the emotions you and your family members experience, and to understand that some people's reactions truly are more sensitive, stronger, and last longer. We also want teach you how you can learn to manage your emotional experiences, even if you do have emotions that happen faster, are larger, and last longer. You can even use your sensitivity to advantage."

If the initial introduction to the biosocial theory can be done in a nonjudgmental and truly transactional manner, it demonstrates an understanding of the youth and the family's circumstances and sets the stage for validation and collaboration.

Parent Involvement in Skills Training and Family Therapy

Parent involvement in both skills training and family therapy can be used in DBT to directly target factors associated with high-risk behavior and to assist with generalization. We next discuss the various ways to provide skills training to family members and then discuss particulars of family therapy in DBT.

Family Skills Training

An unmodified adoption of the adult version of DBT would be to have a teens-only skills training group. But, as mentioned above, when caretakers also learn skills, they can gently serve as skills "coaches" in the home to foster generalization as well as develop their own skills to directly decrease their contribution to family conflict. In practice, nearly all adolescent DBT programs involve caretakers in skills training, although a few DBT programs do not include the parents in any aspect of skills training and instead only involve them in family therapy sessions.

There are many formats used to teach DBT skills to parents. One option is to have each youth bring an adult and join in a multifamily skills training group (MFSTG). Creating an MFSTG allows for family members to learn the behavioral skills alongside their teens. This format depathologizes the teen since many family members are able to acknowledge their own need to learn these skills. The MFSTG format has an advantage over an adolescent-only group because the teens maintain better behavioral control when more adults are seated around the table. Program administrators may appreciate this format because it conserves resources by maintaining one skills group instead of two separate groups for adolescents and adults. Another advantage of the parents joining the multifamily group is that they can enhance attendance by bringing their teens to treatment—

no small thing, as many adolescents attending outpatient treatment rely on these adults for transportation to sessions.

Given that family members attend the skills training group and are expected to learn the material and practice the skills themselves between sessions, a further option is to offer between-session coaching for family members. Thus, similar to their teenager, the family members are encouraged to page one of the skills trainers for coaching on how to apply relevant skills when they are in enough distress to warrant a telephone consultation.

Another option is to offer separate groups, one for teens and another for family members. One perceived advantage here is that teaching skills directly to parents but separately from the teens allows both groups "more space to better express their feelings." However, DBT skills training groups are not process-oriented; rather, the expectation is to learn together in a more didactic setting with a deemphasis on sharing personal information. One significant disadvantage of separate groups is that the adolescent and parents lose an opportunity to observe each other and participate jointly in the learning of the skills. Running separate groups may also require additional staff (two groups instead of one), which may be a practical barrier.

Another option, as in standard DBT, is to offer individualized skills training for the family concurrent with the patient's therapy, with a different DBT therapist for the parents. For example, monthly sessions might be offered in order to address parent training in the areas of contingency management, validation, and problem solving. In residential treatment settings (inpatient and forensic settings), there is often a greater emphasis on milieu therapy as the primary means of facilitating generalization rather than on family skills training. For example, to ensure generalization, all milieu staff apply DBT strategies in every interaction. They provide impromptu validation, skills coaching, behavioral rehearsal, and consultation to the patient as needed throughout the day.

Family Therapy

Another way to directly target factors that influence high-risk behaviors and to assist with enhancing capabilities and ensuring generalization is family therapy. In DBT with adolescents, family therapy sessions can be woven throughout the treatment and often include family behavioral analyses of target behavior, and directly target invalidation, ineffective use of contingency management, and skills deficits particularly in the interpersonal realm (Miller et al., 2002; Woodberry, Miller, Glinski, Indik, & Mitchell, 2002).

For anyone who has done chain analyses exclusively with individuals, it can be quite illuminating the first time a chain analysis is done with a family. Such events bring to mind experiments from social psychology demonstrating the various stories told by multiple witnesses to the same event. While it may be indicated to conduct the analysis with all family members present, some therapists opt to have the adolescent do his or hers in individual therapy, the parents do theirs in another session, and then bring the two different versions of the event together in a joint session. When skillfully handled, such that it doesn't turn into a battle between two different versions of the story, it can be helpful for family members to understand that very different perspectives are at play in a particular event in their lives. It is not uncommon for someone who has harmed him- or herself in response to family conflict to discover that the thoughts and feelings of other family members were very different from what they perceived. On the other hand, it can allow for validation of accurate perceptions of conflict in the family, as well as highlight the consequences of such conflict. At that point, the entire family can engage in the design of skills to target those conflicts.

Another way to meet the functions of structuring the environment and ensuring generalization is to orient the adolescent's support network (e.g., school personnel, case managers, relatives) to DBT treatment goals, objectives, and expectations. As in multisystemic therapy (Huey et al., 2004), the goal is to help orient the adolescent's network to the current problems so that they are involved and assume greater responsibility for helping the adolescent navigate through the next phase of his or her life. This may involve certain people assuming the role of skills coach in the community while others may need to be better able to apply positive and aversive contingencies. A collaborative relationship with other agencies increases a patient's opportunity to gain support in generalization of skills and contingency management across various settings in their different environments (home, school).

One issue to consider when making program decisions about family involvement is what to do if the youth drops out but the family wants to continue. There are cases when even the most skillful therapists have difficulty engaging adolescents who are unwilling to be involved in treatment. In one such instance an adolescent had been involved in therapy, including participation in an adolescent-only skills training group. Prior to entering the DBT program, she had been in a residential facility for substance abuse. When the DBT program decided to shift to skills training with multifamily groups, rather than adolescent-only groups, this young woman began attending with her parents. During the course of the 6-month curriculum the young woman became involved in drugs again and began missing therapy. At the point of four consecutive misses the consultation team was faced with the question of what to do about her parents' involvement in the MFSTG. The parents asked to continue with skills training without their daughter. The consultation team decided, after weighing therapeutic, ethical, and institutional concerns, to allow them to continue. They appreciated the ongoing support from other families in the class, and they focused on learning skills so that they themselves could regulate their emotions and be clear about the contingencies when responding to their daughter.

Directly Targeting Adolescent–Family Dialectical Dilemmas

Another modification to standard DBT when using it with adolescents is to consider directly targeting the common set of adolescent–family dialectical dilemmas and corresponding secondary targets described by Rathus and Miller (2000) that supplement those described by Linehan (1993a) in standard DBT with adults. These central dialectical dilemmas reflect polarized behavior patterns including excessive leniency versus authoritarian control, normalizing pathological behaviors versus pathologizing normative behaviors, and forcing autonomy versus fostering dependence. The secondary treatment targets are aimed at achieving a synthesis between the polarities inherent in each dilemma.

Excessive Leniency versus Authoritarian Control

Parents and adolescents can at times vacillate between being excessively lenient and authoritarian. "Excessive leniency" refers to making too few behavioral demands of adolescents (or, for adolescents, to making too few demands on themselves). With this excessive permissiveness, parents of suicidal adolescents may relinquish many of their rules or standards; many report feeling coerced by their children's suicidality and emotional dysregulation. Adolescents also face similar conflicts with excessive leniency, often pushing their environments to let them live according to their own standards but later facing negative consequences. Following a period of a lack of controls, and the resultant negative consequences, the adolescent, parents, or other involved authority figures (e.g., therapist, inpatient unit staff, teachers) will commonly flip to the other extreme of overly tight controls: a move to the authoritarian control pole of the behavior pattern.

"Authoritarian control" refers to holding tight reins on behavior, by coercive methods of limiting freedom, autonomy, and decision making. Certain adolescents themselves will at times apply harsh restrictions to themselves ("I won't watch any TV after school until after the next marking period so I can get my grades up"). When these extreme methods of exerting control fail, parents and adolescents alike tend to become demoralized and revert to an excessively lenient approach.

The parents' dialectical dilemma here involves vacillating between the extremes of being overly permissive with their adolescents on the one hand and setting overly restrictive limits on the other, often to compensate for a period of perceived overpermissiveness. The first corresponding treatment target involves Increasing Authoritative Discipline while Decreasing Excessive Leniency. This target involves establishing a reasonable degree of parental authority (or self-discipline) while reducing excessive leniency, following an authoritative parenting style (Baumrind, 1991a, 1991b). The second corresponding treatment target involves Increasing Adolescent Self-Determination while Decreasing Authoritarian Control. This target involves establishing a reasonable degree of parental permissiveness without abdicating all parental authority or neglecting the adolescent's needs for external controls.

Pathologizing Normative Behaviors versus Normalizing Pathological Behaviors

Parents and adolescents in treatment vacillate between viewing normal behaviors as pathological and pathological behaviors as normal. Distinguishing between the normal and the pathological may become especially confusing for parents since typical adolescent behaviors include several that overlap with features of borderline personality disorder, such as unstable identity, high-risk behaviors, relationship instability, and emotional lability. Developmentally normative adolescent behaviors include those which are commonly observed within the teenage years (e.g., experimentation with drugs, alcohol, and sexuality; changing goals or self-image; frequent breakups of romantic relationships; interpersonal conflicts, particularly with parents; moodiness), but which *do not* result in self-harm, hospitalization, school dropout, or other life-threatening or severe quality-of-life-impairing consequences. The dialectical dilemma for the parent here involves recognizing and allowing normal adolescent behavior while, at the same time, identifying and addressing those behaviors that are linked to severe dysfunction or negative consequences. For the adolescent, the dialectical dilemma similarly involves recognizing normal versus abnormal behavior, as suicidal adolescents in treatment often fluctuate between second guessing normal behaviors and rationalizing dysfunctional behaviors.

The corresponding treatment targets include Increasing Recognition of Normative Behaviors while Decreasing Pathologizing of Normative Behaviors. Psychoeducation regarding normative behaviors is essential, as is consideration of whether the behavior in question was carried out impulsively or is functionally linked with a target-relevant maladaptive behavior. The second corresponding treatment target is Increasing Identification of Pathological Behaviors while Decreasing Normalization of Pathological Behaviors. This also involves psychoeducation as well as intuitive judgments about the normative nature, comfort level, and risk level of particular behaviors.

Fostering Dependence versus Forcing Autonomy

"Fostering dependence" refers to acting in ways that serve to stifle the adolescent's natural movement toward autonomy. For example, a parent may engage in excessive caretaking, leaving the adolescent unprepared to negotiate the world on his or her own. For the adolescent, fostering dependence may include behavior demonstrated by overreliance on parents. "Forcing autonomy," on the other hand, involves prematurely thrusting the adolescent toward separation and greater self-sufficiency. While adolescents normally increase autonomy, this can occur to the extreme in suicidal, borderline adolescents. Parents of such teens will at times push them toward independence or reject them, often as a result of giving up, feeling exasperated, or burned out. At the same time, adolescents may force their own autonomy by letting go too fast out of an impulsive reaction to conflict or desire to prove themselves. For the parent, the dialectical dilemma here necessitates finding the middle way between clinging or stifling caretaking, and pushing away precipitously. For the adolescent, the dilemma entails achieving a balance between an effective and comfortable degree of relatedness and dependence while working toward an effective and comfortable degree of separation, individuation, and identity formation.

The corresponding treatment targets include Increasing Individuation while Decreasing Excessive Dependence. This target involves teaching parents to balance consultation to their children in how to negotiate their environments with direct environmental interventions. The second corresponding treatment target involves Increasing Effective Reliance on Others while Decreasing Excessive Autonomy. This target involves both parents and adolescents remaining connected enough to enhance effective outcomes for the adolescent. Although adolescents have begun a journey toward separation and individuation from parents, they lack the experience and judgment to negotiate situations entirely on their own. Moreover, adolescents with suicidal behaviors or borderline features lack critical behavioral capacities. Interventions include regulating the amount of distance between parents and adolescents and enhancing communication between parent and child, so that parents can offer and adolescents can ask for guidance. In addition to the newly formulated dialectical behavior patterns (Rathus & Miller, 2000), Miller, Rathus, and Linehan (2007) have added a new skills module entitled "Walking the Middle Path Skills." These additional skills address nonbalanced thinking and behavior among teens and significant others, such as family members, therapists, and friends. These skills involve learning principles of behavior change (e.g., positive reinforcement, shaping, effective punishment), validation (both of self and other), and finding the middle path between common dialectical dilemmas in these interactions with adolescents (as mentioned above).

We now turn to three further topics that, while not a departure from standard DBT, may be given more emphasis with adolescents: creating options for briefer treatment length, the use of booster sessions/graduate groups to further assist generalization, and simplifying the language on skills materials and diary cards.

Length of Treatment and Use of Booster or Continuation Treatment

For adults, data support a 1-year or 6-month outpatient program (Koons et al., 2001). Yet, in our experience, the variability in the needs of adolescents sometimes means that even briefer treatment is sufficient. In practice, among adolescent DBT programs we surveyed, the length of treatment varies from setting to setting. For example, some adolescent outpatient programs offer an abbreviated (e.g., 16 weeks) initial phase of treatment, others a year-long program. (As has been mentioned in the chapters on inpatient and residential/forensic settings, length of treatment in inpatient and residential program varies widely from several days to several months to several years. We will primarily discuss outpatient adolescent DBT here.) On the one hand, some teens with BPD features may not need the longer term treatments that adults with more entrenched personality and behavioral problems require. Further, therapists may more easily "sell" a shorter, 16-week outpatient program than a 6-month or 1-year treatment to adolescents who are not always sure why they need any treatment right now, let alone long-term treatment. Adolescents may also be more likely to remain in treatment when there is a clear end in sight. On the other hand, a shorter length of treatment might not be sufficient to treat those adolescents with severe emotional and behavioral dysregulation and suicidality. Because documented rates of relapse and recurrence among depressed adolescents are high, clinical researchers have recommended either booster or continuation treatment to address this problem in briefer treatments (Birmaher et al., 2000).

One solution to meeting these various needs is to offer an abbreviated 16-week program that can be augmented as needed by offering a continuation phase of treatment (e.g., a graduate or maintenance group or by allowing for a repetition of the program; Miller et al., 2007). For example, the DBT Program at Montefiore Medical Center offers an acute phase of comprehensive DBT that lasts 16 weeks. At the end of 16 weeks four options are reviewed for the adolescent. First, those who are still significantly struggling with Stage 1 targets are invited to repeat a second 16-week acute phase of treatment. Second, adolescents who have successfully completed the acute phase of treatment (i.e., reduced life-threatening, therapy-interfering, and severe quality-of-life behaviors) are awarded a diploma in a graduation ceremony for the MFSTG. These individuals are also invited to join the "Graduate Group" and may choose to discontinue individual therapy. Third, those in the middle, who have made some improvement yet still need more help gaining control of intentional self-injury or substance abuse, have the option of repeating the acute phase of treatment or moving to the Graduate Group while continuing with individual therapy. This decision is made by the treatment team, including the therapist, adolescent, parents, and DBT consultation team. Finally, the fourth choice is to discontinue treatment altogether after 16 weeks.

The Graduate Group comprises adolescent graduates and two therapists. This treatment phase is less time-intensive, consisting of 90-minute groups once per week for 16 weeks with the opportunity to recontract for an additional 16 weeks if the adolescent is able to identify clear treatment goals. While telephone consultation to adolescents is still used in this modality, individual therapy may cease and family members no longer participate in group. Adolescents who do not continue with a primary individual therapist are eligible for as-needed individual or family sessions led by one of the group therapists during enrollment in the Graduate Group. The primary goal of the Graduate Group is to prevent relapse by reinforcing the progress made in the first 16 weeks and to help patients generalize their behavioral skills. The group leaders encourage the adolescents to "consult" with, validate, and reinforce one another, with less emphasis on the therapist, to more effectively manage their current life problems. In fact, each group begins with a different adolescent teaching a skill to his or her peers. An agenda is then set and adolescents use peer coaching and support to address members' current life problems. This group tends to be highly engaging for adolescents, as they come to rely more on one another, depend less on the adult therapists, and build their sense of mastery. These options of repeating the acute phase, moving to a maintenance or a booster phase that focuses on generalization with as-needed access to additional individual or family therapy, provide many ways to tailor treatment length to the adolescents needs. While adjusting the length of treatment or spacing final sessions to ensure maintenance of gains is common practice in DBT with adults, such flexibility may be particularly important in meeting the needs of adolescents in DBT.

Modifying Skills Training

The last modification of standard DBT we discuss is whether one must modify skills training materials and methods of teaching to the age group. With any skills training group, but particularly with a teens-only group, an emphasis on using more experiential and *in vivo* practice exercises *during* group (e.g., role playing, lively discussions related to specific experiences) keeps the groups less didactic and more stimulating for teens. For example, activities like a group juggle can help with the problem of limited attention when impulsive adolescents are required to sit still and also beautifully demonstrates various elements of mindfulness. Similarly, it can be useful to refer to between-session assignments to practice the skills as "practice exercises" rather than as "homework" in order to disassociate this learning from school work, which for many teens (as well as adults!) has a negative connotation.

Another modification often considered in using DBT with adolescents is whether Linehan's (1993b) skills handouts themselves should be modified to make the material easier to understand conceptually as well as to make the content more age-appropriate for teens. While modifications like expanding the pleasant activities list to include playing video games and basketball are noncontroversial, simplifying the language and shortening handouts can become problematic. Besides the obvious problems with modifying copyright-protected materials, changing the skills to make material easier to understand is difficult to do without altering the essence of the skills. Consequently, as a rule, we suggest starting with standard DBT handouts and teaching them to the best of your ability. You can adapt your examples to fit the population you are teaching, whether it be adolescents or families. Finally, evaluate your outcomes, perhaps looking specifically at designing a way to evaluate whether the skills you think need to be simplified actually are "too difficult."

Confidentiality and Treatment of Suicidal Adolescents

A DBT therapist working with adolescents is faced with all of the ethical challenges of working with a high-risk population and then some. Treatment of intentional self-injury in adolescents uses the same protocols and strategies used with adult/standard DBT. Traditional outpatient treatment settings have sent patients to the emergency room when they report serious suicidal ideation. Yet given the absence of data that hospitalization reduces suicidal behavior, DBT favors an approach to managing intentional self-injury on an outpatient basis (for many reasons, including avoidance of reinforcement for escalation of suicidal behavior). This represents a strong shift in thinking that feels threatening to parents and caretakers as well as many clinicians and administrators. Because of patients' age and the likelihood of family involvement in therapy, issues of confidentiality can be more pressing in working with suicidal adolescents using DBT.

One challenge specific to working with adolescents involves the flow of information between the adolescent and his or her family via the therapist, which can be particularly challenging when one person provides both the individual and the family therapy. The first thing to be aware of is the statutory requirement regarding an adolescent's legal right to seek treatment independent of parental consent, as well as the minor's rights regarding privileged information. Due consideration must also be given to variations of parents' rights to seek treatment for their adolescent children, as well as their rights to review the child's record. In the United States, statutory requirements vary by state. In some states, adolescents over a certain age have full rights to invoke privilege. In other states, the parents are allowed liberal access to their child's medical and mental health records. These issues have critical bearing on how information is handled with adolescents and their families who are in treatment with each other. In most jurisdictions there are requirements to break confidence in life-threatening situations. The adolescent must be informed of this mandate.

However, there are many situations where the line about whether something is life-threatening is not clear (as is the case with chronic self-injury that often serves to regulate emotions but is not imminently life-threatening). While intentional self-injury increases the long-term risk for suicide, it does not always create imminent risk of death. Therapeutically, there are no hard and fast rules about communication of self-injurious behavior that is not imminently life-threatening. The guiding principles of dialectics will prove useful. Critical factors include the risk of imminent harm (actual risk based on data vs. perceived risk), the task of responding to high-risk, self-injurious behaviors without intentionally reinforcing them, and managing the risk of liability (e.g., by maintaining a cooperative, open relationship with the family that serves all parties well in the event of serious injury or death).

For example, on the one hand, completely open lines of communication can allow family members to serve a critical role in the analysis of the chain of events leading to self-injury, and family involvement can lead to significant therapeutic gain. Yet, on the other hand, interpersonal conflict is one of the highest ranked precipitants of attempted suicide by adolescents (Miller & Glinski, 2000) and the youth and/or therapist sharing information may itself produce high conflict.

One synthesis can come from adopting a collaborative approach that explicitly outlines ground rules for the sharing of information, limits of confidentiality, and crisis response. For example, in one case a therapist was meeting with an adolescent and her family for the initial treatment planning. This included ground rules for the sharing of information, limits of confidentiality, and crisis planning. As the adolescent became bored with the process she asked, "Why do we have to do all this?" The mother responded, "Because if you kill yourself, I'll sue him." The therapist then responded with direct, matter-of-fact discussion of the risks inherent to therapy so that all family members could give meaningful consent. "Yes, it's important that we all know what we are getting into. You all (indicating all family members) are here because in the past you (indicating the adolescent) have felt suicidal. It is important for you all to realize that no psychotherapy program can stop someone from killing him- or herself if he or she decides to commit suicide. Thus, our treatment program is best thought of as a 'life worth living program,' and not as a 'suicide prevention program.' Today we are talking through how we want to handle crises together, how we will communicate about risks, what actions we will take if you are at risk of killing yourself. Our approach is to provide you with coaching and support in making your life into what you want it to be. In doing that, in making such changes, it can be extremely difficult and stressful. Today's meeting is really about this: we are all in this together. We are all part of your treatment team, and we all manage risk together." Explicit discussions like these help establish a collaborative approach with the adolescent's family and clear expectations about managing suicide risk.

In families where conflict is high around self-injury, it may be recommended that self-injury not be discussed with family members until skills are developed that can help decrease the conflict that might ensue. In such situations it is important for the therapist to remember the high-level trust they are expecting parents to place in a relative stranger, namely the therapist. Given this reality, it is helpful for the therapist to assure the parents of his or her ongoing vigilance regarding the issue and explicitly discuss how intentional self-injury is treated in DBT. Here too the therapist can make it clear that although it may be clinically indicated that the therapist not disclose information, he or she welcomes the parents to provide information to the therapist and makes clear how information provided is shared with the adolescent. This serves the purpose of gathering useful information from the parents, and minimizes the likelihood that the parents will feel cut off from the process. The therapist should also make clear that in situations where information needs to be shared with parents, it is in keeping with the principles of DBT to urge and coach the teen to tell the parents him- or herself to stay true to the consultation to the patient strategy. If the adolescent is unwilling to provide the necessary information to parents, and it is clear that confidentiality needs to be broken, it is often helpful to inform the adolescent of the rationale for disclosing the information, and, unless it is contraindicated, to let the adolescent know beforehand that the disclosure will occur. Direct, explicit negotiation at the onset of therapy regarding the ground rules and agreements regarding confidentiality, sharing information, and handling crises help both parents and the youth to not be caught off guard in distressing moments. Similar explicit agreements about other information that one is not required to report (e.g., substance abuse, eating disordered behavior) and decisions related to disclosure of this information can be made on the basis of what is clinically indicated. Even in jurisdictions that provide the adolescent with a full right to invoke privilege, expectations and roles can be made clear and mutually agreed upon from the beginning in order to open lines of communication. The development of confidentiality agreements and continued consultation with hospital/clinic legal department representatives can also be very important steps to successfully address these concerns.

Many factors make working with chronically suicidal, multiproblem adolescents challenging. DBT offers an alternative to treatment as usual that may reduce intentional self-injury and the use of expensive psychiatric services for this population. It is our belief that by paying particular attention to the functions of generalization and structuring of the environment (e.g., by incorporating caregivers, providing alternative lengths of treatment) DBT can be modified or strategies of DBT emphasized to best meet the needs of adolescents. We hope that this chapter helps you consider how DBT makes sense in your setting and provides useful guidelines as you develop your DBT program for adolescents.

NOTE

1. At least two randomized controlled studies conducted by at least two different research groups (Chambless & Sanderson, 1997).

REFERENCES

Baumrind, D. (1991a). The influence of parenting style on adolescent competence and substance use. *Journal of Early Adolescence, 11,* 56–95.

Baumrind, D. (1991b). Parenting styles and adolescent development. In R. Lerner, AC Petersen, & J. Brooks-Gunn (Eds.), *Encyclopedia of adolescence* (pp. xx–xx). New York: Garland.

Berk, L. E. (2004). *Infants, children, and adolescents* (5th ed.). Boston: Allyn & Bacon.

Birmaher, B., Brent, D. A., Kolko, D., Baugher, M., Bridge, J., Holder, D., et al. (2000). Clinical outcome after short-term psychotherapy for adolescents with major depressive disorder. *Archives of General Psychiatry, 57,* 29–36.

Brown, B. B. (1990). Peer groups. In S. Feldman & G. Elliot (Eds.), *At the threshold: The developing adolescent* (pp. 171–196). Cambridge, UK: Cambridge University Press.

Clarke, G. N., Rohde, P., Lewinsohn, P. M., Hops, H., & Seeley, J. R. (1999). Cognitive-behavioral treatment of adolescent depression: Efficacy of acute group treatment and booster sessions. *Journal of the American Academy of Child and Adolescent Psychiatry, 38,* 272–279.

Dishion, T. J., McCord, J., & Poulin, F. (1999). When interventions harm: Peer groups and problem behavior. *American Psychologist, 54*(9), 755–764.

Halaby, K. S. (2004). Variables predicting noncompliance with short-term dialectical behavior therapy for suicidal and parasuicidal adolescents. *Dissertation Abstracts International, 65,* (06), 3160B. (UMI No. AAI3135769)

Henggeler, S. W., Shoenwald, S. K., Rowland, M. D., & Cunningham, P. B. (2002). *Serious emotional disturbance in children and adolescents: Multisystemic therapy.* New York: Guilford Press.

Huey, S. J., Henggeler, S. W., Rowland, M. D., Halliday-Boykins, C. A., Cunningham, P. B., et al. (2004). Multisystemic therapy effects on attempted suicide by youths presenting psychiatric emergencies. *Journal of the American Academy of Child and Adolescent Psychiatry, 43,* 183–190.

Katz, L. Y., Gunasekara, S., Cox, B. J., & Miller, A. L. (2004). Feasibility of dialectical behavior therapy for parasuicidal adolescent inpatients. *Journal of the American Academy of Child and Adolescent Psychiatry, 43,* 276–282.

Katz, L. Y., Gunasekara, S., & Miller, A. L. (2002). Dialectical behavior therapy for inpatient and outpatient parasuicidal adolescents. *Annals of Adolescent Psychiatry, 26,* 161–178.

Linehan, M. M. (1993a). *Cognitive-behavioral treatment of borderline personality disorder.* New York: Guilford Press.

Linehan, M. M. (1993b). *Skills training manual for treating borderline personality disorder.* New York: Guilford Press.

Linehan, M. M. (2000). Commentary on innovations in dialectical behavior therapy. *Cognitive and Behavioral Therapy, 7*(4), 478–481.

Linehan, M. M., Armstrong, H. E., Suarez, A., Allmon, D., & Heard, H. L. (1991). Cognitive-behavioral treatment of chronically parasuicidal borderline patients. *Archives of General Psychiatry, 48,* 1060–1064.

Koons, C. R., Robins, C. J., Tweed, J. L., Lynch, T. R., Gonzalez, A. M., Morse, J. Q., et al. (2001). Efficacy of dialectical behavior therapy in women veterans with borderline personality disorder. *Behavior Therapy, 32,* 371–390.

Miller, A. L., & Glinski, J. (2000). Youth suicidal behavior: Assessment and intervention. *Journal of Clinical Psychology, 56*(9), 1–22.

Miller, A. L., Glinski, J., Woodberry, K., Mitchell, A., & Indik, J. (2002). Family therapy and dialectical behavior therapy with adolescents: Part 1. Proposing a clinical synthesis. *American Journal of Psychotherapy, 56*(4), 568–584.

Miller, A. L., Rathus, J. H., & Linehan, M. M. (2007). *Dialectical behavior therapy with suicidal adolescents.* New York: Guilford Press.

Miller, A. L., Rathus, J. H., Linehan, M. M., Wetzler, S., & Leigh, E. (1997). Dialectical behavior therapy adapted for suicidal adolescents. *Journal of Practical Psychiatry and Behavioral Health, 3,* 78–86.

Mufson, L., Dorta, K. P., Moreau, D., & Weissman, M. M. (2004). *Interpersonal psychotherapy for depressed adolescents* (2nd ed.). New York: Guilford Press.

Rathus, J. H., & Miller, A. L. (2000). DBT for adolescents: Dialectical dilemmas and secondary treatment targets. *Cognitive and Behavioral Practice*, 7, 425–434.

Rathus, J. H., & Miller, A. L. (2002). Dialectical behavior therapy adapted for suicidal adolescents. *Suicide and Life-Threatening Behaviors*, 32(2), 146–157.

Trautman, P. D., Stewart, N., & Morishima, A. (1993). Are adolescent suicide attempters noncompliant with outpatient care? *Journal of the American Academy of Child and Adolescent Psychiatry*, 32, 89–94.

Trupin, E. W., Stewart, D. G., Beach, B., & Boesky, L. (2002). effectiveness of a dialectical behaviour therapy program for incarcerated female juvenile offenders. *Child and Adolescent Mental Health*, 7, 121–127.

Washington State Institute for Public Policy. (2002). Preliminary Findings for the Juvenile Rehabilitation Administration's dialectic behavior therapy program. Available online at *www.wsipp.wa.gov/rptfiles/JRA_DBT.pdf*.

Webster-Stratton, C., & Taylor, T. K. (1998). Adopting and implementing empirically supported interventions: A recipe for success. In A. Buchanan & B. L. Hudson (Eds.), *Parenting, schooling, and children's behavior* (pp. 127–160). Aldershot, UK: Ashgate.

Woodberry, K., Miller, A. L., Glinski, J., Indik, J., & Mitchell, A. (2002). Family therapy and dialectical behavior with adolescents: Part 2. A theoretical review. *American Journal of Psychotherapy*, 56(4), 585–602.

Woodberry, K. A., Popenoe, E., & Cook, B. (2007). *DBT for suicidal adolescents: A pilot study.* Manuscript submitted for publication.

CHAPTER 10

Dialectical Behavior Therapy for Depression with Comorbid Personality Disorder

AN EXTENSION OF STANDARD DIALECTICAL BEHAVIOR THERAPY WITH A SPECIAL EMPHASIS ON THE TREATMENT OF OLDER ADULTS

Thomas R. Lynch *and* Jennifer S. Cheavens

The primary aim of this chapter is to describe and outline in detail the procedures for an adaptation of dialectical behavior therapy (DBT) for the treatment of depression with comorbid personality disorders. This adaptation of DBT is designed specifically for older adults who meet DSM-IV diagnostic criteria for depression and at least one comorbid personality disorder. This model has been pilot-tested with older adults with depression and comorbid personality disorders, as well as with older adults with depression without Axis II comorbidities. Although these adaptations have focused on older adults (those 55 years of age and older), in our experience the treatment targets and dialectical dilemmas outlined below are likely to be beneficial for many individuals diagnosed with depression and personality disorders, regardless of age.

Following the guidelines for psychosocial treatment development formulated at National Institutes of Health workshops (Rounsaville & Carroll, 2001), we have developed, adapted, and manualized standard DBT to treat older adults with depression and personality disorder (DBT^{D+PD}). Our chapter is organized according to the following topics. First, we briefly review the rationale for applying DBT to depressed individuals with personality disorder and outline the rationale for focusing specifically on older adults. Second, we briefly review two randomized clinical trials that pilot-tested standard DBT with older adults (Lynch, Morse, Mendelson, & Robins, 2003; Lynch et al., in press) that were used as a basis for the current adaptation. Third, we provide an overview of an adapted DBT[D+PD] biosocial model, stages of treatment, targets for treatment, and new dialectical dilemmas for clients with depression and comorbid personality disorders.[1]

Treatment of Personality Disorders and the Issue of Comorbidity

According to the fourth edition of the *Diagnostic Statistical Manual of Mental Disorders* (DSM-IV; American Psychiatric Association, 1994), all personality disorders involve pervasive difficulties associated with two primary areas: emotion/impulse regulation and interpersonal relationships. Personality disorders are associated with significant impairments in health and psychosocial functioning, and, when combined with Axis I disorders (e.g., depression), they have been shown to respond less favorably than Axis I disorders without personality disorders across a variety of empirically supported treatments: psychotherapeutic treatment for depression, antidepressant medications, interpersonal psychotherapy, placebo, and combined medication plus therapy (Duggan, Lee, & Murray, 1990; Hardy et al., 1995; Ilardi, Craighead, & Evans, 1997; Pilkonis & Frank, 1988; Shea et al., 1990; Thase, 1996).

Despite earlier misconceptions that personality disorders "burn out" in late life, an initial meta-analysis (Abrams & Horowitz, 1996) of 11 studies indicated an overall personality disorder prevalence rate of 10% in older adults. In these studies, the most commonly diagnosed personality disorders were obsessive–compulsive, dependent, and "not otherwise specified." The "not otherwise specified" category speaks to the overlap among personality disorders and likely to differences in presentations of personality disorders in later life. An expanded meta-analysis, with an additional five studies, suggests an overall prevalence rate for late-life personality disorders of 20% (Abrams & Horowitz, 1999). Across these studies, the most frequently diagnosed disorders were paranoid, self-defeating, and schizoid. Other studies not included in the meta-analysis or published after it was completed support the initial conclusion that Cluster C personality disorders (i.e., avoidant, dependent, and obsessive–compulsive) are most commonly diagnosed in late life (Kenan et al., 2000; Kunik et al., 1994; Vine & Steingart, 1994), and also support the previous finding of relatively high rates of the "not otherwise specified" category compared with other individual personality disorder diagnoses (Kenan et al., 2000; Kunik et al., 1994). Therefore, reasonable conclusions from the meta-analyses and other studies are that the overall personality disorder prevalence rate is between 10 and 20% of older adults, that the highest prevalence of personality disorders may be in Clusters A and/or C, and that personality dysfunction in older adults may be underestimated by focusing on those who meet full criteria for any one disorder (see Devanand, 2002, for review).

Though supported by fewer completed studies, there is preliminary evidence that late-life depression patients diagnosed with personality disorders share the complicated treatment trajectories similar to their younger counterparts. Personality psychopathology in older adults has generally been associated with poorer response to treatment (Fiorot, Boswell, & Murray, 1990; Thompson, Gallagher, & Czrir, 1988; but not Kunik et al., 1993) and "chronicity" of depressive episodes—meaning relapse or staying continuously dysfunctional (Stek, van Exel, van Tilburg, Westendorp, & Beekman, 2002; Vine & Steingart, 1994). Comorbid personality disorder has been inconsistent in predicting simple depressive relapse, significantly predicting relapse in one study (Brodaty et al., 1993), but not in another (Molinari & Marmion, 1995). In addition, personality disorders in older adults are associated with continued impaired functioning after affective symptoms improve (Abrams, Spielman, Alexopoulos, & Klausner, 1998), impaired social support (Vine & Steingart, 1994), decreased quality of life, suicide, and disability (Lyness, Caine, Conwell, King, & Cox, 1993). Additionally, older adult depressed patients diagnosed with a personality disorder are four times more likely to experience maintenance or reemergence of depressive symptoms than those without personality disorder diagnoses (Morse & Lynch, 2004).

Theorists have observed that the behaviors associated with personality disorders may feel compatible with one's character or sense of self (e.g., Bailey, 1998; Beck, Freeman, & Davis, 2004; Hirschfeld, 1993), and therefore patients are unlikely to seek treatment unless their emotional distress becomes severe due to some environmental event or stressor, the presence of an Axis I disorder, or they are forced to go to treatment by family members or close relations. A notable exception to this observation is borderline personality disorder (BPD), which is experienced as highly problematic by the sufferer, probably due to the extreme affective dysregulation associated with the disorder. Individuals with BPD may seek treatment earlier in life due to the severity of their personal distress or because the severity of criterion behaviors (e.g., suicide attempts or intentional self-injury) result in placement in treatment centers earlier in life.

In our experience, however, many patients with a personality disorder (with the noted exception of BPD) may not seek treatment until later in life. Lack of distress regarding personality style combined with lack of insight regarding the impact of personal behavior on both interpersonal relationships and emotional pain likely reduces help seeking. Individuals with personality disorder may feel increased distress as they age due to the accumulation of damaged relationships and other significant losses related to rigid coping styles associated with their specific personality disorder behavior, and this accumulated stress may eventually lead them to seek treatment. This is one of the reasons we have chosen to take into account developmental issues associated with older adults in our adaptation.

In standard DBT, change is recognized as a potentially distressing event. For older adults such distress may be even greater as many behaviors therapists (and clients themselves) may target are lifelong patterns. Consistent with this, we encourage therapists to entertain the hypothesis that changing lifelong habits (even if these habits are problematic) can be distressing for the patient and will likely be met with some resistance. Thus, as with standard DBT, we start by targeting problems that a patient *is committed* to change while also gently encouraging the patient to examine behaviors he or she is less committed to change that appear to be related to significant impairment (based on functional analysis). This approach from the outset of treatment provides a common ground upon which both patient and therapist can agree is an important area to change (e.g., depression), facilitates alliance, and is one of the reasons our adaptation focuses on treatment of comorbid depression *and* personality disorder pathology. For individuals with personality disorders, motivation for treatment is enhanced and therapeutic change is most likely to occur if the therapist can address therapeutic impasses with nonconfrontational strategies and communicates an understanding of how difficult it is for the client to change (Linehan, Davison, Lynch, & Sanderson, 2006).

Like standard DBT, DBT[D+PD] aims to synthesize several dichotomies within a context that assumes that attachment to the therapist and the development of a therapeutic alliance can at times be difficult to achieve. On the one hand, treatment requires confrontation, commitment, patient responsibility, and the learning of new skills, but, on the other hand, it focuses considerable therapeutic energy on accepting and validating the patient's current condition as it is in the moment. Therapeutic contingencies that reinforce functional behaviors and extinguish or punish dysfunctional behaviors are balanced by efforts aimed at increasing the patient's capacity to emit the requisite functional behaviors. Confrontation is balanced by support. The overarching therapeutic task, over time, is to balance this focus on acceptance with a corresponding focus on change. In the interpersonal terms of Lorna Benjamin (1993), this balance translates into simultaneously giving autonomy and exerting control.

Based on the above observations, we recommend that practitioners not accept patients for treatment when the family is coercing the patient into treatment. For example, in an older adult population, caretakers may communicate to the patient that he or she needs to receive treatment and if he or she does not enter treatment, he or she will have less access to activities or important individuals. In our experience, this will not work. As in standard DBT, patients not committed to changing their behavior at least to some degree are considered to be in pretreatment until the time at which they become committed to some degree to change some problematic behaviors.

Treatment Development and Results from Randomized Clinical Trials

The first issue we faced in modifying DBT for older adults was determining whether a skills-focused approach would be feasible and acceptable to patients. We were specifically concerned about the use of a group setting for behavioral and cognitive skills training. Our feasibility concerns with regard to DBT group skills training were derived from cohort-related attitudinal biases (e.g., Link, Struening, Rahav, Phelan, & Nuttbrock, 1997) that could mitigate willingness to discuss psychological difficulties in front of others, as well as concerns regarding the ability of older adults to routinely come to a "set" group time that could not be rescheduled (due to possible transportation difficulties). Our first study was designed to address these issues in order to determine whether or not older adults would regularly attend a standard DBT skills training group on a weekly basis and utilize phone calls designed to disseminate DBT-based skills.

Study 1

In this study, 34 chronically depressed individuals ages 60+ were randomly assigned to receive 28 weeks of selective serotonin reuptake inhibitor (SSRI) medication plus clinical management, either alone (MED) or in combination with DBT group skills training (MED + DBT) (see Lynch et al., 2003, for additional details on the study and study participants). To be included in the study, participants had to (1) have a score of 18 or higher on the Hamilton Rating Scale for Depression (HAM-D; Hamilton, 1960) *or* 19 or higher on the Beck Depression Inventory (BDI; Beck, Rush, Shaw, & Emery, 1979); (2) be willing to be prescribed antidepressant medication; (3) not meet criteria for bipolar disorder; and (4) be 55 years old or older. The presence of suicidal behavior or personality disorder diagnosis was not considered either an inclusion or an exclusion criterion. Thus, participants were not required to have suicidal behavior or to be diagnosed with a personality disorders but were also not excluded from the study for the presences of suicidal behavior or personality disorder diagnosis. The DBT group skills training consisted of two presentations of a 14-week sequence of DBT skills, for a total of 28 weeks of group skills training. Participants received all four standard skill modules: mindfulness, distress tolerance, emotion regulation, and interpersonal effectiveness. Participants did not receive in-person individual therapy. All participants were provided clinical management of physician choice of antidepressant by a board-certified psychiatrist for the medication component of the treatment.

Results demonstrated that on interviewer-rated depression (i.e., HAM-D scores), 71% of MED + DBT patients met the cutoff for remission classification at posttreatment, in contrast to 47% of MED patients. The relative remission rates were maintained at a 6-month follow-up, with 75% of MED + DBT patients classified as in remission compared to only 31% of MED patients. In addition, only patients in the MED + DBT condition showed significant reductions from pre- to posttreatment on dependency (i.e., sociotropy), perfectionism, self-criticism (i.e., autonomy), and hopelessness (Lynch et al., 2003).

The main objective of this first study was to determine the feasibility of a group intervention with a skills orientation. Based on dropout rates for DBT + MED (N = 1) and anecdotal reports from patients in this condition, we concluded that this treatment format (regularly scheduled group sessions) was acceptable to and feasible for older adults with major depressive disorder (MDD). Encouraged by these findings, we turned our attention to our primary area of interest: depression with comorbid personality disorder among older adults. Our goal in this second randomized clinical trial was to apply standard DBT (both group and individual) to older adults with MDD and personality disorder with a goal of modifying standard DBT and manualizing a new treatment approach designed specifically for this population.

Study 2

This study focused on providing standard DBT (both group and individual sessions following Linehan's [1993a, 1993b] book/manual) with depressed older adults presenting with at least one comorbid personality disorder. For further detail regarding this study, see Lynch et al. (2007). To be eligible for participation, participants were required to be 55 years of age or older, to meet criteria for at least one personality disorder (according to SCID-II criteria; First, Gibbon, Spitzer, Williams, & Benjamin, 1997), and to score 14 or higher on the 17-item HAM-D (Hamilton, 1960). Potential participants were excluded if they were currently receiving electroconvulsive treatment, met criteria for a psychotic or bipolar disorder, refused to discontinue other psychiatric treatments, or evidenced cognitive impairment. Participants were not excluded if they reported suicidal behavior.

Participants participated in two phases of treatment for this study. The first phase of this trial (Phase I) consisted of a standard 8-week medication trial. Participants received physician choice of an SSRI (paroxetine, paroxetine CR, sertraline, or fluoxetine) plus clinical management for 8 weeks. Medications were prescribed by board-certified psychiatrists who met monthly with patients to assess treatment response, monitor any side effects, and adjust dosage as necessary. After 8 weeks of treatment, only 14% of the sample had at least a 50% reduction in HAM-D scores and only 12% were in remission (defined as a HAM-D score of 10 or less). This finding is of considerable importance considering that antidepressant treatment response for older adults without personality disorder is typically 50–70%, supporting findings from prior studies that suggest that comorbid depression and personality disorder do not respond well to standard treatments. In addition, the mean HAM-D score of 14.87 for the sample indicated that participants, on the average, remained quite depressed after 8 weeks of treatment, suggesting the need for more intensive interventions for older adults with both depression and personality disorder.

Those participants who were in remission (HAM-D score of 10 or less) at the end of the 8-week medication trial discontinued the study and the remaining participants were enrolled in the next phase (Phase II) of the study. Thus, those who continued to Phase II had not fully responded to the standard medication trial. For Phase II of the study, all participants continued on antidepressant medication using an algorithm that included three potential medication-switching phases designed to maximize treatment response to antidepressant medication. Participants were randomized to 24 weeks of either medication management alone (MED) or medication management plus standard DBT (DBT + MED). The DBT + MED condition consisted of 24 week of DBT skills training groups plus individual DBT sessions. In keeping with standard clinical practice, therapists were allowed to add individual sessions toward the end of treatment (i.e., taper), but therapists were required to end all individual treatment by 30 weeks after the Phase I medication trial had ended. In both conditions, medication was uncontrolled after Week 24 and all treatment was uncontrolled after Week 30. In addition to assessments over the course of treatment, follow-up data were obtained 6 months after the end of Week 30.

Some of the most relevant findings from the study are presented here. For a more thorough review of the findings related to this study, please refer to Lynch, Cheavens, Cukrowicz, and Linehan (2006). Examination of remission and time to remission findings suggested that the DBT + MED group reached the level of remission more quickly than the MED group. In other words, there were not significant differences in remission rates between MED and DBT + MED at any given time point, but the individuals in the DBT + MED group who reached remission did so more quickly than those in the MED group. The most important findings from this study were related to personality disorder functioning. Using the IIP-PD (Inventory of Interpersonal Problems—Personality Disorders; Pilkonis, Kim, Proietti, & Barkham, 1996), we found significant differences for interpersonal sensitivity and interpersonal aggression between the MED and the DBT + MED groups at posttreatment and follow-up, suggesting that the DBT + MED condition significantly improved personality functioning compared to the MED condition. Interpersonal sensitivity and interpersonal aggression are two constructs that are theorized to be related to interpersonal difficulties often observed in individuals diagnosed with personality disorder.

Overall, results from these two randomized clinical trials suggest that applying group skills training for depressed older adults and *standard DBT* for the treatment of comorbid MDD and personality disorder in older adults has promise. Specifically, results suggest that DBT skills training has utility in effectively treating chronic depression and that standard DBT + MED results in faster remission of depressive symptoms than treatment with MED alone. In addition, standard DBT appears to have promise for modifying personality features such as interpersonal sensitivity and interpersonal aggression compared to medication alone.

As mentioned, the goal of this second study was not only to obtain clinical experience with older adults with both MDD and a personality disorder, but also to determine if standard DBT needed to be modified for this population and, if so, to develop a new treatment manual for the depressed elderly with personality disorders. For the remainder of the chapter we focus on what we have learned for the past 8 years and how we have modified DBT to meet the special needs of this population.

Adaptation of the Biosocial Theory for All Personality Disorders

The biosocial theory in standard DBT was originally formulated to explain the development and maintenance of BPD. As a theory, it is dialectical, in that the theory proposes that the dialectic, or transaction, between a biological tendency toward emotion vulnerability and an invalidating rearing environment produces a dysregulation of the patient's emotional system. In the context of biosocial theory, invalidation is the critical socially mediated etiological process, whereas emotional vulnerability is the key biological factor.

Thus, initially we adapted/expanded Linehan's original biosocial model of BPD to be inclusive of all personality disorders. To review, Linehan (1993a) theorized that a biological predisposition toward emotional vulnerability and an invalidating environmental context transact to produce emotional dysregulation characteristic of BPD. To expand this model to include the development and maintenance of all personality disorders, we have suggested that a biological predisposition toward heightened negative affectivity and an environmental context that reinforces maladaptive forms of avoidance transact to produce cognitive, emotional, and behavioral patterns of personality disorders—particularly in the form of disrupted interpersonal relationships and emotional/impulse regulation difficulties.

For older adults with personality disorders, the biosocial theory must be modified to account for the fact that intense emotion dysregulation in older adults is less likely to be as salient a problem as it is for younger patients with personality disorders. For example, research has shown that compared to younger adults, older adults report decreased frequency and intensity of subjective negative emotional experience, which may be related to the reported greater efforts to control emotions and expression and increased use of effective regulation strategies such as distancing and positive appraisal (Diener, Sandvik, & Larsen, 1985; Gross et al., 1997; Lawton, Kleban, Rajagopal, & Dean, 1992; McConatha & Huba, 1999). Furthermore, there is consensus in the literature based on conclusions from meta-analyses and other studies that the highest prevalence among older adults with personality disorders are in Clusters A and/or C, the less "emotionally expressive" clusters (Abrams & Horowitz, 1999; Morse & Lynch, 2004). Additionally, older adults with MDD and personality disorders also have reported less negative affectivity than their younger counterparts with combined MDD and personality disorders (Cheavens, Rosenthal, Banawan, & Lynch, 2006). It is important to state, however, that although older adults with MDD plus a personality disorder reported less negative affect intensity than younger adults with MDD plus a personality disorder, older adults with MDD plus a personality disorder still reported *significantly more* negative affect intensity than older adults without psychiatric diagnoses. Thus there was an interaction between age and MDD plus a personality disorder that must be accounted for in a biosocial theory.

Applying the Biosocial Model for All Personality Disorders to Older Adults

During the two randomized controls trials (RCTs) previously discussed in this chapter, clinical observations suggested that older adults in treatment presented with difficulties related to being overly rigid and less open to experience, as opposed to difficulties in emotion regulation. Thus, the biosocial model and the resulting DBT model for BPD suggests that individuals with BPD have difficulties with emotional dysregulation such that they often lack the requisite skills to increase or decrease their emotional experiencing to adaptive levels. Our experience suggested that older adults with personality disorders have difficulty moving flexibly from one overlearned "skill" or strategy. Theoretically, this could be related to a longer history of one behavior or set of behaviors being frequently reinforced through the avoidance of negative affect over time.

The theoretical perspective proposed here also is dialectical, in that the theory proposes that the dialectic or transaction between a biological predisposition for negative affect *and* environmental feedback that either disconfirms or confirms the individual's style of emotional responding produces a pattern of rigid maladaptive coping that over time results in the development and maintenance of a personality disorder. In the context of a biosocial theory, environmental feedback resulting in rigid responding is the critical socially mediated etiological process, whereas negative affect is the key biological factor (see Figure 10.1).

From this perspective, it is theorized that older adults with personality disorders develop difficulties via a transaction of a biological disposition for negative affectivity with environmental feedback (disconfirmation of natural responses and/or confirmation of maladaptive rigid responses), resulting in a pervasive rigid, maladaptive way of responding. Thus even though older adults in general report feeling less negative affect than their younger adult counterparts, older adults with MDD plus a personality disorder still report feeling more negative affect than both older and younger adults without MDD plus a personality disorder (Cheavens et al., 2006). This finding suggests that for older adults with personality pathology, negative affect intensity may have decreased over time but remains strong and aversive. Additionally, age impacts the environmental component of the theory by increasing the length of time over which maladaptive styles of coping with negative emotions and feedback from the environment is repeatedly and intermittently reinforced by either temporary reductions in aversive arousal or environmental support (e.g., increased nurturance). Thus, these maladaptive behaviors subsequently become more rigid and difficult to change. Personality disorders in older adults are extremely difficult to treat because maladaptive behaviors have typically been part of the patient's behavioral repertoire for decades (see Figure 10.2).

DBT[D+PD] is a novel treatment model that synthesizes *behavioral skill deficits and deficits in behavioral flexibility* (overly rigid responses, perfectionism, interpersonal difficulties, avoidance behavior, isolation), theorizing that (1) older adults with behavioral dysfunctions secondary to personality pathology lack important interpersonal, self-

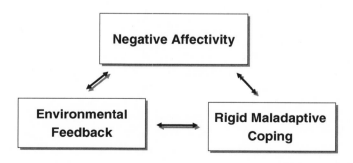

FIGURE 10.1. DBT [D+PD] biosocial theory for all personality disorders.

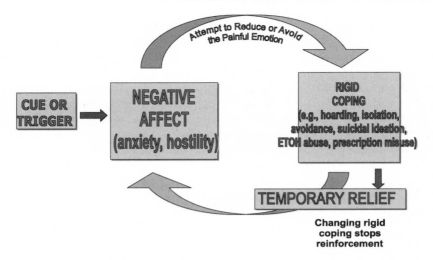

FIGURE 10.2. PD avoidance paradigm.

regulation (including emotion regulation) and acceptance skills; and that (2) personal and environmental factors inhibit the flexible use of behavioral coping skills the individual does have and often reinforce one dysfunctional behavioral pattern. The tension between these two models, *skill deficit* (i.e., the individual does not have the requisite skills) *versus flexibility deficit* (i.e., the individual does have the requisite skills but is not open to using them in new contexts), is one of the fundamental challenges in working with older adults with personality pathology. Thus, therapy must demonstrate and model a balanced stance between change and acceptance in the search for a synthesis.

Negative affect in our modified biosocial theory refers to dispositional negative emotionality that is hypothesized to be a shared etiological feature across all personality disorders and most Axis I disorders. As noted above, all personality disorders diagnoses involve pervasive difficulties associated with emotion or impulse regulation (American Psychiatric Association, 1994). Although Cluster A and Cluster C disorders are presumed to be less emotionally expressive disorders, adults diagnosed with Cluster A and C personality disorders have been shown to include excesses in emotional reactivity (Morey et al., 2002, 2003). Specifically, Cluster C personality disorders have consistently shown heightened experiences of *anxiety* and Cluster A personality disorders have been characterized by an abundance of *hostility* (Hyler, Skodol, Kellman, Oldham, & Rosnick, 1990; Dowson & Berrios, 1991; Schroeder & Livesley, 1991; Klein, Kupfer, & Shea, 1993; Nestadt, Eaton, & Romanoski, 1994; Schotte, DeDoncker, & Vankerckhoven, 1998), while individuals with Cluster B diagnoses present with both heightened *anxiety and hostility* (e.g., Schotte et al., 1998). Our modified biosocial theory places less emphasis on high sensitivity and high reactivity to negative emotions regardless of valence, as proposed for BPD (Linehan, 1993a), but instead emphasizes negative emotionality without the extreme lability or intensity that is often the case in BPD. However, as with emotion vulnerability in BPD, negative affectivity is hypothesized to transact with feedback from the environment that intermittently reinforces maladaptive coping. This pattern becomes progressively rigid over time.

Environmental feedback parallels the invalidating environment that is part of the biosocial theory in standard DBT for BPD; however, the transaction with the environment is not solely experienced as invalidating. As with standard DBT, this approach is based in part on self-verification theory (e.g., Swann, 1997). This concept of self-verification is based on experimental research that has demonstrated that individuals favor information that confirms their self-view over other reinforcers, particularly if that self-view is extreme, and that individuals become anxious or withdraw when they cannot dismiss disconfirming feedback (Giesler, Josephs, & Swann, 1996; Pelham & Swann, 1994; Ritts & Stein, 1995; Swann, 1997; Swann, de la Ronde, & Hixon, 1994). In order to cope successfully with and adapt to changing environments, however, an individual must learn from failure and contradiction; ignoring disconfirming social feedback is hypothesized to exacerbate personality disorder behavior by maintaining ineffective behaviors. It is likely that this is only intensified over time, and thus older adults would have maladaptive strategies more strongly entrenched than they were in their earlier years.

An environmental feedback hypothesis suggests that while a person controls mental and social interactions to avoid aversive feedback, avoidance may reinforce disorder. For example, by repeatedly staying away from interpersonal situations, a female patient with avoidant personality disorder never learns that she can behave adaptively and tolerate her distress in social situations and a male patient with paranoid personality disorder never learns that others are not exploiting or deceiving him in most contexts. In addition, the behavior of a patient can influence the type of feedback received from the environment, which in turn can further exacerbate problems. For example, a patient with obsessive–compulsive personality disorder is often reinforced by his employer for being perfectionistic and rigid in carrying out tasks (e.g., military); however, this positive employer feedback may serve to reinforce problematic behavior in other contexts where the behavior is not adaptive. This style becomes apparent in other environments (e.g., with family and friends) when the individual has difficulty responding flexibly or becomes hostile or moralistic when others prefer to do things differently. Thus, as in standard DBT, from a DBT^{D+PD} perspective, the environment and the patient's style of coping transact to exacerbate problems (often with little insight by the patient).

Rigid maladaptive coping starts with a theoretical premise that considers the patient's attempt to cope with negative affect, not the negative affect itself, as the problem behavior for the patient (similar to standard DBT). Thus from this perspective, maladaptive coping (e.g., isolation, hoarding, avoidance of interpersonal interactions, perfectionistic thinking, suicidal ideation, alcohol abuse, prescription abuse) is seen as an ineffective strategy for dealing with negative affect. The behavior is maintained over time because it functions to provide temporary relief from aversive arousal. For example, by isolating the individual with paranoid personality disorder avoids experiences of hostility and anxiety that can be associated with being around others, or by hoarding the patient with obsessive–compulsive personality disorder reduces the anxiety associated with the possibility of mistakenly getting rid of something valuable. The relief experienced by these avoidant behaviors, however, is only temporary (as cues associated with negative arousal are impossible to fully avoid), functions to increase shame in the patient (e.g., "There must be something wrong with me—other people don't isolate so much"), and reduces opportunities for learning effective ways to regulate negative affect. Importantly, from this perspective, interpersonal and emotional difficulties are secondary to negative affectivity.

Increasing Flexibility
and Reconciling Past Mistakes

DBT^{D+PD} is grounded in theory that directly addresses the challenges facing older adults with MDD plus personality disorder. In our previous work, older adults reported that emotion mind concepts from standard DBT had less relevance in their psychological difficulties than did concepts related to open-mindedness and behavioral flexibility. Thus, one of the primary differences between DBT^{D+PD} and standard DBT is the emphasis on skills designed to maximize openness to and flexibility regarding new experience (e.g., radical openness skills module) and to reduce rigid thinking and corresponding behaviors, as opposed to the primary orientation in standard DBT to emotion regulation (see Figures 10.3, 10.4, and 10.5). *Rigidity* is defined as resistance to changing beliefs, attitudes, or personal habits, and can be divided into cognitive and behavioral components (Rokeach, 1960; Schultz & Searleman, 2002). Related concepts include low openness to experience (McCrae & Costa, 1996) and cognitive inflexibility. Individuals who score higher on measures of rigidity show less creative and divergent thinking (McCrae, 1987), are less likely to become absorbed in pleasurable experiences (Glisky, Tataryn, Tobias, Kihlstrom, & McConkey, 1991), and are less aware of their emotions (Lane, Quinlan, Schwartz, Walker, & Zeitlin, 1990). Both low openness to experience and rigidity have been associated with a number of negative treatment outcomes (Ehrlich & Bauer, 1966; Ogrodniczuk, Piper, Joyce, McCallum, & Rosie, 2002, 2003). In addition, low openness to experience has been associated with increased rates of completed suicide (but not self-reported suicidal ideation) in older adults (Duberstein, Conwell, & Caine, 1994; Duberstein et al., 2000). Moreover, rigidity is a key component in some of the personality disorders most prevalent in older adults (e.g., obsessive–compulsive personality disorder, avoidant personality disorder, and schizoid and schizotypal personality disorders).

DBT^{D+PD} targets rigidity through new targets that are outlined in "Path to Fluid Mind" (see Figure 10.6). First, the patient is oriented to the concept that active avoidance of anything new or challenging and/or continuous repetition of behaviors that "feel safe" leads to reinforcement satiation. Targeting *behavioral avoidance* is hypothesized to broaden, rather than narrow, thoughts and actions and to increase the probability that positive novel experiences will be encountered. For example, research has shown that greater marital happiness is associated with less predictability in couple interactions (Gottman, 1994). Thus, the therapist works on increasing motivation and engagement in new experiences and/or new environments. This can start with the simple act of rearranging the furniture in the patient's house. We also focus on reducing *bitterness*, which often translates into problems with self- and/or acceptance, rigid rules about how life "should" be, and beliefs that one will never obtain one's goals in life. It is not uncommon to believe that others are judgmental and out to cause harm or to harbor beliefs that one "should not" have to put up with, or to cope with, negative experience. Here the treatment focus is designed to increase empathic understanding and self-responsibility and to decrease rigid blaming of others or outside circumstances. We also target *emotion inhibition* that has been shown to mediate the relation between negative affect and both hopelessness and suicidal ideation in depressed older adults (Lynch, Cheavens, Morse, & Rosenthal, 2004). The focus in treatment with this target is to enhance emotional acceptance and nonavoidance of thoughts and feelings, achieved via graduated exposure to relevant cues and mindfulness practice. Finally, we target *rigid thinking*. Here we use primarily cogni-

Basic Principles of RADICAL OPENNESS

- Freedom from feeling "stuck" requires OPENNESS to new behaviors.

- BEING CLOSED to different ways has not worked—otherwise you would not be here.
- Being OPEN does not mean rejecting the past.
- Deciding to be in the moment and staying available to all possibilities is OPENNESS.
- OPENNESS is looking forward without preconception or expectation.
- OPENNESS is looking back without judgment or blame.
- To be OPEN to something is not the same as judging it good.

RADICAL OPENNESS

IS <u>NOT</u>:

    Approval

    Expecting good things to happen

    Being naive

    Always changing

IS <u>NOT</u>:

    Being rigid about being open

WHY BE OPEN TO NEW THINGS?

1. Rejecting and denying that things are different doesn't make it so.
2. Changing reality requires being OPEN to new facts about reality.
3. Old habits have not worked.

Other: _____

FIGURE 10.3. Radical openness handout 1 D+PD.

Pros and Cons of Being Open to New Experience

Name _____ Week starting _____

Make Pros and Cons list for being open to new experience, trying out new things, tolerating the distress of not having an answer or being seen as inexperienced, and Pros and Cons of being closed to new experience and basing decisions on the past.

	Being Open to New Experience	Being Closed to New Experience (describe _____)
PROS	Short term _____ _____ _____ Long term_____ _____ _____	Short term _____ _____ _____ Long term_____ _____ _____
CONS	Short term _____ _____ _____ Long term_____ _____ _____	Short term _____ _____ _____ Long term_____ _____ _____

FIGURE 10.4. Radical openness handout 2 [D+PD].

Name _____   Week Starting _____

FIGURE OUT WHAT YOU NEED TO BE RADICALLY OPEN TO

1st, make a list of three things in your life right now that **you do not want to change but fluid mind knows you should.** <u>Helpful hint</u>: what have caring others told you in the past that would be helpful for you to change but you have resisted? <u>Helpful hint</u>: use adjectives to describe yourself, now list the opposite adjective; these may be clues to what you need to be open to. <u>Helpful hint</u>: what are your "buttons," what can someone say to you that will make you angry? These might be hints to areas that need work on being open.

Then put a number indicating how open you are to trying this new behavior or idea out:

  0 = fixed mind, I am in completely inflexible about and/or unwilling to change . . .

  5 = complete fluid-minded openness

What I need to be open to.   (Openness, 0–5)

1. . _____ (_____)
2. . _____ (_____)
3. . _____ (_____)

REFINE YOUR LIST

2nd, review your two lists above. **Check for judgments.** Avoid good, bad, and judgmental language. Rewrite any items above if needed so that they are **factual and nonjudgmental.**

PRACTICE RADICAL OPENNESS

3rd, choose one item from the list to practice on.

1. _____
2. _____

4th, focus your fluid mind on the new behavior or thought. *Check off* any of the following exercises that you did.

☐ 1. Reminded myself to behave opposite to my old way of doing things

☐ 2. Allowed thoughts of what I have to be open to enter my mind and attended to sensations

☐ 3. Imagined being open to and "loving" any accompanying humiliation

☐ 4. Wrote it out in detail what I need to be open to, not exaggerating or minimizing, factually and without judgment

☐ 5. Relaxed my face and body while imagining being open

☐ 6. Tried out something small that is related to the new behavior or way of thinking

☐ 7. Rehearsed in my mind the things that I would do

☐ 8. Reminded myself that you have to "break an egg to make an omelet"

☐ 9. Other: _____

_____

5th, describe your experiences and what happened next.

1. _____

_____

2. _____

_____

FIGURE 10.5. Radical openness worksheet 3 [D+PD].

DBT Path to Fluid Mind

Decrease **BEHAVIORAL AVOIDANCE**
• staying away from new places or experiences

Decrease **BITTERNESS**
• resentful, distrustful

Decrease **EMOTION INHIBITION**
• thought suppression, don't think, feel, or express it

Decrease **RIGID THINKING**
• assuming the answer is known

Decrease **APPARENTLY UNIMPORTANT BEHAVIORS**
• approaching an area with previous associations to depression/hopelessness
• despair-exacerbating behaviors (e.g., looking only for confirmatory information,
downplaying importance of interpersonal relationships,
alcohol use, prescription misuse)

FIGURE 10.6. Path to Fluid Mind.

tive restructuring techniques designed to help the patient "check the facts" regarding beliefs he or she has formed and provide homework assignments designed to help the patient recognize and challenge his or her own rigid thinking (e.g., Myths of a Closed Mind; see Figure 10.7).

DBT^{D+PD} also differs from standard DBT by emphasizing skills that are specific to reconciling events over the life course through reviewing past events and generating forgiveness. Reviewing and reconciling past experiences has long been theorized to be an important developmental milestone (Butler, 1963; Erikson & Erikson, 1997; Staudinger & Pasupathi, 2000; Webster & Cappeliez, 1993), particularly in the context of moving forward with meaningful goals. In our experience, approximately 45% of older adult patients treated for major depressive disorder and personality disorder reported inhibited grieving regarding a past trauma or perceived mistake. In addition, there is evidence that older adults tend to regulate emotion to a greater degree than younger adults by talking about the past and experience greater positive emotions than younger adults while discussing the past (Pasupathi & Carstensen, 2003). Thus DBT^{D+PD} teaches skills associated with goal adjustment and successful coping with life hassles (Folkman, Lazarus, Pimley, & Novacek, 1987; Meeks, Carstensen, Tamsky, Wright, & Pellegrini, 1989) to older adults who are "stuck" in negative events of the past. We also teach specific skills for dealing with forgiveness of self, of others, and of the environment (see Figures 10.8, 10.9, and 10.10).

Myths of a Fixed Mind

1. Being open means being gullible. Only idiots are open.

   Challenge: _____

2. If you don't have an opinion on how things should be, you'll get hurt.

   Challenge: _____

3. I am too old to try something new.

   Challenge: _____

4. There is a right and wrong way to do things and that's the way it is.

   Challenge: _____

5. Being naïve means being a fool.

   Challenge: _____

6. I have tried everything there is to try. There is nothing new out there.

   Challenge: _____

7. Even if I tried something new, it won't help.

   Challenge: _____

8. You can't teach an old dog a new trick.

   Challenge: _____

9. If I try something new and it works, I was a fool for not trying it before.

   Challenge: _____

10. If I try something new, then it means I was wrong.

    Challenge: _____

11. New things are for gullible young people.

    Challenge: _____

12. Doing something different means giving up my values.

    Challenge: _____

13. It doesn't matter what you say or how things seem, I know I am right.

    Challenge: _____

14. Doing what I always do just feels right.

    Challenge: _____

15. It is more comfortable to do what I have always done.

    Challenge: _____

16. You have to resign yourself to the fact that you can't change.

    Challenge: _____

17. Myth:

    Challenge: _____

FIGURE 10.7. Myths of a Fixed Mind.

**Forgiveness: Letting Go
Goals of Forgiveness**

Reduce Emotional Suffering Tied to the Past
- Let go of emotions from the past
- Radical acceptance of past events

Create Room for New Connections and Experiences
- Focus on present events, relationships, opportunities
- Reduce attention and thought related to hurtful past
  Examples: conveyor belt

Reclaim Your Present Life
- Regain (or gain) a feeling of empowerment and control over life
- Do what needs to be done now, *effectiveness in present*

Allow Other People In Your Life to **Move On**
- Reduce time spent focused on the event
- Increase availability in present relationships

FIGURE 10.8. Interpersonal effectiveness handout 9 D+PD.

**Forgiveness: Letting Go
What Forgiveness Is and Is Not**

Forgiveness is not:
1. Saying that something is "all right, good, OK, not hurtful"
2. Accepting the blame for what happened
3. Blaming someone else for what happened
4. Keeping toxic relationships in your life
5. Repeating something harmful to you

Forgiveness is:
1. Radically accepting *the facts*
2. Living in line with your values
3. Staying focused on the present
4. Bringing a sense of wise mind or peace to your life

FIGURE 10.9. Interpersonal effectiveness handout 10 D+PD.

Steps to Forgiveness

1. **Is there something that happened in the past (e.g., event, decision, hurtful outcome) that you still think about often? Do you have feelings of guilt, anger, sadness?**

   _____

   _____

2. Describe how these feelings and holding on to these feelings influences your life now.

   _____

   _____

3. Figure out who or what you want to forgive:
   a. Forgive yourself for something you did, a decision you made, etc.
   b. Forgive someone else for something he or she did to you or another person
   c. Forgive the environment, higher power, a corporation, another country, etc.

4. **Radically accept that the event happened.** *Go over radical acceptance*

5. **Nonjudgmentally label your feelings associated with the event**
   a. When the event happened: _____
   b. Now: _____

6. **Think of the people involved at the time of the event (including you)**
   a. What was your perspective then? Has it changed?

   _____

   b. What was the perspective of other people involved?

   _____

   c. Any information about the person to be forgiven that you are leaving out?

   _____

   _____

7. **Let go**
   a. Forgive yourself—Practice justified and unjustified guilt skills
   b. Forgive others—What do you want to hear/have done from this person? Can you get this in your life now?
   c. Forgive environment—Work to reduce judgment and increase radical acceptance

8. **Loving Kindness Exercises**

FIGURE 10.10. Interpersonal effectiveness worksheet 4 [D+PD].

Modes of Treatment

The functions and modes of our adaptation parallel standard DBT. A variety of modes can be implemented to fulfill the functions, depending upon the particular setting in which the treatment is provided, but our research to date has focused on the following:

Individual Therapy

Individual therapy is provided to enhance motivation, promote problem solving, and increase the behavioral repertoire and flexibility of the patient to behave in skillful ways. Our research has resulted in recommendations that patients meet for weekly 50-minute sessions with their individual therapist throughout the first 28 weeks of treatment. Following this period, individual session frequency can be gradually tapered if the patient is doing well (we recommend that tapering should occur over an 8-week period or longer). The weekly agenda in DBT^{D+PD} individual therapy is determined by the current maladaptive behavior to be stopped or reduced or by the adaptive behavior to be introduced or increased. As in standard DBT, treatment targets are arranged in a hierarchical order as follows: (1) reduce high-risk suicidal and life-threatening behaviors; (2) reduce therapy-interfering behaviors (e.g., noncompliance, noncollaboration, nonattendance); and (3) reduce quality-of-life-interfering behaviors, with reducing depression and increasing openness to experience as the top priority in DBT^{D+PD} quality-of-life targets. Behaviors to be increased or decreased are tracked daily on a diary card with daily emotions, sleep patterns, and self-care habits (see Figure 10.11). Older adults have successfully completed this card at a high rate during pilot studies (Lynch et al., 2003).

Group Skills Training

We recommend that the DBT^{D+PD} skills training group meet for a minimum of 28 weekly 2-hour sessions. This group emphasizes skills acquisition and the strengthening of previously acquired skills. The treatment manual for DBT^{D+PD} skills training is very similar to that for standard DBT (Lynch et al., 2006) with relatively minor variations for the standard DBT modules distress tolerance, emotion regulation, and interpersonal effectiveness, and more substantial changes for the mindfulness module. In addition, based on specific problems associated with rigidity and lack of openness to change among older adults with personality disorder, we have added a new module entitled "radical openness."

The newly adapted DBT^{D+PD} mindfulness module includes skills related to reducing rigidity and increasing openness to new experience. Thus, in addition to the traditional states of mind (i.e., wise, reasonable, and emotional), we have incorporated fluid, fixed, and fresh states of mind (see Figure 10.12). These states of mind help older adult patients find the synthesis in weighing what they know to be true based on history with what they know to be true based on new information in the present moment. We believe this to be particularly useful for older adults with personality disorders in that much of their experience has been to cognitively shut down and they avoid information that does not fit within an existing framework at all costs.

The new module radical openness focuses on skills related to being more open to new experience (e.g., radical openness worksheets), radical acceptance skills from standard DBT, and skills that target bitterness by focusing on learning to forgive oneself, oth-

Dialectical Behavior Therapy D + PD
Skills Diary Card

Initials/Name _____ ID # _____

Started: Date ___ / ___ / ___

Circle Start Day	Highest Urge To:			Highest Rating for Each Day			Medications				Behavior				
Day of Week	Commit Suicide 0–5	Give Up 0–5	Deactivate 0–5	Emotion. Misery 0–5	Physical Misery 0–5	Joy 0–5	Home Remedy What?	Med as Prescribed Y?N	PRN/Over the Counter #.	What?	Active Y/N	Sleep Hrs #	Skills 0–7	Self-critical 0–5	Tried New
MON															✓
TUE															
WED															
THUR															
FRI															
SAT															
SUN															

USED SKILLS:
0 = Not thought about or used
1 = Thought about, not used, didn't want to
2 = Thought about, not used, wanted to
3 = Tried but couldn't use them
4 = Tried, could do them, but they didn't help
5 = Tried, could use them, helped
6 = Didn't try, used them, didn't help
7 = Didn't try, used them, helped

Openness to New . . . Coming into Session (0–5)		Urge to: Coming into Session (0–5)	
Emotions:		Quit therapy:	
Action:		Give up:	
Thoughts:		Commit suicide:	

Chain Analysis Notes

Med Changes/Other: _____

FIGURE 10.11. DBT skills diary card.

From *Dialectical Behavior Therapy in Clinical Practice*, edited by Linda A. Dimeff and Kelly Koerner. Copyright 2007 by The Guilford Press. Permission to photocopy this figure is granted to purchasers of this book for personal use only (see copyright page for details).

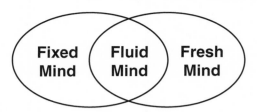

When in **Fixed Mind** you are ruled by the past and rigid rules about how things should be. The desire is not to make a mistake. What worked in the past determines your thoughts, emotions, behaviors. You are rigid, one-minded, rule-governed, and willful. You may be protected but you cannot learn new things.

When in **Fresh Mind**, you are oblivious to dangers that might cause problems. You are overly trusting of others and situations. You are more likely to make decisions without considering consequences and forget or suppress past mistakes. You may be open to new ideas but you are vulnerable.

Both extremes are _problematic_.

Fluid Mind: The safest place to be.
You are open to new experience while honoring the past.
You are able to grow but not always the hard way.

When in **Fluid Mind**, you see and respond to "what is," including the past, present, and future implications. Fluid Mind is that part of you that knows and experiences truth for you. It is where you know something to be true or valid yet do not base this validity solely on the past. It is being peacefully aware of each moment as a new beginning that is based, in part, on previous moments. It is willingness to try something new but not just because it is "new." It is focusing on where you want to go while honoring where you have been. Fluid Mind knows that living effectively requires genuine adjustment to an ever-changing environment over time. What worked once may not now.

One of the greatest skills that a person can learn is to self-correct based on feedback from his or her environment. Self-correcting means you have to balance what you have done in the past and what you want to do in the future with where you are now. Fluid Mind is learning to self-correct in a balanced way. Honor the old while embracing the new.

FIGURE 10.12. DBT $^{D+PD}$ states of mind.

ers, or the environment in general (e.g., natural disasters, God, physical illnesses) for mistakes/grievances that occurred in the past. This module also teaches skills associated with adjusting life goals as a way to let go of feeling "stuck" in negative events of the past or rigidly focusing on attaining a goal that may no longer be possible to attain.

Telephone Consultation

As in standard DBT, brief telephone contact between sessions with the individual therapist is an essential component of treatment. Following standard DBT guidelines, these calls can be for (1) coaching in use of skills in crisis situations and crisis intervention, (2) contact with the therapist to maintain or strengthen the therapeutic relationship, and (3) relationship repair. In our previous research (Lynch et al., 2004; Lynch et al., in press), telephone contact occurred on a relatively rare basis with approximately half of patients using coaching calls and no patient calling more than three times over the course of the study (i.e., three times within approximately 6 months). In particular, older adults in our prior work often stated that they "felt bad about bothering" their therapist. DBT^{D+PD} targets this attitude as therapy-interfering and reorients the patient to believe that calling for consultation demonstrates improvement in skills related to radical openness. At the same time, given that older adults are less likely to present with the intense emotional dysregulation common in younger individuals with BPD, it is likely that telephone consultation will occur less frequently than in standard DBT. It is likely that the first (i.e., crisis help) and third (i.e., relationship repair) functions of coaching calls may be less frequently needed in DBT^{D+PD}.

Team Consultation

As in standard DBT, therapist team consultation is part of the treatment itself, rather than ancillary to the treatment. Therapists meet weekly to assist each other in the implementation of the treatment. As in standard DBT, the consultation team is defined as the treatment of a community of patients by a community of therapists and the treatment of the therapists by the community of therapists.

Family Involvement and Stage 2 Work

To maximize the amount of reinforcement provided by the environment for skillful behavior, family and caregiver sessions are emphasized in DBT^{D+PD} as a means to orient the patient's environment to treatment principles and to increase *in vivo* reinforcement of newly acquired behaviors. In DBT^{D+PD} up to six individual sessions can include family members or caregivers in order to orient them to the treatment approach, provide education regarding problems, and teach skills as needed.

Dialectical Dilemmas

Lynch (2000) articulated four general dialectical tensions, adapted in part from dilemmas defined by Linehan (1993a), that when rigidly adhered to are hypothesized to maintain depression, enhance the likelihood of depressive relapse, and exacerbate personality dysfunction. The goal in treatment is for these extreme stances to be relaxed in favor of more flexible and adaptive responses.

The *first dilemma* relates to acceptance of reality and whether fighting reality or nonresistance have a history of reinforcement during times of stress. Under this dilemma, depression and/or relapse may be more likely when an older adult pervasively refuses to accept loss despite evidence that a desired outcome may be unlikely to be achieved through continued effort (i.e., *Bitter Attachment*) versus consistently acquiescing, nonresisting, and giving up despite evidence that a desired outcome may be obtainable (i.e., *Mindless Approval*).

The *second dilemma* relates to styles of changing reality or solving problems. It is hypothesized that over time individuals develop a characteristic style of either attending to or avoiding problems. Rigid attempts to solve all problems despite evidence that there may not be a solution (*Problem Brooding*) may increase vulnerability to unwanted emotions and depression. Pervasive experiential avoidance and/or unwillingness to problem solve (*Problem Avoidant*) may paradoxically exacerbate distress, reduce the chance that effective change may take place, and increase the likelihood that inhibited or traumatic grief may occur. As with the first dilemma, each style can prove adaptive when followed less rigidly. For example, worry can help orient a person to solving important problems and activate resources, while temporary avoidance can help a person attend to other tasks that require more immediate attention.

The *third dilemma* revolves around issues of how a person manages interpersonal relationships during times of stress. For some this may manifest by withdrawing from potential sources of social support when negative life events occur and communicating that they are not in need of support even though they are (*Apparent Autonomy*). Alternatively, others may single-mindedly demand nurturance and care from others when under stress (*Active Passivity*). Clinically, we have observed apparently autonomous older adults become dysregulated when others try to assist them and to avoid intimate discussions. The actively passive older adult may focus on being cared for, demand support, look to others for solutions, and/or become dysregulated when nurturance is not forthcoming.

The *fourth dilemma* relates to self-validation. One pole consists of wallowing in self-pity and ruminating on thoughts and evidence that life is sad/distressing (*Emotion Vulnerability*). Although wallowing in emotion may have a soothing component, unfortunately doing so may result in stimuli associated with loss becoming more salient, consequently exacerbating depression. The other pole relates to showing oneself no self-understanding, engaging in self-hate, and/or rejecting personal experience (*Self-Invalidation*). A self-deprecating attributional style has been empirically linked to depressive experience and self-invalidation may function to block functional behavior (Linehan, 1993a) and/or to elicit repeated caregiving responses from social supports who eventually burn out (Coyne, 1976).

Diary Cards

Diary cards are completed daily and reviewed weekly by the individual therapist in session. The font size can be increased as needed for an older adult patient and individual targets can be added. See Figure 10.10 for an example of the front side of a DBT^{D+PD} diary card.

Treatment Examples

Our plan in this section is to briefly review several case studies that were derived from our research study examining the use of standard DBT to treat comorbid major depression and personality disorders in older adults. We do not present the treatment trajectory for each case in its entirety, but instead focus on specific elements of the treatment that might explicate some of the adaptations, targets, or skills that served to be useful in working with these patients. In addition, space limitations prevent review of cases associated with each personality disorder.

Paranoid Personality Disorder

Mr. H was a 78-year-old male with a history of chronic depression and an early age of depression onset. He met SCID-II criteria for paranoid personality disorder indicated by pervasive distrust and suspiciousness of others, believing others were exploiting him, holding persistent grudges, and reading demeaning meanings into benign remarks or events that others might say. Mr. H had never married and tended to avoid situations where intimacy was possible; however, he indicated that he would like to develop a new relationship with a woman. The treatment strategy for this problem focused primarily on behavioral exposure to situations that could lead to intimacy combined with skills training in interpersonal effectiveness. In session 14, Mr. H was given a homework assignment to ask a woman friend he knew from church out on a date. At the next session, the therapist checked in on this homework assignment.

THERAPIST: So, how did it go asking Jane out?

MR. H: Oh, I don't know. It didn't seem to work out so good.

THERAPIST: OK, well let's see if we can take a look at what really happened. I'd like to go back and do a chain analysis of this. Would you be willing to do that?

MR. H: Sure.

THERAPIST: OK, so what was the problem behavior? I can see here on your diary card that it looks like you had some increased suicidal ideation on Sunday. Was that the day you asked her out?

MR. H: Yeah, it was. Umm, I just felt so completely miserable after asking her. It just obviously wasn't going to work, that I . . . I don't know, I just got to this place where I just started thinking about maybe I should just end it all.

THERAPIST: OK, so let's go back and see if we can figure out how it is that you got there, because as I recall you and I have done a pretty good job rehearsing how you might go ahead and ask Jane out and it seemed to me that you were more or less ready and willing to do this. So it'd be nice for us to be able to figure out how it is that you moved from planning, to asking, and then ended up thinking about wanting to die. I think that's pretty important.

MR. H: Well, I was actually feeling pretty bad the whole day. I was, umm, I had the night before started worrying about having to do this the next day and started drinking to calm my nerves. I woke up the next day with a hangover and I was feeling really, really ashamed about that.

THERAPIST: As we discussed before, drinking when you are emotional just doesn't seem to work for you. We might want to discuss this later. But for now we know that you started off the day feeling pretty emotionally vulnerable. So, where were you and what time of the day was it when you asked Jane out?

MR. H: Well, I think it was around 3:30 or 4:00. I was at church and I knew that she'd be there. So I decided that, well, even though I was feeling pretty crappy, that I should follow through with our plan. So, without thinking about it much, I just walked right up to her and decided to get it over with.

THERAPIST: What exactly did you say to her?

MR. H: I just said, "Hey, would you like to go out sometime?"

THERAPIST: Ahh, in exactly that tone of voice?

MR. H: Yeah, I figured she wouldn't want to anyway. I was like, well, you know, I don't know, I just wasn't thinking like I really wanted to do this.

THERAPIST: So what did she say when you asked her out?

MR. H: She said, well, she wanted to think about it.

THERAPIST: So what did you do?

MR. H: Well, I just turned away and marched over to the coffee. I didn't say anything more.

THERAPIST: What were you feeling when that happened?

MR. H: I was pissed.

THERAPIST: Is that when you started thinking about suicide?

MR. H: Well, it didn't happen right away, but I was pretty fed up. I was thinking she's cold and calculating, she just wants to hurt me.

THERAPIST: That must have really hurt. Not only to have those thoughts about someone you thought might like you, but to realize that when you asked her out, which is a hard thing to do, you didn't get exactly what you wanted. Although, I must say, she didn't say no, just that she wanted to think about it. So what happened next?

MR. H: I don't know, I went over to the coffee maker and I poured myself a coffee. I just stood in the corner and I started thinking, well, everyone has hidden motives and they are going to manipulate me if given the opportunity. After that, I decided to get out of there. I left the room and sat outside on a bench.

THERAPIST: So when you got outside, what happened next?

MR. H: Well, I sat down, and I then just started thinking about the whole thing and how I was drinking last night and I was sort of screwing up again and I figured, you know, other people are only nice when they want to get something from me or exploit me, just like I am with them. I decided that I'm just doomed for failure and that I'm an evil person. I was thinking that no matter what I do people are gonna always find something wrong with me. I know people don't trust me and I don't trust them. I started thinking about wanting to die.

THERAPIST: At any point during this time or before you left the meeting room did you think of any of the skills that we've been working on?

MR. H: No, and the more I thought about being dead, I don't know, I started feeling better or something. I don't know why and then I just started thinking, you know, this just shows that I'm fatally flawed because I'm feeling better by thinking about killing myself. So, my idea that I am evil must be true.

THERAPIST: So how did you end up not taking any action?

MR. H: For me suicide is always a fantasy. I sat there about 5 minutes, then I thought about you and remembered then that you told me to use opposite action. So I decided that since I wasn't going to really do anything, I might as well take a walk.

THERAPIST: That's a great use of a skill. Now let's see if we can figure out what you might do next time.

The therapist and Mr. H continued with this analysis, focusing on solutions and trouble-shooting potential problems that might occur when trying in the future to use identified solutions. Overall, during treatment repeated chain analyses helped Mr. H gain insight that his anger often was a secondary emotion to fear. Functionally, anger motivated him to be aggressive, and as a consequence his belief that "he is unlikeable or evil" was reinforced because people tended to avoid him when he behaved like that. During individual therapy, emphasis was placed on the use of the GIVE interpersonal skills and increasing nonjudgmental participation, radical openness, and distress tolerance. In addition, metaphor was used frequently. For example, the therapist suggested that Mr. H's way of dealing with intimacy was like a person who desperately desires to go swimming but instead walks endlessly around the swimming pool, never jumping in because he or she can't be certain how deep the water is (i.e., Mr. H is afraid to participate because he is afraid of being hurt again). Dialectical dilemmas for paranoid personality disorder (see Figure 10.13) were reviewed with the patient and specific dilemmas for Mr. H were targeted, including reducing attachment to grudges, reducing brooding, finding a balance between extreme judgmental communications and inhibiting his opinion, and finding balance between blaming himself and blaming others.

Direct challenges of Mr. H's core beliefs (e.g., people will take advantage of him) were found to be less useful. Instead, strategies focused on *reducing ineffective action tendencies linked with hostility and anger* were found to be most effective. We based this on the idea that much of his automatic anger was classically conditioned and therefore less amenable to conscious cognitive change. Thus over time, by behaving more prosocially (i.e., changing his action tendency), he acquired new associations to stimuli associated with intimacy. That is, he learned that bad things do not always happen when he interacted with women. This, after repeated exposures, lead to a change in his beliefs about intimacy. For example, during session 18 Mr. H reported that he had used mindfulness skills to participate without judgment in singing hymns with other church members. Normally he would never do this because he felt it "was stupid." Instead, this time he simply observed thoughts that arose during the singing (e.g., "This is dumb," "Everyone is watching me") while continually turning his mind back to participating in the singing. Over time, Mr. H reported greater success with participation skills. Examples of additional behavioral exposure exercises used with this patient included:

- Interactions in the community with other individuals.
- Interactions with anyone whom he believed to be genuine or trustworthy.
- Practicing confiding in others.
- Increasing prosocial behaviors (e.g., engage in three practices of chitchat per week, say "Thank you" to praise).

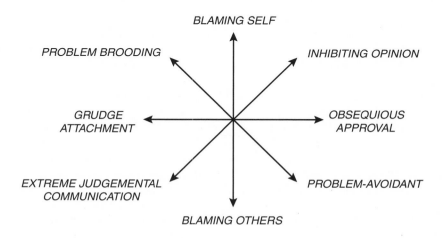

FIGURE 10.13. Dialectical dilemmas for paranoid behaviors.

- Decrease avoidance of situations where positive emotion could occur (e.g., buy a puppy).
- Decrease expectations that all grievances or mistakes made by another person "should" deserve an apology from the other person (e.g., he was instructed to notice the number of times that circumstances prevented him from apologizing when he made what he considered to be an interpersonal mistake).

Narcissistic Personality Disorder

Mr. S was a 61-year-old patient who had never been married and had few relationships. When he was a child he had an invalidating relationship with an alcoholic and demanding father and he was abandoned by his family as a teen. He had a military career and considered himself a risk-taker (e.g., his hobby was motorcycle racing). He sought treatment for chronic depression and met criteria for narcissistic personality disorder. He endorsed feeling superior to others, more intelligent than others, and misunderstood by others. He also reported rarely experiencing joy or strong negative emotions, other than pervasive dysphoria. He was surprised that he had developed very few friends, expressed great loneliness, and experienced intense periods of self-loathing. Therapy started with Mr. S declaring that it was unlikely that the therapist was intelligent enough to help him. Early in therapy, the therapist encouraged the patient to watch sessions on videotape and report back what he observed. When asked about his observations, Mr. S told that he noticed that he (Mr. S) talked a great deal and often interrupted the therapist. When the therapist asked whether Mr. S thought this could cause problems in relationships with others, Mr. S replied: "At first I thought that maybe it could. But then I realized that it is like talking with a great mathematician. When you ask a normal person what 2 + 2 is, if they talked a lot it would be wrong. But for a great mathematician, going to great lengths to explain the facts of 2 + 2 is like sipping a fine wine. So, I ended up deciding this is not a problem."

Therapy revolved around behavioral experiments designed to increase Mr. S's awareness regarding the impact of his behavior on others and improving his ability to judge others interpersonally. The therapist would point out that "unfortunately it appears that your interpersonal style sometimes backfires, despite your good intentions." In other words, his attempts to help others by telling them what to do or pointing out his own expertise often resulted in the other person looking annoyed or walking away. After learning GIVE skills, Mr. S was given homework to notice whether telling others what to do led to longer conversations compared with times when he consciously practiced his GIVE skills. The goal was for him to notice that validation and listening increased positive interactions with others.

Behavioral analyses revealed that social situations often elicited boredom and, less frequently, anxiety. Mr. S reported that talking about himself relieved boredom and reduced anxiety but often was followed by periods of self-loathing, especially if the person he interacted with overtly avoided him. Another major target during therapy was related to helping identify his emotions. Dialectical dilemmas that were found applicable included reducing blaming others, reducing apparent autonomy and increasing his ability to ask for help, looking for balance between self-aggrandizement and self-loathing, and working on ways to increase empathy and reduce solicitation of admiration (see Figure 10.14). Behavioral exposure exercises and other behavioral homework assignments included:

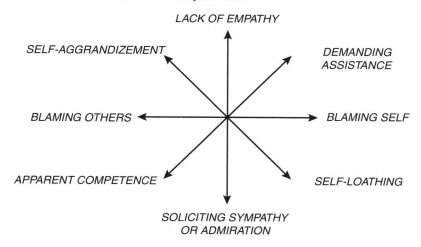

FIGURE 10.14. Dialectical dilemmas for narcissistic behaviors.

- Practicing being treated like other people (e.g., waiting in line rather than cutting in line).
- In-session practice of experiencing criticism without avoidance.
- Spending time with "everyday" individuals.
- Imagining a more average existence.
- Decreasing comparative and superlative language (e.g., monitor each time he said or thought "I'm better than him/her").
- Increasing empathy (e.g., work in soup kitchen, list five empathic statements).
- Increase ability to accurately read emotions of others (e.g., three times in session read emotion of therapist).
- Improve ability to read interpersonal cues by giving rules of engagement (e.g., if someone he is talking with is quiet for more than 3 minutes, assume that he is talking too much and to stop and listen to them at that point).
- Engage in anonymous random acts of kindness.

Obsessive–Compulsive Personality Disorder

Ms. Q presented for treatment to help with long-standing feelings of emptiness, loneliness, and dysphoria. At the beginning of treatment Ms. Q met diagnostic criteria for major depressive disorder and obsessive–compulsive personality disorder. She reported that although some of the depressive symptoms had been long-standing, her current level of distress was significantly increased and had been increased since her retirement approximately 5 years earlier. Ms. Q had retired from a high-powered position in which she was responsible for the day-to-day activities of scores of individuals. Since her retirement, she reported that she was "noticing all the things that have always been wrong." In terms of her obsessive–compulsive personality disorder symptoms, Ms. Q endorsed being preoccupied with rules, lists, and order/organization, excessive devotion to work to the exclusion of important interpersonal relationships, moral/ethical inflexibility, stubbornness, and reluctance in delegating. According to Ms. Q, these behaviors had always disrupted her social and interpersonal functioning but had been reinforced through her occupational trajectory. Ms. Q's goals for treatment included improved relationships with important individuals in her life (including her children), increased leisure activities that did not increase stress and self-judgment, and decreased distress, primarily in the form of less sadness and hopelessness. Although Ms. Q did not specify decreasing judgment as a goal, her therapist believed that this construct was a mediating factor for many of the other goals and introduced this idea to Ms. Q.

Treatment for Ms. Q progressed as would be expected in standard DBT for the most part. Specifically, behavioral activation was introduced to increase leisure activity, and interpersonal effectiveness skills were introduced to target disrupted relationships. Ms. Q reported feeling less distressed and noted progress toward her treatment goals. Most of treatment, however, was focused on increasing fluid mind and working on forgiveness of self and others to reduce judgment and reduce the fluctuations between blaming self and others. In this vein, the therapist and Ms. Q worked together repeatedly to balance "fixed mind" (i.e., a state of mind based on historically relevant information and traditional behavioral responses) and "fresh mind" (i.e., a state of mind based on newness of current information and lack of preconceived behavioral biases) to arrive at "fluid mind" (i.e., a state of mind based on balancing prior knowledge/effective strategies with the possibility of unforeseen opportunities). For example, in the course of utilizing interpersonal effectiveness skills to address damaged relationships with her daughters, Ms. Q would often lament, "Why bother? I know what is going to happen anyway." This thought often preceded feelings of loneliness and hopelessness. Thus, we worked on synthesizing past experiences and honoring what Ms. Q knew to be true in her history with the possibility that something different could occur with the new information of the current moment—including her newly skillful behavior (see Figure 10.15). Other behavioral exposures and homework exercises included:

- Listing all the possible reasons that someone might make a different decision than Ms. Q would make in a given situation.
- Practicing delegation of household chores to others.
- Noticing judgment of other group members and turning attention back to the task at hand.

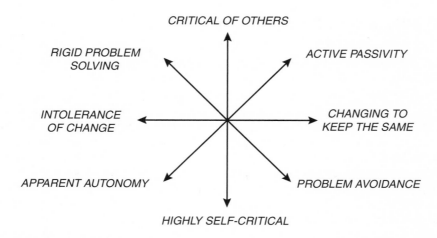

FIGURE 10.15. Dialectical dilemmas for obsessive–compulsive personality disorder.

- In session, changing the agenda without prior warning and practicing flexibility in adapting with fluid mind.
- Participating in leisure events that were likely to evoke judgment (e.g., volunteer organizations being run without "proper" attention to detail).

Conclusions

In conclusion, at this stage of treatment development we have established the feasibility and acceptability of a DBT-based treatment for older adults with major depressive disorder and personality disorder. In addition to the development of significant clinical experience with a undertreated/underrecognized population, we have integrated the existing research literatures from both DBT and geropsychology to develop a treatment manual that targets relevant clinical constructs for older adults with personality disorder and major depressive disorder. We also have completed and refined the first iteration of the DBT^{D+PD} treatment manual that has a new biosocial theory for all individuals with personality disorders, regardless of age, and incorporates new modules focused on increasing behavioral and cognitive flexibility as well as reconciling unresolved grievances from the past. The next step in the continuation of the development and validation of this treatment is to conduct a RCT with the new DBT^{D+PD} treatment manual. We have plans to undertake this project with older adults diagnosed with major depressive disorder and comorbid personality disorder. In addition, future research examining the hypothesized mechanisms of action (e.g., reductions in cognitive/behavioral rigidity) and the utility of these adaptations with younger individuals with personality disorders would add tremendously to the understanding of this adapted treatment. Treatment of individuals with long-standing personality dysfunction is a difficult process for both therapist and patient. We are hopeful that the above adaptations will be found useful by clinicians and we look forward to reporting further results for this approach in the near future.

NOTE

1. We will not cover treatment of borderline personality disorder (BPD) or address in detail treatment strategies used in standard DBT as this has already been clearly explicated by the developer of DBT (Linehan, 1993a, 1993b). This chapter also will not cover in detail basic information about personality disorders, nor present details regarding other treatments for personality disorders. For a critical review of treatments for all personality disorders, interested readers may wish to examine a recent literature review by Linehan, Davidson, Lynch, and Sanderson (2006). Finally, we will not cover DBT adaptations associated with the treatment of depression without comorbid personality disorder, as this has been reviewed in detail in prior publications (see Lynch, 2000; Lynch, Morse, & Vitt, 2002).

REFERENCES

Abrams, R. C., & Horowitz, S. V. (1996). Personality disorders after age 50: A meta-analysis. *Journal of Personality Disorders, 10,* 271–281.

Abrams, R. C., & Horowitz, S. V. (1999). Personality disorders after age 50: A meta-analytic review of the literature. In E. Roscowsky, R. C. Abrams, & R. A. Zweig (Eds.), *Personality disorders in older adults* (pp. 55–68). Mahwah, NJ: Erlbaum.

Abrams, R. C., Spielman, L. A., Alexopoulos, G. S., & Klausner, E. (1998). Personality disorder symptoms and functioning in elderly depressed patients. *American Journal of Geriatric Psychiatry, 6,* 24–30.

American Psychiatric Association. (1994). *Diagnostic and statistical manual of mental disorders* (4th ed.). Washington, DC: Author.

Bailey, G. R., Jr. (1998). Cognitive-behavioral treatment of obsessive–compulsive personality disorder. *Journal of Psychological Practice, 4,* 51–59.

Beck, A. T., Freeman, A., & Davis, D. D. (2004). *Cognitive therapy of personality disorders* (2nd ed.). New York: Guilford Press.

Beck, A. T., Rush, A. J., Shaw, B. F., & Emery, G. (1979). *Cognitive therapy of depression.* New York: Guilford Press.

Benjamin, L. (1993). *Interpersonal diagnosis and treatment of personality disorders.* New York: Guilford Press.

Brodaty, H., Harris, L., Peters, K., Wilhelm, K., Hickie, I., Boyce, P., et al. (1993). Prognosis of depression in the elderly: A comparison with younger patients. *British Journal of Psychiatry, 163,* 589–596.

Butler, R. (1963). The life review: An interpretation of reminiscence in the aged. *Psychiatry, 26,* 65–76.

Cheavens, J. S., Rosenthal, M. Z., Banawan, S. F., & Lynch, T. R. (2006). *Differences in emotional experience and emotion regulation as a function of age and psychiatric condition.* Unpublished manuscript, Duke University Medical Center, Department of Psychiatry.

Coyne, J. C. (1976). Depression and the response of others. *Journal of Abnormal Psychology, 85,* 186–193.

Devanand, D. P. (2002). Comorbid psychiatric disorders in late life depression. *Biological Psychiatry, 52,* 236–242.

Diener, E., Sandvik, E., & Larsen, R. J. (1985). Age and sex effects for emotional intensity. *Developmental Psychology, 21,* 542–546.

Dowson, J. H., & Berrios, G. E. (1991). Factor structure of DSM-III-R personality disorders shown by self-report questionnaire: Implications for classifying and assessing personality disorders. *Acta Psychiatrica Scandinavica, 84,* 555–560.

Duberstein, P. R., Conwell, Y., & Caine, E. D. (1994). Age differences in the personality characteristics of suicide completers: Preliminary findings from a psychological autopsy study. *Psychiatry, 57,* 213–224.

Duberstein, P. R., Conwell, Y., Seidlitz, L., Denning, D. G., Cox, C., & Caine, E. D. (2000). Personality traits and suicidal behavior and ideation in depressed inpatients 50 years of age and older. *Journals of Gerontology, Series B: Psychological Sciences and Social Sciences, 55,* P18–26.

Duggan, C. F., Lee, A. S., & Murray, R. M. (1990). Does personality predict long-term outcome in depression? *British Journal of Psychiatry, 157,* 19–24.

Ehrlich, H. J., & Bauer, M. L. (1966). The correlates of dogmatism and flexibility in psychiatric hospitalization. *Journal of Consulting Psychology, 30,* 253–259.

Erikson, E. H., & Erikson, J. M. (1997). *The life cycle completed.* New York: Norton.

Fiorot, M., Boswell, P., & Murray, E. J. (1990). Personality and response to psychotherapy in depressed elderly women. *Behavior, Health, and Aging, 1,* 51–63.

First, M. B., Gibbon, M., Spitzer, R. L., Williams, J. B. W., & Benjamin, L. S. (1997). *User's guide for the Structured Clinical Interview for DSM-IV Axis II Personality Disorders (SCID-II).* Washington, DC: American Psychiatric Press.

Folkman, S., Lazarus, R., Pimley, S., & Novacek, J. (1987). Age-differences in stress and coping processes. *Psychology and Aging, 2,* 171–184.

Giesler, R. B., Josephs, R. A., & Swann, W. B. (1996). Self-verification in clinical depression: The desire for negative evaluation. *Journal of Abnormal Psychology, 105,* 358–368.

Glisky, M. L., Tataryn, D. J., Tobias, B. A., Kihlstrom, J. F., & McConkey, K. M. (1991). Absorption, openness to experience, and hypnotizability. *Journal of Personality and Social Psychology, 60,* 263–272.

Gottman, J. M. (1994). *Why marriages succeed or fail and how you can make yours last.* New York: Simon & Schuster.

Gross, J. J., Carstensen, L. L., Pasupathi, M., Tsai, J., Skorpen, C. G., & Hsu, A. Y. C. (1997). Emotion and aging: Experience, expression, and control. *Psychology and Aging, 12,* 590–599.

Hamilton, M. (1960). A rating scale for depression. *Journal of Neurological Neurosurgical Psychiatry, 23,* 56–61.

Hardy, G. E., Barkham, M., Shapiro, D. A., Rees, A., Stiles, W. B., & Reynolds, S. (1995). Impact of Cluster-C personality-disorders on outcomes of contrasting brief psychotherapies for depression. *Journal of Consulting and Clinical Psychology, 63,* 997–1004.

Hirschfeld, R. M. (1993). Personality disorders: Definition and diagnosis. *Journal of Personality Disorders, 7,* 9–17.

Hyler, S. E., Skodol, A. E., Kellman, H. D., Oldham, J. M., & Rosnick, L. (1990). Validity of the Personality Diagnostic Questionnaire—Revised: Comparison with two structured interviews. *American Journal of Psychiatry, 147,* 1043–1048.

Ilardi, S. S., Craighead, W. E., & Evans, D. D. (1997). Modeling relapse in unipolar depression: The effects of dysfunctional cognitions and personality disorders. *Journal of Consulting and Clinical Psychology, 65,* 381–391.

Kenan, M. M., Kendjelic, E. M., Molinari, V. A., Williams, W., Norris, M., & Kunik, M. E. (2000). Age-related differences in the frequency of personality disorders among inpatient veterans. *International Journal of Geriatric Psychiatry, 15,* 831–837.

Klein, M. H., Kupfer, D. J., & Shea, M. (1993). *Personality and depression: A current view.* New York: Guilford Press.

Kunik, M. E., Benoit, M. H., Rifai, A. H., Sweet, R. A., Pasternak, R., & Zubenko, G. S. (1994). Diagnostic rate of co-morbid personality disorder in elderly psychiatric inpatients. *American Journal of Psychiatry, 151,* 603–605.

Kunik, M. E., Mulsant, B. H., Rifai, A. H., Sweet, R. A., Pasternak, R., Rosen, J., et al. (1993). Personality disorders in elderly inpatients with major depression. *American Journal of Geriatric Psychiatry, 1,* 38–45.

Lane, R. D., Quinlan, D. M., Swartz, G. E., Walker, P. A., & Zeitlin, S. B. (1990). The Levels of Emotional Awareness Scale: A cognitive-developmental measure of emotion. *Journal of Personality Assessment, 55,* 124–134.

Lawton, M., Kleban, M., Rajagopal, D., & Dean, J. (1992). Dimensions of affective experience in three age groups. *Psychology and Aging, 7,* 171–184.

Linehan, M. M. (1993a). *Cognitive-behavioral treatment of borderline personality disorder.* New York: Guilford Press.

Linehan, M. M. (1993b). *Skills training manual for treating borderline personality disorder.* New York: Guilford Press.

Linehan, M., Davison, G., Lynch, T. R., & Sanderson, C. (2006). Principles of therapeutic change in the treatment of personality disorders. In L. Castonguay & L. Beutler (Eds.), *Principles of therapeutic change that work* (pp. 239–252). New York: Oxford University Press.

Link, B., Struening, E., Rahav, M., Phelan, J., & Nuttbrock, L. (1997). On stigma and its consequences: Evidence from a longitudinal study of men with dual diagnoses of mental illness and substance abuse. *Journal of Health and Social Behavior, 38,* 177–190.

Lynch, T. R. (2000). Treatment of elderly depression with personality disorder co-morbidity using dialectical behavior therapy. *Cognitive and Behavioral Practice, 7,* 468–477.

Lynch, T. R., Cheavens, J. S., Cukrowicz, K., & Linehan, M. M. (2006). *Dialectical behavior therapy for depression with co-morbid personality disorders: An extension of standard DBT with a special emphasis on older adults* [Unpublished treatment manual]. Durham, NC: Duke University Medical Center.

Lynch, T. R., Cheavens, J. S., Cukrowicz, K. C., Thorp, S., Bronner, L., & Beyer, J. (2007). Treatment of older adults with co-morbid personality disorder and depression: A dialectical behavior therapy approach. *International Journal of Geriatric Psychiatry, 22,* 131–143.

Lynch, T. R., Cheavens, J., Morse, J. Q., & Rosenthal, M. Z. (2004). A model predicting suicidal ideation and hopelessness in depressed older adults: The impact of emotion inhibition and affect intensity. *Aging and Mental Health*, *8*, 486–497.

Lynch, T. R., Morse, J. Q., Mendelson, T., & Robins, C. J. (2003). Dialectical behavior therapy for depressed older adults: A randomized pilot study. *American Journal of Geriatric Psychiatry*, *11*, 1–13.

Lynch, T. R., Morse, J. Q., & Vitt, C. M. (2002). Dialectical behavior therapy for depressed older adults. *Behavior Therapist*, *25*, 7–8.

Lyness, J. M., Caine, E. D., Conwell, Y., King, D. A., & Cox, C. (1993). Depressive symptoms, medical illness, and functional status in depressed psychiatric inpatients. *American Journal of Psychiatry*, *150*, 910–915.

McConatha, J., & Huba, H. (1999). Primary, secondary, and emotional control across adulthood. *Current Psychology: Developmental, Learning, Personality, Social*, *18*, 164–170.

McCrae, R. R. (1987). Creativity, divergent thinking, and openness to experience. *Journal of Personality and Social Psychology*, *46*, 919–928.

McCrae, R. R., & Costa, P. T. (1996). Conceptions and correlates of openness to experience. In R. Hogan, J. A. Johnson, & S. R. Briggs (Eds.), *Handbook of personality psychology* (pp. 825–847). New York: Academic Press.

Meeks, S., Carstensen, L. L., Tamsky, B. F., Wright, T. L., & Pellegrini, D. (1989). Age-differences in coping: Does less mean worse? *International Journal of Aging and Human Development*, *28*, 127–140.

Molinari, V., & Marmion, J. (1995). Relationship between affective-disorders and Axis-II diagnoses in geropsychiatric patients. *Journal of Geriatric Psychiatry and Neurology*, *8*, 61–64.

Morey, L. C., Gunderson, J. G., Quigley, B. D., Shea, M. T., Skodol, A. E., McGlashan, T. H., et al. (2002). The representation of borderline, avoidant, obsessive–compulsive, and schizotypal personality disorders by the five-factor model. *Journal of Personality Disorders*, *16*, 215–234.

Morey, L. C., Warner, M. B., Shea, M. T., Gunderson, J. G., Sanislow, C. A., Grilo, C., et al. (2003). The representation of four personality disorders by the Schedule for Nonadaptive and Adaptive Personality Dimensional Model of Personality. *Psychological Assessment*, *15*, 326–332.

Morse, J. Q., & Lynch, T. R. (2004). A preliminary investigation of self-reported personality disorders in late life: Prevalence, predictors of depressive severity, and clinical correlates. *Aging and Mental Health*, *8*, 307–315.

Nestadt, G., Eaton, W. W., & Romanoski, A. J. (1994). Assessment of DSM-III personality structure in a general-population survey. *Comprehensive Psychiatry*, *35*, 54–63.

Ogrodniczuk, J. S., Piper, W. E., Joyce, A. S., McCallum, M., & Rosie, J. S. (2002). Social support as a predictor of response to group therapy for complicated grief. *Psychiatry*, *65*, 346–357.

Ogrodniczuk, J. S., Piper, W. E., Joyce, A. S., McCallum, M., & Rosie, J. S. (2003). NEO-five factor personality traits as predictors of response to two forms of group psychotherapy. *International Journal of Group Psychotherapy*, *53*, 417–442.

Pasupathi, M., & Carstensen, L. L. (2003). Age and emotional experience during mutual reminiscing. *Psychology and Aging*, *18*, 430–442.

Pelham, B. W., & Swann, W. B. (1994). The juncture of intrapersonal and interpersonal knowledge: Self-certainty and interpersonal congruence. *Personality and Social Psychology Bulletin*, *20*, 349–357.

Pilkonis, P. A., & Frank, E. (1988). Personality pathology in recurrent depression: Nature, prevalence, and relationship to treatment response. *American Journal of Psychiatry*, *145*, 435–441.

Pilkonis, P. A., Kim, Y., Proietti, J. M., & Barkham, M. (1996). Scales for personality disorders developed from the Inventory of Interpersonal Problems. *Journal of Personality Disorders*, *10*, 355–369.

Ritts, V., & Stein, J. R. (1995). Verification and commitment in marital relationships: An exploration of self-verification theory in community college students. *Psychological Reports*, *76*, 383–386.

Rokeach, M. (1960). *The open and closed mind: Investigations into the nature of belief systems and personality systems*. New York: Basic Books.

Rounsaville, B. J., & Carroll, K. M. (2001). A stage model of behavioral therapies research: Getting started and moving on from Stage I. *Clinical Psychology: Science and Practice, 8*, 133–142.

Schotte, C. K., DeDoncker, D., & Vankerckhoven, C. (1998). Self-report assessment of the DSM-IV personality disorders: Measurement of trait and distress characteristics: The ADP-IV. *Psychological Medicine, 28*, 1179–1188.

Schroeder, M. L., & Livesley, W.J. (1991). An evaluation of *DSM-III-R* personality disorders. *Acta Psychiatrica Scandinavica, 84*, 512–519.

Schultz, P. W., & Searleman, A. (2002). Rigidity of thought and behavior: 100 years of research. *Genetic, Social and General Psychology Monographs, 128*, 165–207.

Shea, M. T., Pilkonis, P. A., Beckham, E., Collins, J. F., Elkin, I., Sotsky, F. M., et al. (1990). Personality disorders and treatment outcome in the NIMH Treatment of Depression Collaborative Research Program. *American Journal of Psychiatry, 147*, 711–718.

Staudinger, U. M., & Pasupathi, M. (2000). Life-span perspectives on self, personality, and social cognition. In F. I. M. Craik & T. A. Salthouse (Eds.), *The handbook of aging and cognition* (pp. 633–688). Mahwah, NJ: Erlbaum.

Stek, M. L., van Exel, E., van Tilburg, W., Westendorp, R. G., & Beekman, A. T. (2002). The prognosis of depression in old age: Outcome six to eight years after clinical treatment. *Aging and Mental Health, 6*, 282–285.

Swann, W. B. (1997). The trouble with change: Self-verification and allegiance to the self. *Psychological Science, 8*, 177–180.

Swann, W. B., de la Ronde, C., & Hixon, J. G. (1994). Authenticity and positive strivings in marriage and courtship. *Journal of Personality and Social Psychology, 66*, 857–869.

Thase, M. E. (1996). The role of Axis II comorbidity in the management of patients with treatment-resistant depression. *Psychiatric Clinics of North America, 19*, 287–309.

Thompson, L. W., Gallagher, D., & Czirr, R. (1988). Personality disorder and outcome in the treatment of late-life depression. *Journal of Geriatric Psychiatry, 21*, 133–153.

Vine, R. G., & Steingart, A. B. (1994). Personality disorder in the elderly depressed. *Canadian Journal of Psychiatry, 39*, 392–398.

Webster, J. D., & Cappeliez, P. (1993). Reminiscence and autobiographical memory: Complementary contexts for aging research. *Developmental Review, 13*, 54–91.

CHAPTER 11

Dialectical Behavior Therapy for Assertive Community Treatment Teams

Sarah K. Reynolds, Randy Wolbert,
Gwen Abney-Cunningham, *and* Kimberly Patterson

Assertive community treatment (ACT) and dialectical behavior therapy (DBT) are both evidence-based approaches for the rehabilitation of consumers whose severe and persistent mental health problems (e.g., debilitating psychotic and bipolar disorders and borderline personality disorder, respectively) require an intensive level of services. ACT is a model of service delivery that was developed over 30 years ago to extend "hospital-like" services into the community (Stein, Test, & Marx, 1975; Test, 1992). DBT is a comprehensive psychosocial intervention designed more recently for individuals with suicidal behavior and other out-of-control behaviors in the context of borderline personality disorder (BPD; Linehan, Armstrong, Suarez, Allmon, & Heard, 1991, Linehan, 1993a). ACT was designed to provide intensive services in the community for the consumer who has greater needs than can be accommodated by the traditional community mental health system (Allness & Knoedler, 1998). As such, a sizable number of ACT referrals are individuals with BPD who present with chronic suicidality and other extreme behaviors, high use of emergency services, multiple case management needs (e.g., joblessness, inability to manage activities of daily living), and the presence of comorbid diagnoses (e.g., schizoaffective disorder, bipolar disorder) that are typically targeted by ACT services. These referrals are made even though it is unclear that traditional ACT services alone are sufficient for this consumer group (Links, 1998). Ideally, those with BPD would be treated by a specialty program such as DBT, which was specifically designed for this population. Indeed, DBT is the only treatment with substantial efficacy data for chronic suicidality in the context of BPD.

The dilemma ACT teams face, however, is that a referral to DBT is not always appropriate or even possible. A DBT program may not exist in the local community, or the program may be in its infancy with very limited capacity and services (e.g., the DBT "program" consists only of a skills group). In these cases, referral to DBT is either not possible or not likely to have sufficient clinical impact. Furthermore, a DBT team might not always be equipped to deliver all the case management services needed by a particular consumer.

How, then, can an ACT team help their consumers with BPD, whose unique needs are best addressed by receiving DBT instead of, or in addition to, ACT-based services? The present chapter focuses on this question. We begin with a discussion of when and why ACT alone may be insufficient, and different options that ACT teams might have for responding to referrals for consumers with a BPD diagnosis (or suicidal and other extreme behaviors consistent with such a diagnosis). Our approach has been to implement what we will label "ACT/DBT," which consists of a comprehensive DBT "track" within an ACT setting.

Throughout the chapter, we draw upon our experience implementing ACT/DBT within a private, not-for-profit mental health agency and within two countywide public mental health systems, as well as a decade of consulting to ACT teams. Our collective experience includes what could be termed a "bottom-up" effort in which direct care clinicians led the initiative to begin DBT services and gradually expanded the programming, and also a "top-down" approach, in which county administrators and funding agencies mandated that DBT implementation occur in several community agencies and ACT programs. Although systematic data are not available, our own estimate is that the ACT/DBT model has been implemented in systems in at least five U.S. states and one Canadian province. We describe our experience with ACT/DBT and address key issues and challenges to consider when deciding whether to offer DBT within ACT-based services.

Although most readers may be familiar with the ACT model, a remarkable degree of variation exists among programs that self-identify as an "ACT Team" (Deci, Santos, Hiott, Schoenwald, & Dias, 1995; Monroe-DeVita & Mohatt, 2000). To avoid confusion, therefore, we first provide a brief overview and history of the model.

Overview of ACT

ACT is a model of service delivery developed in the early 1970s by Leonard Stein and Mary Ann Test in Madison, Wisconsin. It was designed to serve adults with severe and persistent mental illness (the most common primary diagnosis is schizophrenia). Originally termed "training in community living" (TCL), this approach has also been referred to as "continuous treatment teams" and as the "program of assertive community treatment" (PACT; Test, 1992), and is now most commonly known as ACT. It includes several key elements: a multidisciplinary team approach, instruction and assistance in basic living skills that includes *in vivo* contacts to enhance "real-world" functioning, 24-hour availability of staff, integration of community resources, and an assertive outreach approach to minimize consumer dropout. Services are provided on an ongoing basis and the model is considered a "no discharge" model (Stein & Santos, 1998) in that consumers cannot be terminated from the program and can be guaranteed services for as long as they are necessary.

The ACT model provides an organizational framework for delivering what may be a wide array of mental health services including individual therapy, group therapy, family therapy, vocational services, substance abuse services, health services, medication management, and case management. The particular "package" of services assembled for a given consumer will vary depending on his or her unique needs and goals.

ACT staff function as interchangeable team members to provide the services necessary for community living. Although specialties exist, each staff member is generally expected to provide whatever the consumer may need during a particular community contact. ACT teams share information via daily morning meetings in which each consumer is discussed, including his or her overall progress toward goals and the nature and content of previous contacts. New consumer contact assignments are made for the day. Overall team caseloads are kept small (usually at about 1:10). Staff are available 24 hours a day, 7 days a week to meet consumer needs. ACT teams vary in size from small rural teams containing three or four staff to larger urban teams containing up to a dozen staff.

Research conducted over nearly three decades has shown that ACT successfully meets consumer needs on many fronts (Bond, Drake, Mueser, & Latimer, 2001). Studies have demonstrated that compared to consumers in standard treatment offered in the community, consumers in ACT require less hospitalization, spend more time employed, have improved living conditions, maintain more positive relationships with friends and family, and endorse higher ratings of life satisfaction (Stein & Santos, 1998). The ACT model has proliferated and can now be found in over 35 states and several countries due to its well-documented effectiveness (Phillips, 2001).

Treating Consumers with BPD in a Traditional ACT Setting

While ACT is inarguably effective for many, its success for consumers with personality disorder has been questioned by some ACT experts (e.g., Bond et al., 2001; Jones, 2002). This concern is particularly relevant given that BPD is a relatively common diagnosis among patient groups traditionally referred to ACT: those with psychotic disorders and high utilizers. In U.K. samples, between 30 and 60% of those with psychotic disorders have a coexisting personality disorder (Casey, 2000). In addition, between 9 and 44% of samples of high utilizers typically receive a diagnosis of BPD, with higher prevalence rates among inpatient samples (e.g., Cutting, Cowen, Mann, & Jenkins, 1986) and those with repeated hospitalizations (Woogh, 1986). A large-scale study found that patients with a BPD diagnosis had more extensive histories of both psychosocial and pharmacological treatment than did patients with major depressive disorder (Bender et al., 2001). Further, ample data suggest that the presence of a comorbid personality disorder diagnosis confers poorer long-term outcome among patients with Axis I disorders (e.g., Sanislow & McGlashan, 1998; Pilkonis & Frank, 1988), and a diagnosis of BPD per se is associated with particularly high levels of psychosocial impairment (Skodol et al., 2002). Finally, estimates suggest that up to 10% of individuals with BPD die by suicide, a rate equal to that of schizophrenia and major depressive disorder (Linehan, Rizvi, Shaw Welch, & Page, 2000). Overall, the degree of impairment and the high level of prevalence within the public health system points to the necessity to consider the unique needs of these consumers within ACT teams.

Few studies have examined the effectiveness of ACT for consumers with BPD. However, Weisbrod (1983) found that ACT, when provided to persons with personality disorders, costs *more* than a hospital-based control treatment, in contrast to the *reduced* costs found for those diagnosed with psychotic disorders. Similarly, a series of three randomized controlled trials in the United Kingdom studying "community-focused care programs" (Merson et al., 1992; Gandhi et al., 2001; Tyrer, Manley, Van Horne, Leddy, & Ukoumunne, 2000) also suggested problematic long-term outcomes for personality disorders. Although not explicitly focused on the ACT model, these studies suggested that within their samples of patients with psychotic disorder or affective disorder, the presence of comorbid personality disorder predicted poorer social functioning, higher levels of depressive symptoms, and a greater number of police contacts for consumers in community-focused care programs. In reviewing outcomes from these three studies, Tyrer and Simmonds (2003) concluded that patients with comorbid personality disorder and severe and persistent Axis I diagnoses can be successfully kept out of the hospital with assertive community care, but that "the price of this success is often more impaired social function" and heightened public risk due to criminal behavior (p. 18).

These difficulties are not surprising given that ACT is a model of service delivery, not a psychosocial intervention per se. It was never designed as a primary mode of treatment for BPD, particularly not for the repetitive and chronic suicidal behaviors (i.e., thoughts, threats, attempts, and self-harm) often characteristic of these consumers (e.g., Sansone, 2004; Yen et al., 2003) and also predictive of high service use (Comtois et al., 2003). Indeed, recurrent episodes of suicidal behavior in the context of BPD appear to represent a unique treatment challenge distinct from instances of suicidality that are more acute, unexpected, and circumscribed. Unfortunately, traditional treatment guidelines are geared toward acute episodes of suicidality and typically involve added services and concrete assistance to solve a single problem, an approach that may inadvertently reinforce the behavior (Dawson & MacMillan, 1993; Paris, 2004; Sansone, 2004). In other words, when a consumer's suicide crisis is met by a differential clinician response of increased help and perhaps removal of difficulties (e.g., via hospitalization), that consumer may be more likely to respond to a future stressor with suicidal behavior (Comtois, 2002; Linehan, 1993a). As such, a BPD diagnosis and chronic suicidality signal the need for a specialized treatment approach that teaches the consumer how to handle life stressors in a way other than suicidal behavior.

In our experience, without specialized care that focuses on systematic skill building, overreliance on crisis services, failure to improve, and staff frustration and burnout can result. Those with a comorbid BPD diagnosis often consume a disproportionate amount of staff time, most often in crisis work, external consultation, and the constant revision of treatment plans and contracts. Although standard ACT practice may reduce psychiatric hospitalization rates somewhat in some cases, often there is little improvement in independent functioning over the long term. Furthermore, staff tend to feel helpless and overwhelmed with BPD consumers, often lamenting, "I know I did the wrong thing but I didn't know what else to do." Those with comorbid BPD are often avoided, and typically viewed as manipulative people who simply do not want to get better. Common responses in ACT team meetings include "She keeps 'upping the ante' " and "I'm sick of playing these games." By contrast, the prototypic response to a similar behavior by a patient with schizophrenia without BPD may be much more forgiving: "He's sick, he can't help his behavior." Both the research evidence and these clinical experiences led us to consider other options for consumers with BPD.

Deciding Whether DBT Is Right for Your ACT Setting

If you are considering whether to modify your services, we advise beginning with (1) an assessment of your setting in order to critically evaluate whether changes to services are needed, and (2) then weighing all the available options that may better help this particular consumer subgroup.

Self-Assessment Questions

In characterizing the needs of your setting, it is useful to consider two general questions: First, can you identify a critical mass of patients who are utilizing high-cost services and clearly not benefiting from your current ACT services? In particular, are there individuals with BPD (or subthreshold BPD) who are not showing benefit from ACT services alone and should be offered DBT? Second, what is the burden of this consumer group in terms of both staff time/dollars and staff burnout? Figure 11.1 provides questions that might be used as a guideline to assessing your system. We encourage you to consider what variables are most appropriate for your setting and design your self-assessment tool accordingly. In your initial decision-making phase, consider using such qualitative assessment questions as these to screen for both (1) perception of insufficient and/or unsuccessful services, and (2) provider burnout. Responding "yes" to several questions in each domain may suggest a sufficient level of need to justify modifications to the system. At the next phase, collect numerical data to quantify the need as shown in Figure 11.1. Gathering numerical data will continue to be critically important should you decide to implement a DBT program. Most managed mental health care systems now require such data as a concrete indicator of need prior to allocation of funds for new treatments, and may likewise require ongoing data collection to evaluate effectiveness of a pilot program. Further, gathering data is needed for your own self-assessment to both suggest areas for changing the program and to boost morale by indicating success.

Weighing the Options

If your self-assessment indicates the need to modify your services for consumers with BPD, the next step is to determine whether implementing DBT seems like the best option. (See Chapter 1 for comparison of DBT to other treatments.) Figure 11.2 displays several major alternatives one has for responding to consumers with BPD referred to an ACT team, some of which involve DBT implementation and others of which do not. We reserve a more detailed description of ACT/DBT program models for a subsequent section. Here, we focus on deciding whether DBT is feasible and desirable for you. Hence, we review below what we consider to be the major alternatives to implementing DBT in your setting, followed by a discussion of general issues related to DBT implementation. For illustrative purposes, these options are framed around our own decision-making process where we found ourselves cycling through these various options (separately and in some combination) before undertaking implementation of comprehensive DBT.

Phase I: Qualitative System Screening Questions

Possible Indicators of Insufficient Care "As Usual"

- Does it feel like you're constantly "putting out fires" with the consumers with BPD behaviors?
- Do you receive pressure to reduce your state hospital census, but find that there are few adequate community treatment options?
- Do you find yourself intervening with staff and asking them to provide more services to prevent termination of residential placements, to reduce hospitalizations, or to thwart ongoing complaints (by staff and the consumers themselves)?
- Do you review incident reports on the same consumers over and over?
- Do you get frequent requests for difficult case reviews on the same consumers?
- Do administrators frequently ask, "Why are these consumers not improving when I send staff to workshops?"

Possible Indicators of Provider Burnout

- Do you question why frequent and intense services are provided but outcomes show little improvement?
- Does your staff state they are burned out because they feel they are unable to provide adequate treatment?
- Do you and/or your staff feel uninterested or "hardened" to the emotional pain of consumers with BPD behaviors?
- Do you question whether consumers with BPD even *want* to get better, and perhaps think their most difficult and frustrating behaviors are done to *purposely* frustrate and annoy?
- Are you convinced that these consumers cannot benefit from community treatment and need to reside long term in a state institution due to high-risk self-injurious behaviors?

Phase II: Gather Numerical Data to Quantify System Need

Identify consumers without-of-control behaviors, high utilization	Estimated number in past year	Estimated annual costs	Past/current proposed solutions to reduce costs	Resolved? Yes/No
Consumers in state mental hospital for 90+ days in past 12 months				
Consumers with > three psychiatric and/or substance use admissions in past 12 months				
Consumers with > five crisis/emergency encounters in past 12 months				
Consumers with > one suicide attempt/instance of self-injurious behavior in past 12 months				
Consumers evicted from a community mental health residential program				
Consumers with costly individual wraparound plans or additional supports				

Calculate cost of staff time	Estimated amount in past 3 months	Estimated Annual Costs	Past/current proposed solutions to reduce costs	Resolved? Yes/No
Number of extra meetings that have been held to develop crisis plans and treatment plans				
Amount of staff time each week handling after-hours crisis calls				
Amount of staff time developing individual wraparound plans				
Number of conflicts that have occurred between staff, departments, or external providers regarding how to best manage high-risk behaviors?				

FIGURE 11.1. Sample self-assessment tool.

Accept referral for ACT services?	Level of DBT Integration/Implementation onto ACT Team				
	No DBT	Partial DBT		Facilitate DBT	Comprehensive DBT
Yes	ACT "As Usual"	Gray Zone: Some DBT offered		Outsource to external DBT program in the community (ACT Team may provide DBT coaching)	DBT offered as a "track" within ACT service framework; DBT and ACT delivered with fidelity to each model
		DBT program start-up: elements of DBT offered in start-up phase; intent is comprehensive DBT	New hybrid treatment: only elements of DBT are used or ACT and DBT are blended into new treatment (e.g., DBT-informed ACT program)		
No	• Attempt to refuse BPD referrals on grounds that they cannot be treated on ACT team • Consumer does not need the intensive case management offered by ACT services and is instead referred to DBT program in community (if available)				

FIGURE 11.2. Options for responding to needs of consumers with BPD who are referred for ACT services.

Option 1: Exclude Consumers with BPD from ACT Services

Based on research as well as clinical experience, the logical initial question is whether or not a consumer with BPD is suitable for treatment on your ACT team. Consequently, you may consider excluding consumers with BPD from your program. In our programs, for example, we spent many months refusing to treat consumers with BPD, trying to convince the community mental health (CMH) system that such consumers do not belong on ACT teams, that we were not equipped to treat them, and that BPD referrals should stop. However, CMH continued to firmly believe that if ACT providers saw their consumers with BPD daily to dispense medications, then these consumers with BPD would never overdose or misuse medication, despite ample evidence to the contrary. Similarly, CMH insisted that because these consumers were "burning out" the emergency mental health staff, ACT could offer better service with much less staff frustration.

There are, in fact, ACT programs that have successfully declined to offer services to individuals with BPD. However, consumers with BPD or BPD characteristics usually also have multiple Axis I diagnoses and levels of impairment, which are traditionally appropriate for ACT programs. Similarly, the intensive services and resource-richness of ACT teams seemingly better match the needs of these consumers and lead many in CMH to continue to make the argument that ACT programs "should" and "must" treat these patients. In areas where no DBT programs are available, the reality of the situation is that BPD consumers desperately need treatment and sometimes their only alternative to ACT is long-term institutional care.

Option 2: Offer Standard ACT to Consumers with BPD

Besides the questionable ethical position of failing to offer DBT, a known efficacious treatment, staff offering only traditional ACT services to BPD consumers often find it untenable. For example, our staff were unable to maintain motivation and morale with this approach. As many readers may have also experienced, the rest of the treatment community was also quite judgmental about what they viewed as our incompetent or just plain "wrong" treatment. For example, it was common for emergency room staff and police officers to contact us and insist that we hospitalize a consumer indefinitely. As one frustrated physician told us, "This individual is a real 'nut job' and belongs locked up for the rest of his life! I am not taking the liability for this person and I want him out of my ER now!"

Even efforts to try to improve the situation by "treating" the environment through community treatment plans and the provision of "scripts" for community providers to follow proved insufficient. For example, at InterAct, we distributed elaborate scripts that detailed a response to various scenarios. All scripts began with the following statement:

> "We know that the consumer is behaving inappropriately and we would like the individual to stop acting that way every bit as much as you would. Unfortunately, we are powerless to stop the individual from acting that way—we do believe that if we hospitalize the person the behavior will get worse over time instead of better."

Next, the script provided specific guidelines for how to respond. For example, Script A provided instructions to local police:

> "Has the consumer committed a crime? If yes, please arrest him or her; if not, please ask him or her to go home."

Script B was for emergency room staff:

> "Does the consumer need medical attention for an overdose or sutures?—If yes, treat and release. If not, please ask him or her to go home."

We recommend that teams choosing this option have each new consumer with BPD sign a release form that allows the ACT team to provide scripts to any potential contact in the community. As one might imagine, this procedure is at best cumbersome and sometimes can reach ridiculous proportions; in one instance a consumer in our setting had 13 other providers who attended an ACT team meeting! Be aware, too, that on many occasions providers will not follow the script or a consumer will connect with a new community contact not on the list. For both ethical and practical reasons, therefore, offering only ACT-as-usual is not a good fit for these consumers' needs.

Option 3: DBT Provided via Outsourcing While Your Team Provides ACT Services

Obviously the best option, when available, will be to refer the consumer with BPD to a DBT program. Availability of a CMH DBT program can resolve the problem of meeting consumers needs by having the CMH team provide the majority of treatment for out-of-control behaviors and having the ACT team serve an agreed-upon role. Typically, the case management organization is the ultimate arbiter of treatment, and must agree with the overall treatment plan. The ACT team would also typically need to be involved in decisions regarding consumer hospitalization, even if guided by the decisions of the external DBT therapist. Similarly, as ACT teams are typically available 24/7, they may elect to take crisis calls, in contrast to standard outpatient DBT, in which the individual therapist takes calls. This arrangement will work best if the ACT on-call clinicians can coach DBT skills. The most important *general* point is that the DBT and ACT teams, along with the consumer, develop a clear agreement in advance regarding these issues. Moreover, the agreement should include an ongoing understanding that misunderstandings will be openly discussed as they arise. Minor difficulties with coordination may still exist, but disagreement regarding the fundamental course of treatment may be few given the high consistency of DBT and ACT treatment philosophies. The problem with this option, however, is simply that CMH DBT programs are often unavailable.

Option 4: Offer Additional Non-DBT Mental Health Care in Conjunction with ACT Services

When DBT is not available, another option often considered is to refer the consumer to outside services that exist in the community, such as an individual therapist, a specialized residential setting, or a partial hospitalization program. The primary role of providing therapy would then be conducted by an outside entity and the ACT team would lend support, provide crisis intervention, and also provide case management services. An obvious difficulty to this approach is lack of coordination, as well as disagreement regarding the best course of treatment. One of the most significant problems we faced, for example, were therapists who focused their treatment on childhood trauma with BPD consumers who were already quite dysregulated. This approach typically led to a dramatic increase in suicidal behaviors,[1] in effect igniting a fire that the ACT team then had to extinguish.

Overall, this approach resulted in frequent polarization and anger between ACT team members and external providers, with each blaming the other for crises and/or lack of progress. In fact, there were several occasions in which outside therapists filed complaints against InterAct for not hospitalizing consumers when the therapist believed it was necessary. Finally, we also had the experience that many of our consumers became *more* symptomatic in residential and partial hospital programs, acting increasingly helpless and mentally ill.

Option 5: Provide DBT Services Directly on Your ACT Team

When we (RW & GAC) first grappled with how to better meet the needs of consumers with BPD, we were not aware of the existence of DBT and we experienced repeated failures trying many different approaches. Now, however, there is a growing literature on DBT as an evidence-based approach to treating consumers with BPD. DBT is specifically designed to treat the problem behaviors of the consumers with whom ACT fails: It reduces suicidal behavior, use of crisis services, and inpatient hospitalization, and promotes improved treatment retention relative to usual care in the community (e.g., Lieb, Zanarini, Schmahl, Linehan, & Bohus, 2004; see Koerner & Dimeff, Chapter 1, this volume, for a thorough review of the empirical basis of DBT). DBT is also an attractive approach because it is formalized in a treatment manual (Linehan, 1993a, 1993b), a structured training program is available (*www.behavioraltech.org*), and preliminary data suggest that line clinicians can learn the principles of DBT (Hawkins & Sinha, 1998) after undergoing the structured training program (American Psychiatric Association, 1998; Comtois, Elwood, Holdcraft, Simpson, & Smith, 2006).

In some communities, DBT is offered first through the ACT team, and then in some cases expanded to develop a separate, freestanding DBT program for consumers with BPD who need DBT only (i.e., no ACT services). In other words, DBT can be made available at both levels of care depending on the systems' needs. While ACT as usual is not a reasonable option for meeting the needs of BPD consumers, and outsourcing to non-DBT can be equally problematic, these other options provide a preliminary way for you to think about what's needed in your system. We now turn to the details of planning implementation of DBT in an ACT setting.

Planning an ACT/DBT Program

Described below are some of the initial considerations in setting up your DBT program once you have made the decision to do so. Although presented in a linear fashion, clearly this is an iterative process that is likely to require frequent reevaluation and retooling depending on where you are in your implementation process. The needs assessment that was described in the foregoing section (see Figure 11.1) will provide important information for designing your program, and will also function as data when you are gathering support among reluctant consumers, clinicians, and administrators.

Identify Your Target Population

The ideal candidates for a DBT program are those who meet criteria for BPD (or the subthreshold for the diagnosis of BPD) with numerous hospitalizations, failed efforts at other treatments, and out-of-control behaviors such as suicidal behaviors. (Review the top half of Figure 11.1 for example behaviors.) It is helpful to bear in mind, however, that the common denominator linking seemingly different behavior patterns (e.g., self-injury or fire-setting) and multiple diagnoses is emotion dysregulation (see Korner, Dimeff, & Swenson, Chapter 2, this volume). Consequently, it may be most useful to think of the potential DBT consumer as one who is often emotionally dysregulated and engages in dysfunctional behaviors related to these painful emotions. ACT/DBT consumers must of course also be eligible for ACT, and hence have multiple case management needs and require an intensive level of treatment. (Those not meeting the service selection criteria for ACT are referred to a case manager or outpatient therapist.) In our experience, decisions about who to refer to ACT/DBT are best made on a case-by-case basis and without rule-outs based on clinical diagnosis. Charted diagnoses are often uninformative and even unreliable, with many external factors other than the consumer's presentation determining decisions about diagnosis. For example, many clinicians are loath to use the diagnosis of BPD because of the stigma attached to it and may either omit such a diagnosis or use bipolar affective disorder to refer to the same behavioral phenomenon.

An alternative way to define your target group is to identify individuals who experience dysregulation in at least three of the five following areas of functioning: affective, behavioral, interpersonal, self, and cognitive. Consumers who do not experience sufficient emotion dysregulation would not necessarily benefit from DBT and are typically excluded from such treatment. In practice, most often clients considered for a DBT program experience dysregulation in all five areas of functioning. As with any DBT program, services are entirely voluntary and consumers must want to be in DBT and be willing to agree to DBT-consistent goals for entry. Of course, clinicians work hard to help consumers make this commitment before they enter the program.

Although we do not recommend exclusion based on chart diagnosis, one might exclude consumers with some clear indicator of a significant problem that would preclude them from benefiting from DBT and/or would be therapy-destroying for other DBT program participants. In practice this usually means two characteristics result in exclusion until the consumer behavior(s) are stabilized/shaped up: (1) flagrant psychotic symptoms that would be extremely disruptive for a skills group; and (2) primary substance dependence to the degree that the consumer is unable/unwilling to attend treatment without being extremely intoxicated. Substance abuse/dependence is not an exclusion criteria, as these patients can be readily treated using DBT for substance abusers (DBT-SUD; see McMain, Sayrs, Dimeff, & Linehan, Chapter 6, this volume, for a description of this adaptation). Similarly, in our experience patients with mental retardation and developmental disabilities have also been successfully treated with DBT, although adaptations of the skills may be needed (e.g., addition of a one-on-one skills tutor) and extra efforts are made to ensure that he or she understands things such as the diary card.

Specific entry criteria will vary depending on your unique setting, and may change over time. In the start-up phase, however, it may be most important to identify a small, more homogeneous subgroup of patients who can be treated using standard DBT. If at least 5% of your ACT consumers engage in some of the identified problem behaviors shown in Figure 11.1, you can likely make a strong case for implementing DBT. Even identifying a few consumers is often sufficient to get your foot in the door for starting a program. Our experience suggests that as word spreads that you are offering a DBT program, an increasing number of referrals will materialize.

Gather Support from Administrators

In today's environment of diminishing resources, the efficient use of staff time is critical to a program's survival. The additional challenge is not only to utilize staff time efficiently, but simultaneously to deliver quality services from which consumers benefit. Showing a high level of gaps in services or unmet needs in your system (see Figure 11.1) will indicate that these criteria are not being met, hence signaling the need for change.

Provide a preliminary summary of these data to a supervisor or administrator of services. Consider requesting time for one or more staff to review the literature on DBT as an evidence-based practice and talk to existing programs supporting the integration of DBT and ACT. Then, if possible, have the same staff attend a 1- or 2-day training to receive an overview of DBT. Subsequently, prepare a presentation for agency leadership that includes a summary of the data, the literature reviewed, and the content of the training. The presentation should make a compelling argument for why funding should be allocated for staff training and program development.

You should always keep in mind the "foot in the door" principle: Simply get your administrators to endorse the idea of having a treatment that will cost less and be more efficient. We have found that getting agreement on this point will leave you well positioned to gradually begin making additional requests that are needed for the full program. In short, depending on your unique circumstance, it may not be effective to start by requesting that administrators "provide funds to start a DBT program." Depending on the political landscape, you may need to be strategic. And, on the other hand, sometimes it's worth "shooting for the moon"! If the facts are that your system is failing to meet the needs of some consumers and inadvertently expending tremendous resources on ineffective treatment, outlining a proposal to launch a full, comprehensive DBT program may be exactly the right first step. The principle here is the same as using the commitment strategies with clients: Get what you can take and take what you can get. Link your requests with the administrators' goals, and propose how your envisioned DBT program can move the agency toward them.

Address Differences between ACT and DBT

For ACT staff and consumers to adopt and adapt DBT requires consideration of similarities and differences between current practice and the proposed new program. Early in the transition process, program leaders should orient staff and consumers to key differences in order to ensure a successful transition to ACT/DBT. (See Table 11.1 for a review of key orienting points.)

TABLE 11.1. ACT and DBT: Important Orienting Points for New Staff and Consumers

	DBT	ACT
	Model similarities	
• Developed for consumers with severe, chronic, and complex problems; typically with history of multiple treatment failures		
• Treatment delivered in community and strong efforts to keep consumers out of hospital (e.g., provision of phone coaching)		
• Rehabilitation-oriented		
• Team-based treatment		
• Strong emphasis on keeping consumers committed and engaged in treatment		
• Emphasis on practical, problem-solving approach for solving problems in the "here and now"		
	Model differences[a]	
Behavior change focus	Skill building is specific and systematic treatment target; done in group setting and woven throughout interactions with individual therapist and all other providers	Present to some degree, but formal psychosocial intervention component not necessarily part of standard ACT service delivery
Modal case management approach	Provider acts as "consultant-to-the-consumer"; teaches patient to intervene on own behalf	Providers more likely to intervene and act as advocate on consumer's behalf
Voluntary nature of treatment	DBT begins with "orienting and commitment" phase in which therapy expectations are discussed and consumer is asked to give voluntary "informed consent" for treatment. Consumer viewed as in pretreatment phase until commitment is made.	Explicit commitment not typically requested of consumer
Treatment duration	Programs often time-limited, and specific protocols exist to keep consumer engaged and actively working in therapy (e.g., "four-miss rule")	Care provided "as long as needed"
After-hours phone coaching	Provided with instruction to call for coaching *before* problem escalates to emergency; systematic efforts to ensure consumer does not associate extra services/help with crises (e.g., "24-hour rule")	Also provided, often with emphasis placed on using phone coaching *if* a crisis occurs
Development of treatment plan	Done in collaboration with one person (usually individual therapist), with rest of team working to support that dyad.	Done in collaboration with entire team; each team member strives to be interchangeable vis-à-vis consumer

[a] Most differences are of *emphasis* rather than polar opposites.

Similarities

Fortunately, DBT and ACT share numerous commonalities that make DBT resonate with ACT workers. First, ACT and DBT are both geared toward treatment of refractory consumers. Usually a prerequisite for ACT involvement is a failure of the rest of the system to treat the individual with less intensive services. Similarly, DBT consumers have typically had multiple treatment failures before coming to DBT. Second, both models emphasize rehabilitation of the consumer so that he or she can remain out of the hospital and work actively and effectively with community providers. Third, both ACT and DBT are community-based programs in which clinicians work actively to develop and maintain treatment engagement among consumers. Both view treatment dropout not as a failure of the consumer, but as a failure of the treatment provider or the treatment system. Fourth, both treatment approaches offer after-hours phone consultation for consumers. Fifth, both approaches are a team-based treatment; each consumer is treated by the entire team, and the team is there to keep staff motivated, to provide consultation, and to ward off burnout. Finally, both programs emphasize a practical, problem-solving approach to treatment, and the need for practice and generalization of life skills to the "real world" in which the consumer will need them.

Differences

Nonetheless, there are also areas of "cultural dissonance" that require extra orienting and problem solving to effectively integrate the models. The central distinction is a stronger and more systematic emphasis on behavior change within DBT. This overarching difference underlies the majority of ACT-DBT differences in clinician strategy and response toward the consumer. Although both models are oriented toward consumer rehabilitation, the aim of DBT is to help consumers develop a life worth living *independent* of the mental health system. Consumers are viewed as inherently capable of exiting the system if they learn the necessary skills and have sufficient motivation to do so (both of which are targeted in DBT). Given this overarching treatment goal, every interaction with the consumer is treated as a chance to teach/coach skills, whether formally (e.g., during skills group) or informally (e.g., during case management interactions), and many DBT programs are time-limited. In contrast, ACT has historically emphasized that many of their consumers could require services for life, and treatment is thus offered "as long as needed" (e.g., "cradle to grave"; Bond et al., 2001). Although there has been more recent discussion of the merits of a shift *away* from a uniform policy of time-unlimited ACT services (Salyers, Masterton, Fekete, Picone, & Bond, 1998), it is safe to say that systematic skill building in order to graduate out of the mental health system is not typically an explicit target in traditional ACT settings. Hence, although ACT teaches problem-solving skills depending on consumer need, behavior change is not as comprehensive or as "front and center" as is the case in DBT.

A particular point of departure for traditional ACT teams is in the DBT "consultation-to-the-patient-strategy" used for case management needs. A DBT clinician typically takes the role of "consultant" to the consumer in helping him or her manage basic needs (e.g., obtaining housing, managing finances) and in managing his or her treatment network. That is, the DBT clinician teaches the consumer how to actively solve his or her own problems and manage his or her own treatment network. This contrasts with the traditional approach to case management which more often involves intervening directly in the environment *for* the consumer (i.e., "environmental intervention strategy"), an approach used much less frequently in DBT, and then only under certain, very limited, prescribed circumstances, as it represents a missed opportunity for skill development and runs the risk of reinforcing a passive problem-solving style often characteristic of consumers with BPD. When adopting DBT in an ACT context, this philosophy should guide ACT contacts for DBT consumers; clinician and consumer must adopt the outlook that "every problem is an opportunity to practice skills." ACT workers may recognize the value of this approach, but may nonetheless struggle with the often slow process of *teaching* the consumer "to fish," when *giving* them the fish is much easier in the short term.

The emphasis on change is also seen in how DBT and ACT differ somewhat in their approaches to phone coaching. Although provided in both models, DBT phone coaching emphasizes the need to call for coaching *before* a problem escalates out of control, so that consumers can receive assistance in how to solve it before engaging in a dysfunctional behavior such as self-injury. This contrasts somewhat with the ACT model, in which staff and consumers are oriented to thinking that these are "crisis calls" and so are to be used only in the case of an emergency.

The notion of offering this degree of phone availability can make even ACT workers balk. Thus, it's important to thoroughly orient team members regarding the philosophy and purpose of the calls in order to promote their willingness to take them. Even so, your team members will undoubtedly worry that consumers will misuse phone coaching. Be reassured that this kind of anxiety will drop significantly as you teach team members how to handle these calls. For example, it's useful to immediately and explicitly counter the mind-set of "*crisis* calls" by using the terms "*coaching* calls" and "phone consultations." This is extremely important for consumers as well, who must likewise be educated about the purpose and approach to phone calls. At InterAct, each team member was already sharing on-call duties as part of their job responsibilities. When DBT was introduced into the program, the expectation became that every staff member would have sufficient knowledge of the DBT skills to provide phone coaching. To facilitate the transition, both consumers and staff unfamiliar with DBT are given an InterAct "DBT Coaching Sheet" that orients them to the phone policy and guides the clinician in how to do DBT phone coaching (see Appendix 11.1).

For consumers who continue to struggle with problematic phone call behavior, it can be helpful to have them complete the coaching sheet *prior* to calling. The consumer is then asked to review the coaching sheet during the phone call, and to problem-solve skills to be used when the call has ended.

Similarly, some of the roles team members play may shift as DBT is added. For example, whereas in ACT team members are relatively interchangeable, in DBT one person serves as individual therapist and plays the central clinical role of treatment planner, working with the patient on progress toward all goals, and helping to consolidate what is learned in other treatment modes (e.g., skills training). A strong relationship is formed with this individual therapist, which can serve as an important reinforcer (and at times is the only reinforcer) for the consumer to stay engaged and working in treatment. Other providers on the team work to support the dyad of consumer–individual therapist.

The role of the team and the manner in which team meetings are conducted can also vary between DBT and ACT models. In DBT, as in ACT, the ongoing support offered by a team is considered an integral part of treatment. The goals of the DBT team are to improve capability and motivation to do DBT and to keep each other adherent to the treatment "frame" (i.e., the philosophies, principles, and protocols of the DBT model) in treating consumers. There is strong attention to signs of burnout and emotional reactions, members are asked to be vulnerable and nondefensive, and encouraged to point out any unspoken "elephant in the room." When running optimally, the consultation team functions like group therapy for the therapist. In short, while providers are applying DBT to consumers, the consultation team applies DBT to the providers. In contrast the ACT team meeting is run in much more of a traditional, case-report style in which there is a "round-robin" report on individual cases, associated treatment plans, and administrative issues. Thus it may take a significant cognitive shift as well as strong commitment in order to stay the DBT course. Certainly, simple case reporting can be more comfortable! The InterAct DBT team struggled with the DBT team approach for some time, with members frequently "reverting" to the ACT team mode with little focus on issues related to burnout and motivation. The problem was intensified since all of the DBT team members were also part of a traditional ACT team. Having some team "leaders" to model DBT-consistent behaviors can be very useful for a new team, particularly in modeling vulnerability and self-disclosure.

Another difference ACT staff and consumers may find challenging is that DBT programs are often time-limited, they have clear targets, and there are contingencies in place to try to keep consumers engaged and working toward the ultimate goal of a life worth living free from mental health system. That is, entering and keeping your place in a DBT program is not entirely unconditional and contingencies are actively structured to reinforce clinical improvement. Providers work collaboratively with consumers to try to gain commitment to DBT goals (e.g., reduction of suicidal behavior), but consumers are of course free to decline such treatment goals. This contrasts with ACT services, which typically allow unconditional entry and continue indefinitely without termination.

To best help consumers transition to a new program, you need to advertise the new program such that consumers can clearly evaluate how the DBT program will meet their needs, and you also must keep participation voluntary. The key is to determine the consumer's own goals and then to demonstrate how DBT will assist the consumer in meeting those personal goals. Providers sometimes have no awareness of consumers' goals; they may never have asked. Other providers make the common mistake of formulating goals *for* the consumer, which are actually DBT treatment targets. The other essential element is highlighting consumer choice. You want these consumers to enter voluntarily into the DBT program and freely commit to the goals of DBT. A consumer who enters under coercive conditions is very likely to drop out, or at best be unengaged in treatment. To have a choice, the consumer must have an alternative treatment, which in this case is treatment as usual, provided by ACT only.

One of the likely stumbling blocks for reluctant ACT consumers will be fear of committing to the ultimate goal of DBT: independence from the mental health system. This is very understandable since many ACT consumers have virtually been raised and socialized, so to speak, in the public mental health system. It may be inconceivable for them to imagine anything else. Validating fears and generating hope are essential. Staff continually works on commitment strategies with this group to increase the likelihood of eventual participation. Once a program has its own DBT "old-timers" who have experienced success in their lives, these consumers become powerful role models for what is possible.

If selecting consumers for your new program, consider the strategies used at InterAct. For their initial group of consumers, they pursued those with whom they already had established relationships and hence were likely to commit to treatment. The five consumers selected were also quite severe, so when their extreme behaviors were reduced the improvements seemed all the more remarkable. The program immediately became a "success story" and hence more in demand by staff and consumers.

Overall, we cannot overemphasize the importance of using orienting and role-induction strategies for both prospective consumers and staff who are transitioning to a new ACT/DBT program. Without sufficient orienting that genuinely speaks to consumer needs and freedom of choice, enrollment and retention will suffer. Likewise, ACT staff will transition much more smoothly and willingly if they also have advance warning and explanation for key differences between models. Given the substantial compatibilities between ACT and DBT, orienting such as this mitigates any problems that may arise from model differences.

Decide ACT/DBT Program Structure

When considering how to set up your program, we recommend aiming for a comprehensive model that addresses all five functions of DBT (see Koerner, Dimeff, & Swenson, Chapter 2, this volume). These functions can be flexibly applied to fit the unique needs of your treatment setting. If resources are scarce, start with partial implementation that incorporates some of the principles and components of DBT while working systematically, step by step, toward a long-term plan to implement a comprehensive DBT program.

The best model for implementing DBT in an ACT setting, in our opinion, is a "DBT track" model, in which DBT is a specialized program within the ACT service framework that offers treatment to a subgroup of consumers with BPD. Although a simplified description, it is useful heuristically to regard DBT and ACT as separate from each other within the track model, such that each service approach retains most of its "traditional" elements. In contrast, you will see in Figure 11.2, that we have also presented an alternative that represents a "gray zone": a new hybrid treatment that is DBT-informed. This gray zone typically arises through efforts to accommodate various pressures in the system or personal preferences (e.g., "Given productivity pressures, we don't have time for a DBT consultation team, so let's drop that" or "I like the skills group idea, but I can't see doing individual therapy"). The resulting modifications to DBT or ACT potentially deviate from the empirically supported models (see Koerner et al., Chapter 2, this volume, for fuller discussion of these issues). So, for example, as a team begins implementing DBT, resources may be such that only certain elements of DBT can be offered at first (say a skills training group but no individual therapy) or that morning report is used to learn DBT and consequently less time is put toward discussion of ACT contacts. Such temporary way stations may be necessary as part of the step-by-step route to ACT/DBT, where the ultimate outcome is a comprehensive version of DBT offered in the context of high-fidelity ACT services. However, if partial or blended implementation is the stopping point, then this moves to a gray zone: a new treatment approach that may appear quite different from either traditional outpatient DBT or ACT. A partial implementation of DBT or ACT may inadvertently leave out elements responsible for good client outcomes. Attempts to blend ACT and DBT may become a hodgepodge without coherence.

On the other hand, a partial implementation may represent a streamlined version that's equally effective yet easier to deliver. A fully integrated/blended version of DBT and ACT, if systematically developed and carefully evaluated, could represent an improvement to either approach alone. Such creative tinkering may make a treatment better fit a service setting or better serve a consumer's needs. The problem, however, is that in these gray zones one can't *assume* that the clinical outcomes are better—they could be worse! The development of a new treatment model requires a thorough knowledge of *both* DBT and ACT principles such that each can be flexibly adapted and integrated yet maintain their integrity (i.e., this requires the team to be expert in both approaches). Deviating from fidelity means one must assess and evaluate which particular modifications do or do not have the intended effects. Because most of us are not in a position to carry out this degree of careful treatment evaluation and development, we strongly recommend adoption of the DBT track model. Particularly if DBT is new to you and your team, we recommend that you learn how to deliver the *standard* outpatient model within a track model before you undertake the substantial modification that may be needed with a hybrid approach. Also note that reimbursement for services is becoming increasingly tied to documented adherence or fidelity to the particular evidence-based practice being delivered, and consequently partial or blended models that are untested may be ineligible for reimbursement.

DBT "Track" within an ACT Structure

A DBT track program looks similar to an outpatient DBT program in a CMH setting (see Table 11.2). Consumers receive all modes of standard DBT and commit to the Stage 1 target hierarchy (see Koerner & Dimeff, Chapter 1, this volume, for a complete description). DBT individual therapy and skills groups are delivered by DBT "specialists" on the ACT team who also continue to treat non-DBT consumers in traditional ACT work. All other staff are DBT "generalists," that is, they must learn at least a sufficient amount of DBT to provide skills coaching during an after-hours call, which is rotated among team members. All staff (both DBT specialists and generalists) attend the daily morning ACT team meeting, while only DBT specialists attend the weekly DBT consultation team meeting.

An important orienting point for all ACT staff and administrators is the difference between the DBT consultation meeting and the ACT morning report. Consistent with standard DBT, the consultation team serves the function of reducing burnout and maintaining fidelity to the DBT model among the DBT/ACT specialists. Team members use DBT strategies, techniques, and principles on each other in order to enhance their own effectiveness with consumers. In this way, the team meeting is *therapist-centered* (rather than being a round-robin report centered on consumers) and is essentially therapy for the DBT specialists. As such, there should not be regular attendance by non-DBT specialists (e.g., administrators, outside clinicians), and the team should never become a watered-down DBT seminar or class.

Regular ACT contacts for ACT/DBT consumers may be conducted by any team member, including those who are DBT generalists. To maintain fidelity to DBT, consultation-to-the-patient strategy is the modal approach among DBT specialists conducting ACT case management contacts. This approach is also encouraged for DBT generalists. In fact, through informal "diffusion," the consultant strategy and many other elements of DBT invariably become part of the repertoire of the ACT generalists and thus arise naturally with every consumer—whether in the ACT/DBT track or the ACT-only track. Our experience suggests that though many ACT workers may not be interested in becoming DBT specialists, most view the DBT philosophies and specific skills as useful tools in their general approach to consumers. As such, ACT contacts within the track model likely appear much more DBT-informed and skills-oriented than in traditional ACT, or ACT "as usual."

A great deal of *in vivo* DBT coaching can occur during ACT contacts, which makes it an ideal opportunity to promote generalization of DBT skills to daily life. For example, a staff person is assigned to assist a consumer in grocery shopping during their contact. While at the grocery store, the consumer becomes frustrated while waiting to check out. It is taking unusually long and there are still several people ahead of the consumer before

TABLE 11.2. Comparison of Program Prototypes for Providing Comprehensive DBT to ACT Consumers

	DBT provided via outsourcing to external agency	ACT/DBT: DBT services provided directly on ACT team
Level of DBT implementation	Full implementation; all DBT functions and modes	Full implementation; all DBT functions and modes
Eligible ACT consumers?	ACT team refers those with BPD/emotionally dysregulated behavior patterns	Subgroup with BPD/emotionally dysregulated behavior patterns
Which staff trained to deliver DBT?	No ACT staff trained to deliver DBT; all outside agency staff provide DBT.	Some division of labor; interested staff subgroup trained as "DBT specialists"; all staff trained to function as "DBT generalists" (e.g., do DBT skills coaching)
Who handles ACT contacts/case management?	ACT team; DBT providers view case management as ancillary	Entire team; although may make efforts to avoid scheduling contacts between DBT individual therapist–consumer pairs.
What do ACT contacts look like?	Traditional ACT services	Informal "diffusion" of DBT strategies influence ACT contacts; individual DBT therapist coaches consumer to interact with ACT workers "DBT-style"
Who collaborates with consumer to develop treatment plan?	DBT individual therapist, with secondary plan developed with ACT team	DBT individual therapist is an ACT team member, who serves as consultant to rest of ACT team regarding case management needs
DBT team attendance versus ACT team attendance?	Two separate meetings with no overlapping team members	Two separate meetings: all staff attend daily ACT meetings; only DBT specialists attend separate weekly DBT consultation meeting
Who handles after-hours calls?	Often the ACT team but depends on prior agreement; requests for hospitalization usually require ACT team	Entire ACT team rotates
Who handles individual therapy?	DBT therapist at agency	A DBT specialist on team
Who is skills trainer/coach?	DBT skills trainer at agency	DBT specialists run skills group; all staff use skills coaching during routine ACT contacts
How is DBT termination/treatment vacation handled?	Consumer remains with ACT services	Consumer remains with ACT services and contact with DBT individual therapist on team ceases; if reentry possible, then DBT therapist "pines" for return

they can check out. The consumer becomes more and more frustrated and has the urge to "just forget it and leave." The ACT staff would coach the consumer on utilizing a skill taught in his or her weekly skills group such as distress tolerance (e.g., distract by looking at a magazine from the display case). In cases where ACT staff (DBT generalists) are consistently failing to use skills coaching during ACT/DBT case management activities, a target for the individual DBT therapist is to coach the consumer to take an active stance in his or her own case management and to interact with ACT staff "DBT-style."

One situation that requires careful consideration is when ACT/DBT consumers drop out of their DBT services or in rare circumstances when they may lose the services by being placed on a DBT "vacation" as a contingency management strategy (i.e., an aversive consequence in this case). In both instances, the consumer loses contact with his or her DBT specialists, and particularly his or her individual therapist, but retains the ACT-only services. A therapy vacation is the cessation of therapy for a specified period of time and is used only after all lower level contingencies and problem-solving strategies have been tried. (A comprehensive discussion of "vacations" is beyond the scope of this chapter; readers are urged to consult the DBT manual [Linehan, 1993a] for detailed guidance on how to effectively use therapy vacations in DBT.)

In our experience, DBT vacations within ACT teams most often occur because the consumer has violated the DBT attendance contract to which he or she has agreed upon entry into the DBT program. (See p. 325 for additional information regarding this contract.) That is, the consumer has missed four consecutive scheduled DBT sessions (either four skills groups or four individual therapy sessions). Importantly, the cessation of DBT services should be of sufficient length and aversiveness to achieve its purpose: to encourage consumers to modify their problem behavior and to act skillfully in order to regain DBT services. On our ACT teams, consumers who lose treatment due to missing four sessions are placed on the bottom of the waiting list for DBT services, which typically means a minimum vacation period of 8 weeks. Further, contact with the DBT individual therapist should be avoided during the vacation, and perhaps contact with other DBT specialists (e.g., the skills leaders) to whom the patient is emotionally attached. At the same time, any ACT team members who have contact with the consumer can coach and assist him or her in how to negotiate for reentry once the vacation is over. Further, the DBT individual therapist might make occasional brief contacts with the consumer, encouraging completion of required tasks so that he or she can reenter ("I am *so* looking forward to working with you again once you have made your repairs"). It is also very important to remember that when a consumer is in the smallest danger of being placed on vacation, the DBT team (as well as DBT generalists on the ACT team) must mobilize to assist the consumer in problem solving so that a vacation can be prevented if at all possible.

Behavior change required for reentry should be linked to the problem that led to the vacation in the first place. Efforts to solve the problem should begin as soon as the vacation begins. We recall a consumer who, despite the best efforts of his DBT team, missed four skills groups in a row and was put on vacation. After he had missed just one group, his DBT individual therapist oriented him about the danger of vacation. A chain analysis of the incident revealed that a pivotal problem was that the consumer had a pattern of using drugs on group day, in part because of his social anxiety related to group attendance. Ultimately he would avoid the group when intoxicated due to shame and fear of detection. Once placed on vacation, he was required to develop a behavior plan for how he would remain abstinent on group days (a minimal goal), and make a verbal commitment to the plan as well as demonstrate his ongoing commitment to the DBT team by a series of steps: demonstrate progress with his social anxiety by going to the public library several times a week, go to ACT contacts scheduled at the same day/time of DBT skills group while staying sober, and doing a DEAR MAN with the skills group and his individual therapist to regain entry, including an explanation of what he was doing to address his social anxiety and substance use. The consumer was out of skills group for 10 weeks; twice during that interval his individual therapist sent him a card that "pined" for his return to DBT.

On occasion, ACT contact with the DBT individual therapist during a DBT vacation may be unavoidable. For example, the therapist may be on-call, and be asked to go to the emergency room to conduct an assessment for possible hospitalization of his or her consumer on vacation. The principle in such situations is to be matter-of-fact, cool, and focused on the specific task at hand. The therapist should keep the contact as brief as possible to complete the task and orient the consumer to the nature of the contact (e.g., "I know this is difficult, but I am here as the ACT staff on-call right now, strictly to conduct this assessment"). Extraneous conversation should be limited or avoided completely, and it can be quite useful to remind the consumer that the relationship will be renewed once the consumer completes the steps to reenter (e.g., "Remember, I really want to get you back into treatment with me too, just as soon as you do what you need to do to get back in. And I know you can do it!"). The overarching point is to limit warmth and contact whenever possible, and to link consumer behavior change to a return to DBT services and a renewal of the therapy relationship (i.e., to "pine" for the consumer's return).

A common perceived problem with the track model is that without a unified approach, inconsistency can result for both consumers and clinicians. For the DBT consumer, there may be times when an ACT worker (generalist) fails to use skills coaching or perhaps overuses environmental intervention. These occasional instances can inadvertently reinforce passive problem solving on an intermittent basis and slow the efforts of the DBT individual therapist who is continually pushing client toward active problem solving. As noted earlier, an essential target for the individual DBT therapist is to coach his or her consumers to take an active stance in his or her own case management and interact with all ACT staff "DBT-style." In other words, when viewed dialectically, these inconsistencies can be a significant asset of the track program because they provide a terrific opportunity to practice skills and work on not engaging in dysfunctional behavior despite reinforcement for those old behaviors being available. Such practice opportunities can greatly facilitate generalization.

Similarly, the ACT team member who is required to function as both a DBT individual therapist to a consumer at one point and to do ACT-style case management at other points may sometimes experience role confusion. For example, you may be trying to conduct a medication assessment on a consumer who becomes angry at you because he or she is reminded of something you said during your previous individual DBT session. Problems can arise when the consumer is insistent that you discuss the issue at length until you reach resolution, while your main task is to conduct a medication assessment in a limited amount of time. One approach is to try to avoid scheduling such contacts between DBT individual therapist and consumer pairs. Nonetheless, when unavoidable, bear in mind your role/targets as interactions change and also orient the consumer to the change in roles as well. A good general strategy is to maintain a collaborative stance and to offer soothing and validation of any consumer frustration, coupled with suggestions for skills coaching when needed (e.g., "I know this is frustrating, but our main goal here right now has to be this med assessment. How about we try to hurry up and get it out of the way, and then we can talk for 5 minutes about yesterday's session? What skills would help you now?").

Thorough training in how to conduct individual therapy in DBT can help to mitigate some of these problems. This highlights another challenge to address: A track program requires a cadre of skilled individual DBT therapists in order to ensure treatment success. This is a difficulty for any agency, but perhaps more so for ACT teams given that many ACT workers do not have extensive prior training in individual psychotherapy skills. At a minimum, the person serving in the role of individual therapist should have adequate formal training in psychotherapy such that he or she can effectively implement the four change procedures in DBT (exposure-based procedures, contingency management, skills training, and cognitive restructuring).

Nonetheless, we recommend this model above all others because it closely parallels the standard outpatient DBT program as described in the treatment manual (Linehan, 1993a), allowing new practitioners to become skilled in the standard format before undertaking a modification. Similarly, standard outpatient DBT has undergone the greatest amount of empirical scrutiny, and hence has the greatest amount of data supporting its use. Doing anything else is not evidence-based. Second, the potential inconsistencies mentioned above can be well accommodated within a dialectical framework that argues that inconsistency, polarities, and change are an inevitable part of life. Hence, when they crop up in the treatment context, consumers can be coached in how to manage and approach such change as well as on how to search for a synthesis between the potentially conflicting approaches among the DBT providers and the ACT workers.

Finally, since not all ACT workers need to be trained as DBT "specialists," administrators and program planners can train only those who volunteer for the role, which affords clear advantages in terms of motivation and commitment to the lengthy and time-intensive process of learning and practicing DBT.

It is important to remember that implementing ACT/DBT is a major undertaking that requires long-term planning and a system-level perspective to survive over time. As such, consider advocating for a DBT training that will involve not only ACT team(s) in your system but also a team of clinicians from a local community mental health center. Consumers requiring few case management needs can then be referred to an external agency for a comprehensive DBT program, and ACT teams can work to develop their own ACT/DBT program for consumers with substantial case management needs. Such an approach allows for flexibility and recognizes that you may be uncertain at the outset *which* type of program to develop. Further, the landscape, and hence your plans, can change over time.

An Example of Implementing DBT in an ACT Setting: InterAct of Michigan

To illustrate the foregoing points, we briefly describe the DBT implementation process at InterAct, a private, not-for-profit agency that provides outpatient mental health services through a contract with Kalamazoo Community Mental Health. InterAct started a pilot DBT program in 1995. At that time, the agency consisted of five ACT teams and one case management team. Several staff members became interested in DBT after reviewing the empirical literature in a desperate search to better serve their consumers with BPD. Eventually, six staff members (including the third author, G. A. C.) attended a 2-day overview training in DBT. They returned very excited and sought the support of administration to begin a pilot program to assess the effectiveness of providing DBT for their consumers.

They gained the interest and approval of the InterAct clinical director (second author, R. W.), who authorized the pilot program.

They elected to begin a comprehensive DBT program within their ACT services that would consist of all DBT treatment modes (individual therapy, group skills training, phone consultation, peer consultation meeting for providers). The consultation team included five of the original group of staff members along with the clinical director, who met together weekly for 50 minutes of peer consultation and 45 minutes of training. While only the five DBT team members attended the consultation meeting, all staff members were invited to the training portion of the team and some team supervisors required all their staff to attend. The five DBT team members rotated the teaching responsibilities for the training portion.

As described earlier, InterAct solicited five consumers (one from each of five teams) for entry into the pilot program, with each of the five clinicians on the team acting as an individual DBT therapist for one consumer. Each consumer had a history of extreme, out-of-control behaviors that are consistent with BPD criterion behaviors, including impulsive self-injury, frequent utilization of after-hour on-call services, frequent presentation at various community resources (ER, hospitals, jail), history of treatment dropout and failure, and/or staff endorsement of a high level of frustration and helplessness in treating them. Two consumers had current difficulties with substance abuse/dependence and one had limited cognitive functioning. Selecting the most difficult cases was politically advantageous because the ACT team members felt grateful for the assistance and were more understanding about staff time spent in DBT-related activities. The five consumers who were "courted" for DBT were already engaged in ACT services. Thus staff had some rapport with the consumers, which facilitated their decision to begin a new treatment.

Consistent with the DBT model, consumers received a great deal of orienting about what the "new treatment" would entail so that they could make a decision in advance about whether they wanted to enter treatment. The orienting process is particularly important when starting an entirely new program (see Table 11.1), and in particular clinicians should be very explicit regarding DBT rules related to attendance at DBT services (the "four-miss rule") and cessation of unscheduled phone contacts in the 24 hours following suicidal behavior (the "24-hour rule"). Please see the treatment manual (Linehan, 1993a) for a comprehensive discussion of these rules.

Obtaining commitment from this initial set of consumers was readily possible because of our previous rapport, as well as the fact that they were giving up nothing to enter treatment (they were not giving up any of their ACT team providers or a previous therapist), but were instead getting the addition of new and specialized services. Nonetheless, over time we have refined our orienting/commitment phase, and have incorporated a written contract which consumers review with their prospective DBT therapist during the initial treatment sessions. This brief contract (see Appendix 11.2) reviews the major orienting points of DBT (including the 24-hour rule and the four-miss rule), and can include other individual plans and consumer "life-worth-living" goals as well. We work collaboratively with our consumers to come up with a productive activity plan. This contract is for 1 year and is renewable. Rather than taking it for granted that the consumer will begin treatment, consumer goals are elicited and the "terms" of the contract are discussed for the first several sessions so that the consumer has time to gather information about the treatment, evaluate his or her chemistry with the clinician, and is empowered to make an informed treatment decision before fully committing to treatment.

To examine program outcomes, data were collected for the five consumers prior to program entry, and thereafter at regular intervals throughout treatment. Given heavy work demands, feasibility of data collection should always be a first priority. Thus, efforts were made at InterAct to collect simple variables that where possible were already recorded in the chart. These included incidents of self-injury/suicide attempts, number of hospital days, on-call use, unscheduled during- and after-hours contacts, and emergency room use.

Once the program began, unscheduled treatment contacts began to decline. Consumers who prior to DBT showed up at the ER on a daily or weekly basis were no longer going to the ER. As consumers showed progress, staff became less demoralized and more interested in learning about and implementing DBT. All staff were invited to the training portion of the DBT consultation team. An increasing number began to attend. Some team supervisors began to require that their staff attend. Community agencies noticed an improvement in consumer behaviors. Despite the program's initial success, it became clear that more in-depth training was needed, and thus several staff attended an intensive training program led by Linehan. These staff members were charged with the duty to provide DBT in-services to other staff members as well as to the community.

It was very encouraging when all five individuals who were in the 12-month pilot project completed the DBT program. Based on initial success, InterAct began to expand their DBT program within ACT, adding more consumers and clinicians. They also continued their heavy emphasis on training, arranging to have a local 2-day DBT training from an outside DBT expert, and also received in-depth consultation from her. By 1998, the program was in full swing with approximately 17 staff members treating 36 consumers; there were two consultation teams for providers and three skills groups and one advanced skills group for consumers. In 1999 InterAct started a separate, comprehensive outpatient DBT program for non-ACT consumers (adults and adolescents), while also maintaining the DBT "track" within the ACT program. Both programs run concurrently today. There are strong advantages to utilizing DBT at both of these levels of care. Many consumers are appropriate for DBT, but don't need the full array of ACT services. The outpatient program also appears to prevent many consumers from further decline to the point that they require the intensive level of ACT services.

Program Outcomes

Program evaluation data from InterAct collected as part of routine clinical care showed improved consumer outcomes in psychiatric hospitalizations and vocational functioning in the years following DBT implementation. Between 1995 and 2003 InterAct averaged 26 ACT consumers per year in the DBT program. In the 12-month period prior to admission to the InterAct DBT program, consumers spent an average of 32.7 days in the hospital. By contrast, during the 12 months following admission to the DBT program, consumers spent just 3.2 days in the hospital. Beginning in 1998 data were also available regarding the number of consumers who were involved in structured vocational activities (yes/no distinction). Vocational activities were defined broadly to include structured work-related activities that had a contract or role with clearly defined expectations such as a specified task-set and time commitment. As such, this category included not only paid employment but also volunteer and school/training activities that fit the foregoing description. Prior to entry into the DBT program, an average of 18.2% of consumers were involved in vocational activity; after 12 months in the program, 60.4% were involved. In addition, systematic qualitative interviews conducted with 14 DBT program participants at InterAct indicated a high degree of consumer satisfaction with DBT (Cunningham, Wolbert, & Lillie, 2004).

Finally, additional data suggest that DBT has been helpful to staff from InterAct as well as to staff members from other Michigan ACT teams practicing ACT/DBT. Wolbert, Cunningham, and Boerman (2002) reported significantly lower levels of clinician burnout in a group of 10 ACT/DBT clinicians (five from InterAct, five from another ACT agency in Michigan with a DBT track program similar to InterAct) in comparison with clinicians practicing ACT alone in two traditional ACT teams. Burnout was assessed with the widely used Maslach Burnout Inventory (MBI; Maslach, Jackson, & Leiter, 1996). In addition, on a structured telephone interview, this group of ACT/DBT practitioners was more likely to rate their consumers as "improved" and more likely to rate themselves as "helpful" to their consumers.

Although these data are uncontrolled and must be viewed as preliminary, we find the positive outcomes very encouraging. Further, our collective years of clinical experience developing, managing, and consulting to ACT teams, and functioning as a mental health administrator to a team leader, have clarified many issues for us. Questions such as "Can our organization afford to train our ACT teams to provide treatment to individuals diagnosed with BPD?" and "Do our ACT teams *really* need to do something different for the consumer with BPD?" are no longer viable. Rather, the question is, "If our ACT teams are serving individuals with BPD, who have exhausted all other available treatment options, then how will our teams provide effective treatment to this target population?" In our experience, incorporating DBT into ACT represents the best synthesis.

NOTE

1. To avoid this possibility, DBT specifically refrains from exposure-based treatment of childhood trauma until the consumer has stabilized—that is, until suicidal and other extreme behaviors are under control and the consumer reliably copes with emotional pain with skillful behaviors.

REFERENCES

Allness, D. J., & Knoedler, W. H. (1998). *The PACT model of community based treatment for persons with severe and persistent mental illnesses: A manual for PACT start-up.* Arlington, VA: National Alliance for the Mentally Ill.

American Psychiatric Association. (1998). Gold Award: Integrating dialectical behavioral therapy into a community mental health program: The Mental Health Center of Greater Manchester, New Hampshire. *Psychiatric Services, 49,* 1338–1340.

Bender, D. S., Dolan, R. T., Skodol, A. E., Sanislow, C. A., Dyck, I. R., McGlashan, T. H., et al. (2001). Treatment utilization by patients with personality disorders. *American Journal of Psychiatry, 158,* 295–302.

Bond, G. R., Drake, R. E., Mueser, K. T., & Latimer, E. (2001). Assertive community treatment for people with severe mental illness: Critical ingredients and impact on patients. *Disease Management and Health Outcomes, 9,* 141–159.

Casey, P. (2000). The epidemiology of personality disorders. In P. Tyrer (Ed.), *Personality disorders: Diagnosis, management, and course* (pp. 71–79). London: Arnold.

Comtois, K. A. (2002). A review of interventions to reduce the prevalence of parasuicide. *Psychiatric Services, 53,* 1138–1144.

Comtois, K. A., Elwood, L., Holdcraft, L. C., Simpson, T. L., & Smith, W. R. (2006). *Effectiveness of dialectical behavior therapy in a community mental health center.* Manuscript submitted for publication.

Comtois, K. A., Russo, J., Snowden, M., Srebnik, D., Ries, R., & Roy-Byrne, P. (2003). Factors associated with high use of public mental health services by persons with borderline personality disorder. *Psychiatric Services, 54,* 1149–1154.

Cunningham, K., Wolbert, R., & Lillie, B. (2004). It's about me solving my problems: Clients' assessments of dialectical behavior therapy. *Cognitive and Behavioral Practice, 11,* 248–256.

Cutting, J., Cowen, P. J., Mann, A. H., & Jenkins, R. (1986). Personality and psychosis: Use of the Standardised Assessment of Personality. *Acta Psychiatrica Scandinavica, 73,* 87–92.

Dawson, D., & MacMillan, H. L. (1993). *Relationship management of the borderline patient: From understanding to treatment.* New York: Brunner/Mazel.

Deci, P. A., Santos, A. B., Hiott, D. W., Schoenwald, S., & Dias, J. K. (1995). Dissemination of assertive community treatment programs. *Psychiatric Services, 46,* 676–678.

Gandhi, N., Tyrer, P., Evans, K., McGee, A., Lamont, A., & Harrison-Read, P. (2001). A randomized controlled trial of community-oriented and hospital-oriented care for discharged psychiatric patients: Influence of personality disorders on police contacts. *Journal of Personality Disorders, 15,* 94–102.

Hawkins, K. A., & Sinha, R. (1998). Can line clinicians master the conceptual complexities of dialectical behavior therapy?: An evaluation of a state department of mental health training program. *Journal of Psychiatric Research, 32,* 379–384.

Jones, A. (2002). Assertive community treatment: Development of the team, selection of clients, and impact on length of hospital stay. *Journal of Psychiatric and Mental Health Nursing, 9,* 261–270.

Lieb, K., Zanarini, M. C., Schmahl, C., Linehan, M. M., & Bohus, M. (2004). Seminar section: Borderline personality disorder. *Lancet, 364,* 453–461.

Linehan, M. M. (1993a). *Cognitive-behavioral treatment of borderline personality disorder.* New York: Guilford Press.

Linehan, M. M. (1993b). *Skills training manual for treating borderline personality disorder.* New York: Guilford Press.

Linehan, M. M., Armstrong, H. E., Suarez, A., Allmon, D., & Heard, H. L. (1991). Cognitive-behavioral treatment of chronically parasuicidal borderline patients. *Archives of General Psychiatry, 48,* 1060–1064.

Linehan, M. M., Rizvi, S. L., Shaw Welch, S., & Page, B. (2000). Psychiatric aspects of suicidal behaviour: Personality disorders. In K. Hawton & K. van Heeringen (Eds.), *International handbook of suicide and attempted suicide* (pp. 147–178). London: Wiley.

Links, P. S. (1998). Developing effective services for patients with personality disorders. *Canadian Journal of Psychiatry, 43,* 251–259.

Maslach, C., Jackson, S. E., & Leiter, M. P. (1996). *The Maslach Burnout Inventory* (3rd ed.). Palo Alto, CA: Consulting Psychologists Press.

Merson, S., Tyrer, P., Onyett, S., Lack, S., Birkett, P., Lynch, S., et al. (1992). Early intervention in psychiatric emergencies: A controlled clinical trial. *Lancet, 339,* 1311–1314.

Monroe-DeVita, M. B., & Mohatt, D. M. (2000). The state hospital and the community: An essential continuum for persons with severe and persistent mental illness. In W. D. Spaulding (Ed.), *The role of the state hospital in the twenty-first century* (New Directions for Mental Health Services, No. 84). San Francisco: Jossey-Bass.

Paris, J. (2004). Is hospitalization useful for suicidal patients with borderline personality disorder? *Journal of Personality Disorders, 18,* 240–247.

Phillips, S. D. (2001). Moving assertive community treatment into standard practice. *Psychiatric Services, 52*(6), 771–779.

Pilkonis, P. A., & Frank, E. (1988). Personality pathology in recurrent depression: Nature, prevalence, and relationship to treatment response. *American Journal of Psychiatry, 145,* 435–441.

Salyers, M. P., Masterton, T. W., Fekete, D. M., Picone, J. J., & Bond, G. R. (1998). Transferring clients from intensive case management: Impact on client functioning. *American Journal of Orthopsychiatry, 68,* 233–245.

Sanislow, C. A., & McGlashan, T. H. (1998). Treatment outcome of personality disorders. *Canadian Journal of Psychiatry, 43,* 237–250.

Sansone, R. (2004). Chronic suicidality and borderline personality. *Journal of Personality Disorders, 18*, 215–225.

Skodol, A. E., Gunderson, J. G., McGlashan, T. H., Dyck, I. R., Stout, R. L., Bender, D. S., et al. (2002). Functional impairment in patients with schizotypal, borderline, avoidant, or obsessive–compulsive personality disorder. *American Journal of Psychiatry, 159*, 276–283.

Stein, L. I., & Santos, A. B. (1998). *Assertive community treatment of persons with severe mental illness.* New York: Norton.

Stein, L. I., Test, M. A., & Marx, A. J. (1975). Alternative to the hospital: A controlled study. *American Journal of Psychiatry, 25*, 669–672.

Test, M. A. (1992). Training in community living. In R. P. Liberman (Ed.), *Handbook of psychiatric rehabilitation.* New York: Macmillan.

Tyrer, P., Manley, C., Van Horn, E., Leddy, D., & Ukoumunne, O. C. (2000). Personality abnormality in severe mental illness and its influence on outcome of intensive and standard case management: A randomised controlled trial. *European Psychiatry, 15*, 7–10.

Tyrer, P., & Simmonds, S. (2003). Treatment models for those with severe mental illness and comorbid personality disorder. *British Journal of Psychiatry, 182*, 15–18.

Weisbrod, B. A. (1983). A guide to benefit–cost analysis, as seen through a controlled experiment in treating the mentally ill. *Journal of Health Politics, Policy, and Law, 7*, 808–845.

Wolbert, R., Cunningham, K., & Boerman, K. (2002, November). *DBT: As helpful for the therapist as it is for the client?* Poster presented at the 36th annual meeting of the Association for the Advancement of Behavior Therapy, Reno, NV.

Woogh, C. M. (1986). A cohort through the revolving door. *Canadian Journal of Psychiatry, 31*, 214–221.

Yen, S., Shea, T., Pagano, M., Sanislow, C. A., Grilo, C. M., McGlashan, T. H., et al. (2003). Axis I and Axis II disorders as predictors of prospective suicide attempts: Findings from the Collaborative Longitudinal Personality Disorders Study. *Journal of Abnormal Psychology, 112*, 375–381.

APPENDIX 11.1. DBT Coaching Sheet

The following is a checklist to assist with providing DBT coaching. Check the steps you used and briefly answer each question. Teams have found it useful to review in morning meeting. It can also be helpful to give a copy to consumer.

The goal is to assist the person in identifying and committing to using skills instead of engaging in suicidal and/or other impulsive behaviors. **FOCUS of coaching is applying skills.

Date _____ Consumer _____ Time Called __ to __ Staff _____

☐ **1) Problem definition**:

    What is going on?   Event _____

                       Thought/feelings _____

    When did it start? _____

    ☐ **Assess for suicidal lethality and/or harm to others.**

☐ **2) Assess for vulnerabilities:** ☐ Physical illness ☐ Eating, when ate last

    ☐ Mood-altering drugs (caffeine, alcohol, marijuana . . .)

    ☐ Sleep, too much, not enough ☐ Any physical activity

☐ **3) What skills have you tried ?** _____

    **Label skills you see client trying even if he or she doesn't identify them as skills.

    ☐ Reinforce effort.

    ☐ Trouble-shoot noneffort and coach on need of effort—remind goal is to reduce impulsive behaviors.

☐ **4) Generate alternative skills**:

Core mindfulness

☐ Wise Mind ☐ Nonjudgmental stance

☐ Observe ☐ One-mindfully in-the-moment

☐ Describe ☐ Effectiveness: focus on what works

Emotion regulation

☐ Reduce vulnerabilities _____

☐ Build mastery _____

☐ Build positive experiences _____

☐ Opposite action _____

Distress tolerance

Distracting: Wise Mind accepts

☐ Activities (task that will help distract)

☐ Contributions (i.e., do something for someone else)

☐ Comparisons (compare to yourself or someone else)

☐ Emotions (an event that creates different emotions)

☐ Pushing away (i.e., put pain on a shelf)

☐ Thoughts (count to 10, read, puzzles)

☐ Sensations (ice in hand, squeeze rubber ball, walk briskly)

Self-soothing

☐ Vision (look at something pretty)

☐ Hearing (music, hum, listen to nature)

☐ Smell (potpourri, candles, bake)

☐ Taste (have a meal or sip favorite tea)

☐ Touch (wrap up in blanket, bath, pet cat)

Improve the moment

☐ Imagery (imagine a relaxing safe place)

☐ Meaning (find or create some purpose)

☐ Prayer (meditation)

☐ Relaxation (hot bath, breathing exercise)

☐ One thing in the moment

☐ Vacation (get in bed for 20 mins)

☐ Encouragement (Cheerlead yourself: "I can stand this!")

    Interpersonal effectiveness

☐ Objective effectiveness: DEAR MAN

☐ Relationship effectiveness: GIVE

☐ Self-respect effectiveness: FAST

☐ Pros and cons

☐ Radical acceptance

*Skills coached on phone (i.e., breathing exercise) _____

*List skills committed to using _____

☐ **5) In case plan doesn't work, troubleshoot a plan B** _____

6) Plan a check-in on outcome of skills tried ☐ Scheduled call ☐ Discuss at next contact

ACT/DBT agrees to provide a qualified DBT therapist for weekly 1:1 psychotherapy.

ACT/DBT agrees to provide group or individual skills training by qualified skills trainer(s).

ACT/DBT agrees to provide therapist with weekly peer consultation.

ACT/DBT agrees to provide phone consultation to _____.

_____ agrees to attend scheduled therapy sessions.

_____ agrees to attend scheduled skills training group.

_____ agrees to disclose information regarding other therapies currently receiving and agrees to terminate on a schedule negotiated with his or her individual therapist.

ACT/DBT providers and _____ are committed to making treatment effective and agree on the following treatment targets:

1. To decrease suicidal, parasuicidal, and self-harm activities.
2. To decrease therapy-interfering behavior.
3. To decrease quality-of-life-interfering behaviors.
4. To increase interpersonal effectiveness.
5. To increase the ability to tolerate stress.
6. To increase the ability to manage strong emotions.
7. To increase core mindfulness skills.
8. Others as agreed to by _____ and DBT therapist.

ACT/DBT providers and _____ agree to give each other 24 hours' notice if an appointment is going to be missed or needs to be rescheduled.

Missing four consecutive sessions of individual therapy or four consecutive skills training groups means _____ may not remain in ACT/DBT treatment.

If _____ engages in suicidal behavior, _____ agrees to the contingency that there will be no contact aside from assessment of lethality for 24 hours, or as agreed upon.

_____ agrees to structure _____ hours per week of time participating in an activity negotiated between _____ and _____ by _____.

This agreement is valid for the period of 1 year or as negotiated. Starting from __ to __ . At the end of the agreed-upon time, this agreement can be renewed, revised, or terminated.

_____ Date / /

_____ Date / /

DBT Primary Therapist

CHAPTER 12

Evaluating Your Dialectical Behavior Therapy Program

Shireen L. Rizvi, Maria Monroe-DeVita,
and Linda A. Dimeff

To date, nine randomized controlled trials (RCTs) and numerous quasi-experimental studies support the efficacy and effectiveness of dialectical behavior therapy (DBT; see Chapter 1, this volume). In spite of all the research evidence, the question that you or your administrators may be asking is: Will it work in our setting? This is particularly relevant if your program differs from the original structure of standard DBT. Although DBT functions may be achieved in new, creative ways that absolutely address the overarching function or principle, they have nonetheless not yet been tested empirically. The primary purpose of this chapter is to aid you in your effort to collect data in your own unique setting so that you can determine for yourself the extent to which your DBT program is working and to answer a variety of evaluation questions that will help you continue to implement your program as intended. A further aim is to make what can be a daunting process one that is accessible, enjoyable, and straightforward, so that even clinicians with little to no research experience will feel more confident in moving forward to collect, analyze, and present data on your DBT program.

There are many reasons to collect data from your DBT program—that is, to conduct a *program evaluation*. First and foremost, it is important to know whether DBT is actually achieving good outcomes in your program. Many researchers and clinicians alike have fallen prey to positive illusions and hold the absolute belief that a client is improving or a treatment is working in the absence of any empirical evidence that either conclusion is accurate. The opposite scenario is often true when working with your most challenging clients, including individuals with borderline personality disorder (BPD): the therapist and the team become convinced that there has been no change, and as a result they get discouraged and demoralized, when in fact there has been quite a bit of change that has gotten lost in the hurricane of client out-of-control behaviors.

Of course, there many other equally important and compelling reasons to collect data on your DBT program. Here are just a few:

- *Gaining additional resources and support from administrators.* Often the best way to convince the "powers that be" (from program directors to high-level administrators) of the need for greater resources, training, and/or support is to use objective evidence to make the case. Many programs, for example, have received considerable funding for extensive DBT training by demonstrating the cost savings if DBT were to work with one client who is currently costing the system hundreds of thousands of dollars annually in repeated, lengthy hospital stays. Other DBT programs use program evaluation data to demonstrate their success in the service of gaining additional support. For example few, if any, administrators would consider cutting or rolling back a successful treatment program that is saving the system considerable dollars, dramatically improving client outcomes, and improving staff morale (which translates behaviorally to decreased use of sick leave and staff turnover rates).
- *Convince potential clients and colleagues to make a commitment to DBT.* One of the most effective ways to increase client referrals to your DBT program is to have a track record of client success. In response to a potential client wondering why in the world he or she should give up severely dysfunctional behaviors (e.g., intentional self-harm, suicide attempts, substance abuse), you are able to communicate with conviction, "If what you want is a life worth living, I am your person and we are your team." You have the data to back it up. Similarly, all things being equal, there is no better way to attract the most motivated, talented, and devoted colleagues than to demonstrate that you are a team that means business and you have the data to prove it.
- *Use as leverage for reimbursement.* It is not uncommon for behavioral health organizations to initially limit reimbursement of different DBT outpatient services. (Comtois et al., Chapter 3, this volume, describe a number of strategies to address this specific problem.) Presenting process, outcome, and cost data from your DBT program to the behavioral health organization at the time that you negotiate a new payment rate can provide a powerful leveraging tool, as data from a well-implemented DBT program are likely to show significant cost savings tied directly to client improvements.
- *To treat yourself.* There is nothing like objective data to provide reassurance that you are, in fact, an effective DBT therapist—particularly during rough and rocky periods with a particular client who has you convinced that just the opposite is true.

We need to offer three comments before getting started with the nitty-gritty details: First, our intent is to provide the rudimentary tools that will allow programs to begin to collect data right now. It is not our intent to make you, our keen reader, an *expert* in program evaluation (nor is it important that you be an expert in order to collect, interpret, and present important data about your DBT program). Second, with the advent of HIPAA (the Health Insurance Portability and Accountability Act of 1996), as well as a concern for the rights of your clients and their confidentiality, states and institutions have developed different policies regarding informed consent and the extent to which use of data for evaluation is included within the consent form. Thus, it is essential that you review these policies and talk them over with your administration before you begin your project. Doing so will ensure that you are mindful of both the ethical and the legal issues involved with conducting research and will minimize potential risk to your clients. Third, *get started*! We have watched a number of very bright, competent teams wait months to years before beginning to collect data. Some were waiting to know more. Others were waiting for approval to receive funding to hire a researcher. Others waited until they were sure their outcomes would be positive. We encourage you to start now, as there is no better (or worse) time. The data will be what the data are. You will learn what you need to learn in the context of *doing*. By rigorously collecting data, you will ultimately strengthen and solidify your DBT program.

How This Chapter Is Organized

In this chapter, we provide you with tips and a structure for starting your own program evaluation. Specifically, we offer some defining features of program evaluation, touch upon how to tailor your evaluation to your own specific needs, and offer principles to follow as you begin to collect data. Furthermore, some suggestions for standard measures to use will be given, as well as a brief tutorial on alternative data collection options, such as case studies and single-subject designs. Finally, tips for how to present your data are included to ensure that all your hard work pays off through a meaningful final report.

What Is Program Evaluation?

Program evaluation is a systematic procedure for examining the activities, characteristics, and impact of a program on the target population for the purpose of improving the program, examining its overall effectiveness, and and/or making decisions about future programming (Patton, 1997; Wolfe & Miller, 1994). Program evaluation can help answer many questions relevant to you and your DBT program, such as: Do our clients improve in the outcome areas we would expect (e.g., decreases in suicide attempts and self-injurious behavior; reductions in inpatient hospital days, emergency room visits, and other crisis services)? Are our DBT therapists and skills trainers delivering the treatment as intended? Are total service costs decreasing for our clients who are receiving DBT?

Two Overarching Purposes of Evaluation

Program evaluation can be divided into two broad categories based on their differential purposes: formative evaluation and summative evaluation (Scriven, 1991b).

Formative evaluation is typically conducted to answer questions regarding *program improvement*. That is, the purpose is to use the evaluation findings to continue to shape and enhance the program. Most services researchers and agency administrators conduct some form of formative evaluation, even if they do not refer to it as such. For example, it is not uncommon for treatment developers to conduct formative evaluation as they begin developing their treatment (e.g., vetting new strategies or skills to be included, soliciting expert reviews of treatment handouts) and before they conduct a clinical trial to evaluate its impact (i.e., with a summative evaluation). Similarly, most agencies have a quality improvement (QI) program in place, which is essentially a form of formative evaluation. Examples of formative evaluation questions are included in Table 12.1.

TABLE 12.1. Sample Formative Evaluation Questions

Overarching question: How can we make our program work better?

Examples of specific questions:

- How can we change our program to ensure that it targets a decrease in client use of inpatient hospital services, emergency room services, and other crisis services?
- Should we add telephone consultation within our program rather than outsource it to a mobile crisis program?
- How can we make our program more cost-effective?
- What are the characteristics of the clients we are treating? If they are our target population, how can we better meet their needs based on any new information on their characteristics (e.g., a relatively high percentage are minorities, a subset don't have a high school degree or GED)?
- What are the specific training needs of our staff to ensure that they can competently deliver DBT?
- How can we most efficiently offer comprehensive DBT within our setting (e.g., create a specialty DBT team or require that all staff learn, know, apply DBT)?

In contrast, *summative evaluation* is typically used to render judgment about overall *program effectiveness*. It focuses on the "bottom line" or how the program "sums up" (Wolfe & Miller, 1994). Summative evaluation is essential in determining whether the program is resulting in the desired outcomes and whether the program should be continued (or, in the case of funders, whether the program should continue to be funded). Table 12.2 includes several sample summative evaluation questions.

One metaphor to consider in distinguishing these two types of program evaluation is "When the cook tastes the soup, that's formative; when the guests taste the soup, that's summative" (Scriven, 1991a, p. 169). Both types of evaluation are important, and the two are *not* mutually exclusive. In fact, many programs include a little bit of both formative and summative evaluation. For example, a program may have an ongoing quality improvement program in which they examine how the program is performing and whether any improvements need to be made (i.e., formative evaluation), and then produce an annual report to their board or their funding agency regarding the overall effectiveness of the program (i.e., summative evaluation).

TABLE 12.2. Sample Summative Evaluation Questions

Overarching question: How well does our program work?

Examples of specific questions:

- Does the program help clients get better? To what extent do clients in DBT show a decrease in self-injurious and/or suicidal behavior?
- Does the program result in a reduction in client use of more expensive services? To what extent do inpatient hospital days, emergency room visits, and crisis beds decrease for clients in the DBT program compared to the year prior to their inclusion in the program?
- Was the DBT program implemented as intended? Is it comprehensive DBT?
- Did staff receive the training necessary to competently deliver DBT services?
- Do the benefits of DBT outweigh the costs of the program?

Common Evaluation Questions and Methods for Answering Them

While there are many types of evaluation questions to consider, the most common questions include:

1. Is the program operating as planned (addressed by *process evaluation*)?
2. What is the impact of the program on the target population (addressed by *outcome evaluation*)?
3. Is the desired impact of the program attained at a reasonable cost (addressed by *efficiency evaluation*; Rossi, Freeman, & Lipsey, 1999)?

Remember, each type of question and the evaluation method for addressing them can be used for the purposes of either formative evaluation or summative evaluation. It all depends on the overarching purpose of your evaluation (i.e., whether you want to improve how your program is "working" or to determine whether it "works").

Process evaluation addresses questions related to the activities, services, and overall functioning of the program (i.e., the "process" within the program). Process evaluation is also typically called "program monitoring" when used for formative evaluation or quality improvement purposes. Process evaluation may include, for example, assessment of whether the services are in alignment with the goals of the program, whether the services are delivered as intended, the extent to which the program is meeting its intended client population, and/or whether program staffing or training are sufficient. Many programs already collect much of these data because they are necessary for day-to-day administrative processes (e.g., billing, administrative reporting). Example process evaluation questions are included in Table 12.3.

Providers are typically most familiar with *outcome evaluation* since it focuses primarily on the extent to which a program produces the intended benefit for the clients who receive services from that program. Outcome-related questions typically assume a set of operationally defined criteria or measures of success (Rossi et al., 1999). These may include instances of self-injurious behavior or urges to use alcohol or drugs, or they may be based on client or therapist reports on an assessment scale such as the Beck Depression Inventory (BDI). Examples of outcome evaluation questions are included in Table 12.4.

Efficiency evaluation is focused on program cost, cost–benefit considerations, and cost effectiveness of the program. This type of evaluation is often the most convincing and essential to funding agencies and policymakers who will want to know whether the

---

TABLE 12.3. Sample Process Evaluation Questions

- Is the DBT program being implemented as intended? (E.g., if the intent was to implement comprehensive DBT, does it include all of the functions of comprehensive DBT?)
- Are DBT services delivered to a level of adherence and/or competence?
- Is DBT being delivered to the intended population? (E.g., adults with BPD only? Clients with suicidal behavior? Adolescents with behavioral problems?)
- What is the rate of staff turnover on the DBT team compared to rates agencywide or in other service areas (countywide, national trends)?
- Are clients in the DBT program satisfied with their treatment?

TABLE 12.4. Sample Outcome Evaluation Questions

- To what extent do inpatient hospital days, emergency room visits, and crisis beds decrease for clients in the DBT program compared to the year prior to their inclusion in the program?
- To what extent do client outcomes maintain or improve 1 year after completion of the DBT program?
- What is the dropout rate for clients in the DBT program in comparison to dropout rates in other programs agencywide?
- What percentage of clients are no longer on psychiatric disability? Of that group, what percentage have jobs or are enrolled in school upon completion of DBT? What percentage are volunteering/contributing in the community?
- Do client outcomes improve when a DBT advanced group is added to our program in the second year? To what extent do client outcomes hold steady or continue to improve when an advanced group is offered during the second year?

program is essentially worth the cost of its implementation. Table 12.5 includes sample questions related to efficiency evaluation.

Again, for any given program, you may use a combination of these types of evaluation and they may differ depending on whether you're conducting a formative or a summative evaluation. For example, for your annual report to your agency's board (i.e., summative evaluation), you may decide to report on the extent to which all DBT modes and functions are being delivered, therapist adherence to DBT (i.e., process evaluation), and the extent to which clients showed improvement in self-injurious behaviors, suicide attempts, and use of inpatient and crisis services (i.e., outcome evaluation). However, in your quality improvement program (i.e., formative evaluation), you may focus on data that relates to identified areas of weakness in your particular program (e.g., new therapist training in DBT during times of high staff turnover).

Before You Get Started: Deciding Where to Begin

The beauty of program evaluation is that it can and should be designed in a fashion that allows you and other program stakeholders to answer the most relevant questions linked to your most important goals. For example, if your goal is to determine whether the costs of conducting DBT are justified by the savings to your system, your program evaluation will naturally involve collecting client data involving utilization of resources (e.g., emer-

TABLE 12.5. Sample Efficiency Evaluation Questions

- If there was a reduction in utilization of inpatient hospital and crisis services for clients in the DBT program, how much money was saved in total treatment costs?
- Do the benefits of the DBT program outweigh the costs? What is the net benefit per client?
- What is the return on investment of the DBT program (e.g., clients in DBT returning to the workforce)?
- Would alternative treatment approaches yield equivalent benefits at a lower cost?
- Would the DBT program be equally effective and less costly if staffed by intensively trained bachelor's-level clinicians rather than master's- and doctoral-level therapists?

gency rooms, psychiatric hospitalization, destruction of waiting room property, professional staff sick leave). If your initial goal is to develop a DBT program that has a very positive valence to staff and clients alike (i.e., clients and clinicians view the program quite favorably, and as a result clinicians refer their clients with BPD and clients opt voluntarily to receive services), then your evaluation may focus instead on staff and client attitudes about DBT.

An individually tailored approach to evaluation design ensures that the evaluation is produced in a manner that is realistic and practical given the allotted resources, while providing credible findings that are useful to DBT program stakeholders. In order to tailor your evaluation individually, you need to know a variety of details about your program and the purposes of your evaluation. We offer the following list of questions to help you to focus your evaluation to fit your program's goals and needs:

At What Stage of Implementation Is Your DBT Program?

The stage of implementation of your DBT program may have a huge impact on how you design your evaluation. Take a look at the following implementation stages (adapted from Fixsen, Naoom, Blasé, Friedman, & Wallace, 2005) and determine which stage best fits with the current status of your DBT program:

- *Exploration and adoption*: At this stage, program stakeholders begin exploring the possibility of implementing a DBT program. Typically, planning groups come together to examine which programs fit their needs and then they make decisions about whether to adopt, adapt, or pass on a particular program.
- *Early implementation*: This stage includes both the early planning for implementing the program (e.g., securing space, enlisting personnel) as well as the initial program operation where staff are in place and clients are now receiving services. This stage typically occurs within the first year of implementing the program, but can take longer depending on how long it takes for the program to obtain all of its necessary implementation resources and staff.
- *Full implementation*: By now, the program staff are completely trained and the program is fully functional. Training, supervision, evaluation, daily operations, and administration are routinized.
- *Sustainability*: This stage typically occurs anywhere between 2 and 4 years after full implementation. By this time, the program has survived some turnover in staff and administration and has successfully recruited, trained, and retained new personnel. During the sustainability stage, the program is focused on long-term survival and continued effectiveness in the context of many internal (e.g., staffing, administration, referral base) and external changes (e.g., public policy, funding priorities).

Once you have identified the implementation stage of your DBT program, you're ready to answer the remaining questions below. Please note that if you're in the exploration and adoption stage, you may first want to consider conducting a formal or informal assessment of the *need* for a DBT program (i.e., a "needs assessment"). In many cases, the need for DBT has already been established informally and the reason for the program is obvious (e.g., high utilization rates of expensive services, high staff turnover rates due to difficulty with working effectively with clients with BPD). However, even if the need for DBT has been identified, it is not uncommon for programs to have to go the extra mile to convince their administration that a *comprehensive* DBT program versus, say, a program that implements only DBT skills training is needed, or that intensive training and ongoing consultation are needed to effectively implement this treatment. While it is not within the scope of this chapter to walk you through how to conduct a needs assessment, it is important to keep this in mind. A useful resource for conducting a needs assessment can be found in an evaluation reference manual published by the World Health Organization (2000).

Who Are the Primary Stakeholders?

Stakeholders, sometimes called "constituents," are people and/or organizations who have a vested interest in the program, such as clients, their families, clinicians, and program directors. You need to ask yourself, Who are the people who are both interested in and who will make use of the evaluation findings? This answer will provide guidance regarding which key players should be included in the evaluation design and potentially the ongoing oversight of the evaluation (e.g., an evaluation advisory board), as stakeholder involvement is one of the best ways to ensure that evaluation findings are both informative and useful (Patton, 1997). Knowing your program stakeholders will also help you to determine which evaluation questions to include (see below: "What questions do you want your evaluation to answer?"). Evaluation data may be useful to any combination of the following DBT stakeholders:

• *Clients:* Is my life better in identifiable ways (e.g., decreased self-injurious behavior, hopelessness, depression)?
• *Families:* Is the life of my family member (who is being treated) better? Is there a positive change in my own life (e.g., reduced family burden, fewer crisis calls) because my family member's life is better?
• *Therapists and skills trainers:* Is our DBT program helping our clients? Am I delivering this therapy in the way in which it was intended to be delivered? Am I feeling effective and enthusiastic about our program?
• *Program supervisors and directors:* Are our DBT therapists adherent to DBT? Are clients and therapists in our program satisfied with their services?
• *Program funders:* Is the DBT program actually delivering DBT so that we can justify reimbursement/payment? Is the DBT program resulting in positive outcomes?
• *High-level administrators:* Is the program resulting in reduced costs and/or reduced risk of liability, compared with alternatives?

What Is the Overarching Purpose of the Evaluation?

Is the purpose to provide feedback on how the program is doing and what changes need to be made in order to continue to enhance and improve upon the program? Is the purpose ultimately to render judgment on whether the program is effective? Or is it both? Most evaluations within community programs focus on quality and program improvement at the very least. In fact, available resources to conduct the evaluation (see below: "What resources are available for the evaluation?") often determine the extent to which program effectiveness can be assessed with much methodological rigor.

Another consideration in deciding the purpose of your evaluation is how it relates to your program's implementation stage. If your program is in the early stages of implementation, you may want to consider doing a formative evaluation with a focus on program improvement instead of a summative evaluation. This is because some of your evaluation findings may be disappointing at this early stage and you wouldn't want to inadvertently communicate to decision-making stakeholders (e.g., state mental health directors, funding agencies) that the program is ineffective by doing a summative evaluation at this stage. Disappointing findings may be due to any number of things that are simply part of being a young program: poor initial implementation, a small sample size due to the fact that you only have so many slots available as your program starts out, and assessment of outcomes that typically take some time to show any sort of effect (e.g., by clients returning to work). Instead, a formative evaluation can help you identify relative strengths and weaknesses in your program and will help you to target efforts to improve the latter.

What Resources Are Available for the Evaluation?

Unfortunately, there usually are little to no resources devoted to program evaluation. Even when start-up costs are provided, it is important to consider what resources are available for the day-to-day management of collecting the data, cleaning it, analyzing it, and providing the results in a timely manner. If fewer resources are available, make sure that the evaluation isn't too large and doesn't require more person power than is realistic.

What Questions Do You Want the Evaluation to Answer?

In order to use your evaluation findings, you must be sure that the evaluation is measuring the kind of data important to your DBT program. This question overlaps considerably with "Who are the primary program stakeholders?", since these questions may differ based on the stakeholders identified and the extent of their involvement in the evaluation process. For example, clients and families may tend to focus on the extent to which the program helps them, whereas program funders and high-level administrators may be interested in whether the program is cost-effective in addition to whether it has a positive impact on clients and their families. Furthermore, the stage of implementation may also play a significant role regarding the types of evaluation questions you ask. Programs in the later stages of implementation (*full implementation* and *sustainability*), that have been collecting data for a longer period of time, may have more to say about whether the program is cost-effective or whether clients achieve longer term gains such as employment or sustained decrease in self-injurious behaviors.

Now that you know the various types of program evaluation and you have had a chance to answer the five questions above to further fine-tune where to begin with your evaluation, we turn to teaching you how to conduct your evaluation.

Conducting Your Evaluation: Principles for Data Collection

The most typical method for evaluating a program is to measure a number of variables (e.g., incidents of self-injurious behavior, psychiatric symptoms, employment status) on a regular basis and examine how these variables change over time, which is a type of *outcome evaluation*. With these data, you can chart changes on a micro- or individual-client level, on a day-to-day basis (as with daily diary cards), or at a global level such as assessing how clients in an entire program are doing before, during, and after participating in the program (also known as a "pre–post" assessment). That is, with the latter, you can measure a number of variables of interest when a client first enters treatment and then measure these same variables when he or she ends treatment, or on a routine basis like every 3 months or every 6 months. For novice researchers, this task can seem overwhelming even after all the questions about tailoring your evaluation have been answered. Therefore, we have developed seven principles to help you get started with data collection on your DBT program. These principles are illustrated in Table 12.6 and described more fully below.

Keep It Simple

It is easy to get bogged down by collecting too much data too quickly. It is preferable by far to collect reliable information on just a few variables of interest than to collect a lot of data that is of little interest or use to the program, or to be so ambitious that you get overwhelmed by the task before you're out of the gate. As a general guideline, think about collecting data on eight or fewer variables of interest. For example, in Table 12.6, the primary variables of relevance for the standard DBT and the adaptations described throughout this book are listed.

Keep It Consistent

Measure the same items for all clients in your program. Although it might be tempting to collect different data for different subtypes of clients (e.g., measuring urges to self-harm only with clients who already have a self-harm history or measuring urges to drink only with those individuals who have an alcohol problem), measuring different variables for each unique subset of your population will undoubtedly complicate your evaluation and give you headaches in the long run. Keeping the variables of interest consistent will allow you to combine your data across clients and will give you clearer results later. One fairly easy way to do this is to use a standard diary card (see example in Chapter 4, this volume) for all clients in your program that includes a set number of variables of interest while allowing for a couple of variables to vary across clients. For example, you might decide to measure instances of self-harm and drug use, urges to self-harm and use drugs, and suicide ideation for all of your clients, but might measure hours of sleep only for those individuals whom you are directly targeting for better sleep hygiene. Furthermore, be sure that you are comparing "apples to apples" with each period of data collection. That is, when examining "baseline" data (also known as "pretreatment" or "pre-DBT" data), be sure that you are comparing data from the same timeframe for *each* client on *each* measure. For cost and service utilization data (e.g., inpatient hospitalizations, use of crisis services), a common convention among outpatient programs is to collect data on each client 6 months to 1 year prior to entering treatment. Baseline measurement for outcome data (e.g., number of self-injurious behaviors, symptoms of depression) typically takes into account symptoms and behaviors that occurred 30 days prior to each client's admission to the program. See Table 12.6 for typical timeframes for data collection across various DBT adaptations and treatment settings.

Keep It Useful

Think about what variables matter to the key program stakeholders: you, your clients and their families, your administration, and potentially any policymakers who may have ultimate control over continued program funding. Measure behaviors for which changes

TABLE 12.6. Relevant Outcome Variables for DBT Adaptations

DBT adaptation	Population of interest	Setting	Top five to eight outcomes	How each outcome can be measured
DBT in outpatient settings	Chronically suicidal individuals with BPD	Outpatient weekly individual and group therapy	1. Number of suicide attempts, number of nonsuicidal self-injurious behaviors 2. Psychiatric admissions and length of psychiatric inpatient hospitalization 3. Months receiving psychiatric disability payment 4. Engagement in work, school, volunteer work	1. Diary card; SASII 2. Number of days over specified period of time (e.g., monthly) 3. Client self-report of income; diary card; verification through SSDI 4. Diary card (record average hours per month at work, in school, volunteering) *All data collected for each client at baseline and every 6 months.*
DBT in inpatient units	Hospitalized individuals with BPD	Inpatient therapy	1. Self-harm behaviors 2. Violent acts toward others 3. Use of medications for behavioral or emotional control 4. Attendance at unit groups and modalities 5. Length of stay 6. Skills practice	1. Hospital staff reports of "incidents" 2. MAR (medication administration record) or hospital pharmacy data 3. Chart notes; attendance sheets 4. Chart notes; medical records 5. Diary card *All data collected on each client at hospital admission and discharge. Best if some type of follow-up data can be collected postdischarge.*
DBT for substance use and BPD	Individuals with substance use disorders and BPD	Outpatient individual and group therapy	1. Substance use 2. Self-injurious behaviors 3. Treatment retention 4. Anger 5. Symptom distress 6. BPD symptomatology	1. Urine screens—conducted randomly monthly/Addiction Severity Index (ASI; McLellan, Luborsky, O'Brien, & Woody, 1980; McLellan et al., 1992) 2. Suicide Attempt Self-Injury Interview (SASII; Linehan, Comtois, Brown, Heard, & Wagner, 2006) 3. Treatment History Interview (THI; Linehan & Heard, 1987) 4. State–Trait Anxiety Inventory for Adults (STAXI; Spielberger, 1996) 5. Symptom Checklist 90—Revised (SCL-90-R; Derogatis, 1977) 6. Zanarini Rating Scale for Borderline Personality Disorder (ZAN-BPD; Zanarini et al., 2003) *Other than urine screens, measures administered to each client at baseline and every 4 months.*
DBT for eating disorders	Individuals with bulimia nervosa or binge-eating disorder	Outpatient weekly group therapy	1. Frequency of binge episodes 2. Frequency of purge episodes 3. Weight change	1. Eating Disorders Examination (EDE; Fairburn & Cooper, 1993) 2. EDE 3. Balance beam scale, no shoes

(continued)

TABLE 12.6. *(continued)*

DBT adaptation	Population of interest	Setting	Top five to eight outcomes	How each outcome can be measured
DBT for eating disorders *(cont.)*			4. Emotional eating 5. Depression	4. Emotional Eating Scale (EES; Arnow, Kenardy, & Agras, 1995) 5. Beck Depression Inventory (BDI; Beck et al., 1961) *Data collected at baseline, posttreatment, and follow-up.*
	Individuals with anorexia nervosa	Outpatient weekly individual or group therapy; intensive outpatient program; partial hospital program	1. Frequency of binge episodes 2. Frequency of purge episodes 3. Weight change 4. Emotional eating 5. Depression	1. Eating Disorders Examination (EDE; Fairburn & Cooper, 1993) 2. EDE 3. Balance beam scale, no shoes, after voiding 4. Emotional Eating Scale (EES; Arnow, Kenardy, & Agras, 1995) 5. Beck Depression Inventory (BDI; Beck et al., 1961) NOTE: All measures are referenced in Telch, Agras, and Linehan (2001).
DBT for adolescents	Suicidal adolescents with borderline personality features	Outpatient	1. Suicide attempts 2. Inpatient admissions 3. Outpatient treatment compliance 4. Suicidal ideation 5. Depression 6. Global psychiatric symptomatology	1. Self-report/diary card 2. Medical chart 3. Medical chart reports of completion of 12-week (2x/week) treatment 4. Harkavy–Asnis Suicide Survey (HASS; Harkavy-Friedman & Asnis, 1989a)/ Suicidal Ideation Questionnaire (SIQ; Reynolds, 1988) 5. Beck Depression Inventory (BDI; Beck et al., 1961) 6. Symptom Checklist 90—Revised (SCL-90-R; Derogatis, 1977) *All data collected for each client at baseline, after each skills group module, and at posttreatment. Best if some type of follow-up assessment could also be completed.*
DBT with couples and families	Couples	Outpatient	1. Validating and invalidating responses 2. Aggression and domestic violence 3. Relationship quality 4. Individual distress	1. Observational ratings using the Validating and Invalidating Behaviors Coding Scale (VIBCS; Fruzzetti et al., 1995, 2005) 2. Conflict Tactics Scale 2 (CTS2; Straus, Hamby, Boney-McCoy, 7 Sugarman, 1996) 3. Dyadic Adjustment Scale (Spanier, 1979) or Quality of Marriage Index (Norton, 1983) 4. Symptoms Checklist 90—Revised (Derogatis, 1977)

(continued)

TABLE 12.6. *(continued)*

DBT adaptation	Population of interest	Setting	Top five to eight outcomes	How each outcome can be measured
DBT with couples and families *(cont.)*				*Measures administered to each client at baseline, posttreatment, and follow-up. The VIBCS can be used more frequently (often with each session).*
	Victims of domestic violence	Outpatient	1. Distress 2. Depression 3. Social adjustment 4. Safety/revictimization	1. Symptoms Checklist 90—Revised (Derogatis, 1977) 2. Beck Depression Inventory (Beck et al., 1961) 3. Social Adjustment Scale—Self-report (Weissman & Bothwell, 1976) 4. Conflict Tactics Scale 2 (CTS2; Straus et al., 1996)
				Measures administered to each client at baseline, posttreatment, and follow-up. The VIBCS can be used more frequently (often with each session).
	Parents of adolescent children	Any	1. Validating and invalidating responses 2. Safety/revictimization 3. Adolescent's family satisfaction	1. Observational ratings using the Validating and Invalidating Behaviors Coding Scale (Fruzzetti et al., 2005) 2. Conflict Tactics Scale 2 (parent–child version; Straus et al., 1996) 3. Adolescent Family Life Satisfaction Index—Parent Child Subscale (Henry, Ostrander, & Lovelace, 1992)
				Measures administered to each client at baseline, post-treatment, and follow-up. The VIBCS can be used more frequently (often with each session).
DBT in highly restricted and long-term settings	Adults adjudicated not guilty by reason of insanity (NGRI)	Forensic Inpatient	1. Physical self-harm 2. Physical other-harm 3. Staff burnout 4. Psychiatric symptoms 5. Depression 6. Coping skills	1. Hospital incident reports 2. Hospital incident reports, seclusion and restraint reports 3. Maslach Burnout Scale (MBI; Maslach & Jackson, 1981) 4. Brief Symptom Inventory (BSI; Derogatis & Melisaratos, 1983) 5. Beck Depression Inventory (Beck et al., 1961) 6. Vitaliano's Revised Ways of Coping Scale (WCCL-R; Vitaliano, Russo, Carr, Maiuro, & Becker, 1985; Vitaliano, Maiuro, Russo, & Becker, 1987)

(continued)

TABLE 12.6. *(continued)*

DBT adaptation	Population of interest	Setting	Top five to eight outcomes	How each outcome can be measured
DBT for assertive community treatment (ACT)	Individuals with severe and persistent mental illness (SPMI) who have BPD-consistent behaviors	Community/ outpatient— ACT team	1. Days in psychiatric hospital, jail, or crisis residential 2. Number of ER visits for parasuicidal behaviors 3. Work, school, volunteer work or other structured or scheduled activity 4. Program retention rate 5. Disposition of client after discharge 6. Client living situation 7. Individual distress	1. Chart notes or program incident reports 2. Chart notes or program incident reports 3. Chart notes (percentage of DBT clients who are working and average hours involved in a structured activity including work each week) 4. Chart notes/attendance records 5. Disposition plan/chart notes 6. Chart notes 7. Brief Symptom Inventory (BSI) score (Derogatis & Melisaratos, 1983) *For #1 and #2, data collected on each client 2 years prior to program entry, during treatment at regular intervals (e.g., every 4–6 months), and at 1-year follow-up if possible.* *For #3–7, data collected for each client at baseline and posttreatment.*

are meaningfully and directly linked to goals (both your program's goals and your clients' goals). Get clear beforehand about what information would be most revealing to you and your team 6 months from now. What data will help "sell" your program to those whom you need to convince?

Keep It DBT

Think about what your primary targets are for the population of clients that you treat. Include variables that are on your primary target list, as these are anticipated to change after applying DBT. Table 12.6 describes the primary outcomes for several adaptations of DBT. The outcomes tie specifically into the primary targets of each adapted intervention. For example, in evaluating DBT for substance-abusing individuals with BPD, one of the outcomes is substance use as measured by urine screens and the Addiction Severity Index (ASI; McLellan et al., 1980, 1992).

Keep It Behaviorally Specific

Measure discrete, recurring behavior that you can count and observe. For example, when measuring suicidal behavior, collecting data on the number of emergency room visits due to suicide attempts and number of self-harm episodes is more behaviorally specific than asking clients to report whether they were suicidal. Similarly, if you're interested in measuring depression, using a psychometrically sound rating scale such as the Beck Depression Inventory (BDI; Beck, Ward, Mendelson, Mock, & Erbaugh, 1961) will glean more behaviorally specific data than simply asking clients whether they feel depressed.

Keep It Scientific

Be guided by existing research and don't measure items that you have no reason to believe would change. For example, if your program consists of an intensive 2-week inpatient program for recent suicide attempters, there may be a number of variables that you would expect to change as a result of the targets of the intervention, such as degree of hopelessness, level of suicidal ideation, or medication compliance. However, given the length of the program, there is no reason to expect that issues that may take longer to address, such as chronic PTSD symptoms or quality of life, would change as a result of the 2-week stay.

Keep It Manageable

Don't do (much) more than you have to. While there may be data that you do not currently collect on a routine basis but would like to, try to also use data that you are already collecting for other purposes. The best and most accessible data may come from the diary cards, chart notes, or even billing paperwork regarding services delivered. If your chart note does not include information on variables of interest (e.g., days of hospitalization, emergency room visits, days in jail), and either it would be inappropriate to modify the note or it's simply not possible to do so, generate an additional note that is to be completed once monthly. Some therapists have generated a calendar for the year for each client and recorded significant events associated with variables of interest (e.g., marking the period of time the client was hospitalized, missed individual therapy sessions or groups, period where half-time work began). Similarly, much process evaluation data can be pulled directly out of billing reports that show number of hours of treatment provided, attendance numbers, and even type of treatment provided.

Choosing the Right Measures and Comparison Groups

Now that we have made a clear recommendation to keep things simple and straightforward, you may be saying to yourself, "But what about using well-established, validated research measures and research designs like those used by Linehan and others in large research trials? How important is it to include these sorts of measures in our evaluation and an appropriate comparison or control group?" The decision about whether to use these sorts of measures and whether to add a control condition all depends on your goals as well as your resources. Although collecting data in a similar fashion as the large research trials is impressive and offers many other positive rewards and directions (e.g., it is another means to compare your outcomes with those found in other RCTs or it may increase the odds that your data could be written up and published in a scientific professional journal), there are also many potential negatives to starting such a huge research effort launched primarily by clinicians and other key stakeholders. For starters, such an effort can be resource-heavy in many ways. Larger-scale research projects typically require more time from clients (to complete the more lengthy measures) and staff (to organize and systematically administer the assessments and to enter and analyze the data). Similarly, a number of measures cost money for each administration (e.g., the BDI, and the Symptom Checklist–90—Revised [SCL-90-R]; Derogatis, 1977). Furthermore, such large-scale research efforts, particularly if random assignment is involved, would require human subjects or some type of institutional review board (IRB) approval. Comparing your treatment to some other treatment (or treatment as usual) also requires twice as many clients and usually twice as many therapists, thus requiring even more financial resources. One way to cut down on this particular resource drain, rather than to have another treatment condition, is to instead compare data from your new program to data from your program prior to the implementation. In other words, using chart review or other records, you can measure how outcomes have *changed* as a result of the addition of your new treatment program.

We have one important suggestion in terms of how to start: If your answer to the question, "Will collecting data like those in the published RCTs interfere with our efforts to begin collecting *any* data on our program," is "Yes," then we suggest an alternate route. Start simple first. Get a straightforward program evaluation effort off the ground before considering whether to enter the "big leagues." If you do, make sure it's in addition to your ongoing, existing efforts to gather simple data well.

Alternative Methods of Gathering Data: Case Studies and Single-Case Designs

There are many instances in which it may not make sense or it isn't feasible to conduct a program evaluation as described in this chapter. Perhaps the "program" you wish to evaluate serves only one or two clients; or your program is still in the early phases of implementation, in which modes are gradually added to create a comprehensive DBT program; or your system administration decides it wants to take a few well-trained therapists and provide comprehensive DBT "by the book" for only the highest of high-treatment utilizers. In all these scenarios, given the size of the program and the small number of clients with whom you want to apply DBT, it may make more sense to consider other methods intended to evaluate single cases at a time. This section describes some alternative methods for evaluating the success of your treatment, namely, case studies and single-case designs.

In addition to being more appropriate for a smaller group of individuals, case studies and single-case designs offer many advantages over other types of research designs. First, this type of research is more practical especially for a novel research idea or hypothesis. In some research design methodologies, only one person is needed for a study. Even with other methodologies, such as multiple baselines across subjects (described below), a study can be completed with three to 10 participants. Therefore, it is easier to recruit participants, takes fewer resources to conduct the research, and can be completed in a relatively short period of time (depending on the length of the intervention to be studied). Second, as compared with large-scale outcome studies, there is no need for a wait-list/no treatment control group. Third, as opposed to larger treatment outcome studies in which you might have several "rule-out" criteria in order to make your group more homogenous (e.g., in order to study if DBT is effective for comorbid PTSD and BPD, you might have to rule out all individuals who also meet criteria for depression), in single-subject designs you can treat a more heterogeneous set of individuals. Finally, because of the fine-tuned attention to incremental changes within the person, single-subject designs and case studies allow for the ability to look at within-person variability, a topic usually of great interest to clinicians, and also to explore clinical course as well as mechanisms of change more readily. For example, if you are conducting skills training with an individual client and notice a significant decrease from one week to the next in terms of depression scores, you can then look at what happened in the session prior to the decrease and attempt to understand what caused the depression to remit that week, even if it is only temporary. Table 12.7 lists some of the pros and cons for these alternative evaluation methods.

TABLE 12.7. Advantages and Disadvantages of Case Studies and Single-Case Designs

Case studies	Single-case designs
Advantages	
• Only need one client • Does not require much more resources than writing up an account of what you are doing in treatment • Options exist for publishing in case study journals	• One or more clients, depending on which design you use • Can systematically determine the causal effects of your intervention • If done well (i.e., effectively following the principles), can publish in a scientific journal
Disadvantages	
• Does not allow you to make causal inferences about your treatment • May not provide a lot of weight if you're trying to demonstrate that your intervention will work for more than one person	• Requires that you be very structured in your approach • May take more time on the front end because you'll need to study the various types of designs and decide the best design for your study

Case Studies

Although its relative use has decreased in recent years as greater emphasis has instead been placed on large treatment outcome studies, it may be important to remember that the case study method was the standard for clinical investigation up until the mid-20th-century (Barlow & Hersen, 1984). A *case study* is the documentation of procedures used to treat a person with emotional and/or behavioral problems and, regardless of whether it is written for publication in a journal or book, it is the necessary first step in evaluating any new intervention. That is, every new treatment begins with the treatment of one person (sometimes referred to as a "pilot case") in which new techniques are applied and the effects of this technique are observed. In fact, the development of DBT occurred within the process of Linehan noting that standard cognitive-behavioral therapy (CBT) was not working for chronically suicidal and self-harming individuals (described in Linehan, 1993). A team observed her sessions with a series of pilot cases as she added new techniques to the standard CBT treatment. Through this iterative process, she identified the strategies that appeared effective. These early observations were then translated into a treatment manual and were eventually evaluated in large clinical outcome research trials. The beauty of a case study is that every client presents as an opportunity for assessing the impact of your treatment.

With the advent of new journals devoted solely to publishing case material (e.g., *Clinical Case Studies* and the electronic journal *Pragmatic Case Studies in Psychotherapy*), it is not difficult to find examples of case studies in the literature, including examples of case studies using DBT or DBT principles. Swenson and Linehan (2003), for example, discuss the implementation of DBT with a highly suicidal individual who spent the greater part of her adult life in inpatient settings. The authors provide an extensive personal history of the client and a DBT case formulation and treatment plan based on the target behaviors. Then a sample behavioral chain analysis is described and information about how this client fared in treatment is given. What is notable about this case study is that it is thorough and provides a compelling rationale for using DBT with clients such as this one; however, it contains no inferential statistical analyses, did not require a sample of more than one person, and was simply a record of what was occurring in therapy. Other case studies, like Becker (2002), do include descriptive statistics to provide objective data for changes over the course of treatment. In this case study, Becker describes an integrated behavioral treatment for a complex case with BPD, obsessive–compulsive disorder, and PTSD, using elements of DBT, exposure therapy, and response prevention. Becker administered various self-report measures to the client throughout treatment and also utilized chart review in order to gather data, which she then presented in graphs to demonstrate the client's progress in treatment.

There is no set standard for how to conduct and write up a case study, but here are some guidelines for information you would want to gather and provide (see also Table 12.8). Like any case conference presentation you might make, demographic details, a full diagnostic picture, information about relevant history, and presenting problems (i.e., what initially brought this client to see you) generally help to set the stage. A detailed assessment of the client's goals and problem areas is also necessary. The frame of DBT provides an advantage here because you can describe your hierarchy of targets and explain why you organized the targets in a particular way, according to the DBT model. The emphasis in DBT on constant assessment and linking to goals is also consistent with what is required in a case study. Case conceptualization is central in a case study, and time and effort should be placed in spelling out specifically what you think contributes to the development and maintenance of disorder in this client and how your treatment plan will address these factors in a substantive way. Next, you want to provide a detailed description of the course of treatment and client progress over time. If you have data, you might want to present it in graphic form in this section to pictorially represent change over time. Finally, you need to discuss how the treatment ended, any follow-up information you may have about the client, and concluding comments with your opinions about the treatment. Sometimes authors of case studies also provide suggestions for doing similar work with other clients, thus transferring their knowledge learned from the experience to other clinicians.

An important note: The nature of case studies is such that you are including specific and personal information about a particular client whom you have treated. If you are writing up the case for publication in a journal or another outlet, you are going to want to ensure that there is *no* possible way for others to identify the client based on your writing. Changing particularly unique pieces of information and other details that don't significantly affect the accurate description of your treatment is necessary in order to protect the client. *The client's welfare should always outweigh the benefit for you of your name in print.*

Single-Case Designs

As mentioned earlier, one potential downside to case studies is the lack of experimental control to account for other non-treatment-related factors that may be responsible for the clinical changes. Without the most rigorous experimental controls, it is never possible to

---

TABLE 12.8. Necessary Ingredients for a Case Study

• Demographic information	• Client's goals
• Diagnostic assessment	• Case conceptualization
• Relevant history	• Course of treatment (include data if you have it!)
• Treatment history	• End of treatment
• Presenting problem	• Follow-up information
• Other problem areas	• Suggestions/guidelines for other clinicians

determine fully whether the treatment was responsible for changes in the target behavior, or if the change occurred due to other factors, such as natural change due to maturation or simply the lapse of time or other random factors (e.g., the client's much-sought-after divorce had finally transpired). In contrast to the case study approach, single-case designs are intended to provide the same level of experimental rigor as controlled studies to address alternative, competing explanations for why the target behavior has changed. Rather than needing a large number of individuals to test hypotheses, sometimes only one client is needed, thus making this method an easy, efficient way to evaluate the effectiveness of your intervention.

In single-subject design studies, the effects of the intervention are examined by observing the influence of the intervention on previously measured baseline behavior, that is, behavior that occurred prior to the start of the intervention. There is a heavy reliance on repeated observations over time. Measurement of variables of interest should begin before the intervention is applied and then continue throughout the course of the intervention so that you can note whether the behavior changed when, and only when, the intervention was applied. There are several types of single-subject experimental designs that have several common elements and varying degrees of complexity, including AB design; ABAB, or reversal, designs; and multiple-baseline designs. In general, "A" indicates baseline or no-treatment phases and "B" indicates a treatment phase. Before describing in more detail each of these types of interventions, some common elements to all single-subject designs are outlined:

1. *Identification of a specific target behavior.* Before the study is begun, a specific behavior that can be reliably and validly measured must be identified.

2. *Continuous measurement.* The foundation of single-subject designs rests on its measurement. In these types of designs, the same measurement must be applied on a regular basis so that you can accurately assess both subtle and not-so-subtle changes over time.

3. *A baseline period* ("A"). A baseline period during which data is gathered on the target behavior before any intervention is applied is necessary in order to truly test the effects of your intervention. Without a baseline phase, there is no way of knowing whether your intervention had any true effect.

4. *Stability of the specific target behavior.* In order for the effects of your intervention to be the most clear, you want to demonstrate that the target behavior changes *only* when your intervention is applied. If your target behavior is unstable and vacillates widely before the intervention is applied, then it becomes increasingly difficult to demonstrate that your intervention has had any effect.

5. *Systematic application of intervention.* Once a baseline period has been established and you decide to apply your intervention, you must do it in a systematic and conscientious manner. For example, if you want to show that the application of interpersonal effectiveness skills has an effect on quality of social interactions (as measured by a self-report instrument on relationship satisfaction administered weekly), then you must figure out a way to have the client practice the skills in a methodical and consistent way. If he or she only practices DEAR MAN once every 3 weeks, then your single-subject design will not be able to demonstrate the intended effect.

These elements are used in various formats to create the different designs. For example, in the simplest AB design, a baseline period, "A," is followed by an intervention period "B," and then the effects of the addition of the intervention are assessed. In an

ABAB design, also known as a "withdrawal design," following a specified period of intervention (the first "B"), treatment is then withdrawn and the effects on the behavior are documented. If a treatment is what is causing the change in the behavior, then, in many instances, you would expect that the targeted behavior will regress to initial levels during the second "A" period. Finally, the treatment is applied again with the hypothesis that the behavior will again decrease as a result of the treatment.

For example, say you wanted to directly test the effects of positive reinforcement on maintaining eye contact with the therapist in a client who has been shut down and withdrawn for all of the previous sessions (with the client's informed consent, of course!). During the initial baseline period, you would not positively reinforce the client at all and you, or your research assistants, would be coding the amount of time the client makes eye contact. This continues for several sessions while you establish a baseline. Next, you apply your positive reinforcement intervention for several weeks, again coding each session for amount of time the client makes or maintains eye contact. If you notice positive changes, that is, if your client shows greater amount of time with maintained eye contact, then you can move into a second baseline period and again withdraw positive reinforcement. Assuming that your initial hypothesis is correct and that reinforcement increases eye contact, then withdrawing reinforcement will cause the client to stop making eye contact. Finally, after a few sessions of this withdrawal phase, you can once again become your naturally reinforcing self and document the resulting changes.

Of course, as you might be noting, there are some ethical concerns with using a withdrawal design. This concern is heightened when working with vulnerable or at-risk populations. If an intervention is working and the client is improving, then it would be very difficult to justify withdrawing the intervention in order to measure its effects. Your ability to use an ABAB design depends in large part on the client, the type of intervention, and the target behavior. Having suicidal behavior as your target, for example, should be a good indication to you that withdrawing treatment in order to see if your client reverts back to being more suicidal would be highly unethical.

Multiple-baseline treatment requires taking repeated measurements on clients for differing lengths of time to create a "baseline" with which the intervention will be compared. This allows you to study specifically how the introduction of your specific intervention changed the baseline behavior. For example, say, you want to examine how the DBT mindfulness skills affect clients' urges to use drugs. If you were doing a multiple-baseline design, you might randomize three clients to three different baseline periods, perhaps of 2 weeks, 4 weeks, and 6 weeks in length, and then monitor their urges to use drugs on a daily basis on a 0–10 scale, using diary cards. After their individual baseline period, you teach the clients the seven skills of mindfulness and ask them to practice these skills every day for 4 weeks. You continue to monitor their urges to use drugs on a daily basis for this 4-week period, at which point you can compare how the mindfulness skills influenced their urges to use drugs. In multiple-baseline designs, graphs are used to indicate the changes that occur. Figure 12.1 is an example of some ideal outcome data using this design.

Single-subject design studies are abundant in the clinical psychology literature. It does not take long to find numerous examples. (An excellent resource for descriptions and instructions for these types of design is Kazdin, 2001; anyone seeking to begin a single-subject design study is strongly encouraged to read this manual.) Relevant to BPD, for example, Nordahl and Nysaeter (2005) applied schema therapy to six clients with BPD, using an AB design. Rizvi and Linehan (2005) utilized a multiple-baseline design across subjects to test the effectiveness of a particular component of DBT, the skill of "opposite action," for the treatment of maladaptive shame in five individuals with BPD.

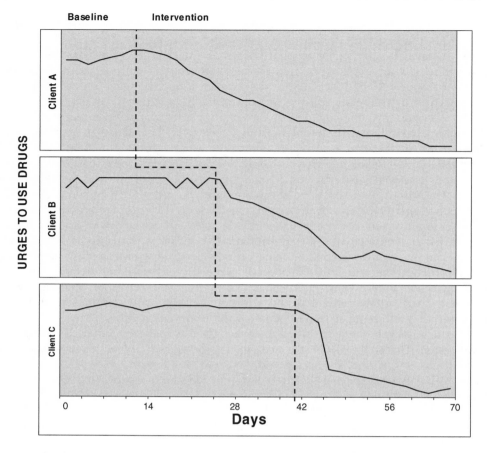

FIGURE 12.1. Example of hypothetical results from a mutiple-baseline design.

In summary, in addition to the program evaluation guidelines of the previous section, we have also provided you with some information on alternative evaluation methods, including case studies and single-case designs. Each method has its own unique advantages and disadvantages. It will be up to you and your team to determine what is right for you at this time. But because there are so many options available to you, it's our hope that nothing will stop you from getting started on an exciting data-collection process now, whether it be with one client or 100 clients. Now that you know how to collect your data, we'll teach you some strategies for presenting your data in the most accurate and appealing way.

Presenting Your Findings

It's never too early to begin thinking about how to present your evaluation findings. In fact, thinking about what your findings may look like as you design your evaluation can help to verify that you are collecting the data most important to you and your program. Whether your goal is to present your data in a one-page executive summary to your administration or at a conference to dozens of scientists, there are many items to consider when determining how to best present your data.

- *Tailor your presentation to your audience.* How you choose to present your data invariably depends on who comprises your audience. In many cases, particularly as you report formative evaluation results, it is likely that your audience will be key program stakeholders who may not have much background in data, evaluation, or statistics. In these cases, it is essential to make sure that you present your findings in the most straightforward and clearest way possible, perhaps avoiding more complicated tables and figures in order to best present "the bottom line." In the case of presenting your findings to a scientific audience, however, a more formal presentation of key results and statistics is often necessary. If you are less experienced in this domain, it may be important for you to consult with others who have given similar presentations so that you have appropriate models. You may even want to contact a local university to see whether a student with experience in statistics might be willing to consult to your program for course credit or a small fee.

- *Stick to the data.* It's not surprising that you would be excited to find results suggesting that DBT had a positive impact on the outcome variables of relevance. This is what we want! However, it's important to be vigilant about not inferring more than what is actually demonstrated by the data. For example, many program evaluations are designed in a manner that does not allow you to ultimately say that DBT was responsible for or caused the positive outcomes. Most program evaluations do not control for other variables that may actually have had an impact on these findings (e.g., lack of randomization to different conditions). In these instances, what you can report is that positive change occurred after the DBT program was implemented (not that DBT "caused" these changes) and that findings suggest a positive trend in x, y, and z. Also, be sure to acknowledge limitations to your evaluation in order to keep you and your program honest.

- *Link the data to your goals.* Remember the questions we reviewed earlier as you design your evaluation: At what stage of implementation is your program? Who are the primary stakeholders? What is the overarching purpose of the evaluation? What resources are available for the evaluation? What questions do you want the evaluation to answer? The answers to these questions will not only help you to design your evaluation, they will also help to solidify what findings are most important to report and to whom. For example, if the overarching purpose is formative evaluation, report your findings in a manner that highlights the extent to which your program has improved in these targeted areas over time.

- *Put your best foot forward.* Where have you found positive findings? Highlight these by picking the top three or four salient findings, perhaps using the DBT targets to prioritize the data or prioritizing based on what is most relevant to your audience (e.g., presenting cost savings to an audience of administrators).

- *Be fair with your presentation.* Results do not always turn out the way we anticipate they will! Be sure to describe important discrepancies in data or places where your hypotheses did not pan out as you had hoped. Offer explanations for why this may be the case, if you know. While negative or neutral findings can be disappointing, they can also provide valuable information, particularly if your purpose is formative evaluation and identifying areas in need of improvement in your program.

- *Place your findings in context.* Results are difficult to interpret without some basis for comparison. There are several ways by which you can incorporate your findings into a broader context that will make them more meaningful and relevant. One, you could compare your program's evaluation findings with results from research studies on DBT. When you do this, it may be important to note how your program differs from your point of comparison, which might explain any differences in results. Two, you could compare your program's findings to those of programs that are very similar to yours (e.g., similar training of staff, same target population, and same setting). Third, you can compare your own program's outcomes now to those of the previous year(s), including outcomes reported before the DBT program was implemented to illustrate changes that have occurred as a result of the implementation of DBT.

Don't forget: A picture is worth a thousand words. The best presentations are those that include simple and easy-to-read graphs and charts that accurately depict the results. This may require that you or someone on your team become a bit of a master at using Excel or PowerPoint graphs and charts to illustrate your points. Of course, it's easy to overdo this—sometimes presentations are so flashy that all people can remember at the end were the "tricks" instead of the data. Striking a balance is necessary in order to effectively communicate your findings in an accurate and stimulating manner.

Conclusions

In this chapter, we have striven to provide you with enough background information and resources to help you launch your DBT program evaluation. It should be obvious by now that the possibilities are virtually endless in terms of questions you can answer and the methodologies you can employ. If you are reading this book and this chapter, it is clear that you are passionate about your work and interested in increasing the quality of life of your clients. So why not demonstrate with hard evidence that you can do this? We encourage you to jump right in, using the advice from this chapter, and obtain some solid information about your program that will help prove that your efforts are paying off or suggest areas for improvements or refinements.

REFERENCES

Arnow, B., Kenardy, J., & Agras, W. S. (1995). The Emotional Eating Scale: The development of a measure to assess coping with negative affect by eating. *International Journal of Eating Disorders, 18,* 79–90.

Barlow, D. H., & Hersen, M. (1984). *Single case experimental designs: Strategies for studying behavior change* (2nd ed.). Boston: Allyn & Bacon.

Beck, A. T., Ward, C. H., Mendelson, M., Mock, J., & Erbaugh, J. (1961). An inventory for measuring depression. *Archives of General Psychiatry, 4,* 561–571.

Becker, C. B. (2002). Integrated behavioral treatment of comorbid OCD, PTSD, and borderline personality disorder: A case report. *Cognitive and Behavioral Practice, 9,* 100–110.

Derogatis, L. R. (1977). *SCL-90: Administration, scoring, and procedure manual for the R (revised) version.* Baltimore: Johns Hopkins University School of Medicine.

Derogatis, L. R., & Melisaratos, N. (1983). The Brief Symptom Inventory: An introductory report. *Psychological Medicine, 13,* 595–605.

Fairburn, C. G., & Cooper, Z. (1993). The Eating Disorder Examination (12th ed.). In C. G. Fairburn & G. T. Wilson (Eds.), *Binge eating: Nature, assessment, and treatment* (pp. 317–360). New York: Guilford Press.

Fixsen, D. L., Naoom, S. F., Blasé, K. A., Friedman, R. M., & Wallace, F. (2005). *Implementation research: A synthesis of the literature.* Tampa, FL: Louis de la Parte Florida Mental Health Institute Publication #231.

Fruzzetti, A. E. (1995). *The Closeness–Distance Family Interaction coding system: A functional approach coding couple interactions.* Coding manual, University of Nevada, Reno.

Fruzzetti, A. E., Shenk, C., Lowry, K., & Mosco, E. (2005). *Defining and measuring validating and invalidating behaviors: Reliability and validity of the Validating and Invalidating Behaviors Coding Scale.* Unpublished manuscript, University of Nevada, Reno.

Harkavy-Friedman, J. M., & Asnis, G. M. (1989a). Assessment of suicidal behavior: A new instrument. *Psychiatric Annals, 19,* 382–387.

Harkavy-Friedman, J. M., & Asnis, G. M. (1989b). Correction. *Psychiatric Annals, 19,* 438.

Henry, C. S., Ostrander, D. L., & Lovelace, S. G. (1992). Reliability and validity of the Adolescent Family Life Satisfaction Index. *Psychological Reports, 70,* 1223–1229.

Kazdin, A. E. (2001). *Behavior modification in applied settings* (6th ed.). Belmont, CA: Wadsworth.

Linehan, M. M. (1993). *Cognitive-behavioral treatment of borderline personality disorder.* New York: Guilford Press.

Linehan, M. M., Comtois, K. A., Brown, M., Heard, H. L., & Wagner, A. (2006). Suicide Attempt Self-Injury Interview (SASII): Development, reliability, and validity of a scale to assess suicide attempts and intentional self-injury. *Psychological Assessment, 18,* 303–312.

Linehan, M. M., & Heard, H. L. (1987). *Treatment History Interview.* Seattle: University of Washington.

Maslach, C., & Jackson, S. E. (1981). The measurement of experienced burnout. *Journal of Occupational Behaviour, 2,* 99–113.

McLellan, A. T., Kusher, H., Metzger, D., Peters, R., Smith, I., Grissom, G., et al. (1992). The fifth edition of the Addiction Severity Index. *Journal of Substance Abuse Treatment, 9*(3), 199–213.

McLellan, A. T., Luborsky, L., O'Brien, C. P., & Woody, G. E. (1980). An improved evaluation instrument for substance abuse patients: The Addiction Severity Index. *Journal of Nervous and Mental Disease, 168*(1), 26–33.

Nordahl, H. M., & Nysaeter, T. E. (2005). Schema therapy for patients with borderline personality disorder: A single case series. *Journal of Behavior Therapy and Experimental Psychiatry, 36,* 254–264.

Norton, R. (1983). Measuring marital quality: A critical look at the dependent variable. *Journal of Marriage and the Family, 45,* 141–151.

Patton, M. Q. (1997). *Utilization-focused evaluation* (2nd ed.). Beverly Hills, CA: Sage.

Reynolds, W. M. (1988). *Suicidal Ideation Questionnaire, professional manual.* Odessa, FL: Psychological Assessment Resources.

Rizvi, S. L., & Linehan, M. M. (2005). The treatment of maladaptive shame in borderline personality disorder: A pilot study of "Opposite Action." *Cognitive and Behavioral Practice, 12,* 437–447.

Rossi, P. H., Freeman, H. E., & Lipsey, M. W. (1999). *Evaluation: A systematic approach* (6th ed.). Thousand Oaks, CA: Sage.

Scriven, M. (1991a). Beyond formative and summative evaluation. In M. W. McLaughlin & D. C. Phillips (Eds.), *Evaluation and education: At quarter century, 90th yearbook of the national society for the study of education* (pp. 18–64). Chicago: University of Chicago Press.

Scriven, M. (1991b). *Evaluation thesaurus* (4th ed.). Newbury Park, CA: Sage.

Spanier, G. (1979). The measurement of marital quality. *Journal of Sex Marital Therapy, 5,* 288–300.

Spielberger, C. D. (1996). *Manual for the state–trait anger expression inventory* (STAXI). Odessa, FL: Psychological Assessment Resources.

Straus, M. A., Hamby, S. L., Boney-McCoy, S., & Sugarman, D. B. (1996). The revised Conflict Tactics Scales (CTS2): Development and preliminary psychometric data. *Journal of Family Issues, 17*(3), 283–316.

Swenson, C., & Linehan, M. M. (2003). Borderline personality disorder. In I. B. Weiner (Ed.), *Adult psychopathology case studies* (pp. 29–52). Hoboken, NJ: Wiley.

Telch, C. F., Agras, W. S., & Linehan, M. M. (2001). Dialectical behavior therapy for binge eating disorder. *Journal of Consulting and Clinical Psychology, 69*(6), 1061–1065.

Vitaliano, P. P., Maiuro, R. D., Russo, J., & Becker, J. (1987). Raw versus relative scores in the assessment of coping strategies. *Journal of Behavioral Medicine, 10,* 1–18.

Vitaliano, P. P., Russo, J., Carr, J. E., Maiuro, R. D., & Becker, J. (1985). The Ways of Coping Checklist: Revision and psychometric properties. *Multivariate Behavioral Research, 20,* 3–26.

Weissman, M. M., & Bothwell, S. (1976). Assessment of social adjustment by patient self-report. *Archives of General Psychiatry, 33,* 1111–1115.

Wolfe, B. L., & Miller, A. L. (1994). *Program evaluation: A do-it-yourself manual for substance abuse programs.* Albuquerque: Dept. of Psychology, University of New Mexico. Retrieved June 6, 2006, from *casaa.unm.edu/download/programeval.pdf*

World Health Organization, United Nations International Drug Control Programme, & European Monitoring Center on Drugs and Addiction. (2000). *Needs assessment: Workbook 3. Evaluation of psychoactive substance use disorder treatment.* Geneva: WHO. Retrieved June 6, 2006, from *whqlibdoc.who.int/hq/2000/WHO_MSD_MSB_00.2d.pdf*

Zanarini, M. C., Vujanovic, A. A. Parachini, E. A., Boulanger, J. L., Frankenburg, F. R., & Hennen, J. (2003). Zanarini Rating Scale for Borderline Personality Disorder (ZAN-BPD): A continuous measure for DSM-IV borderline psychopathology. *Journal of Personality Disorders, 17*(3), 233–242.

Index